COMPLEMENTARY AND INTEGRATIVE THERAPIES FOR CARDIOVASCULAR DISEASE

WILLIAM H. FRISHMAN, MD, FACC, FAHA, MACP
Rosenthal Professor and Chairman of Medicine,
Professor of Pharmacology,
New York Medical College;
Director of Medicine,
Westchester Medical Center,
Valhalla, New York

MICHAEL I. WEINTRAUB, MD, FACP, FAAN
Clinical Professor of Neurology and Medicine,
Departments of Neurology and Internal Medicine,
New York Medical College,
Westchester Medical Center,
Valhalla, New York

MARC S. MICOZZI, MD
Director, Center for Integrative Medicine,
Thomas Jefferson University Hospital,
Philadelphia, Pennsylvania

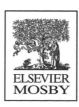

ELSEVIER
MOSBY

ELSEVIER
MOSBY

11830 Westline Industrial Drive
St. Louis, Missouri 63146

COMPLEMENTARY AND INTEGRATIVE THERAPIES FOR
CARDIOVASCULAR DISEASE   ISBN 0-323-03002-5
Copyright © 2005 by Mosby, Inc.
All rights reserved.

NOTICE

Complementary and integrative medicine is an ever-changing field. Standard safety precautions must be followed, but as new research and clinical experience broaden our knowledge, changes in treatment and drug therapy may become necessary or appropriate. Readers are advised to check the most current product information provided by the manufacturer of each drug to be administered to verify the recommended dose, the method and duration of administration, and contraindications. It is the responsibility of the licensed prescriber, relying on experience and knowledge of the patient, to determine dosages and the best treatment for each individual patient. Neither the publisher nor the author assumes any liability for any injury and/or damage to persons or property arising from this publication.

Publishing Director: Linda Duncan
Acquisitions Editor: Kellie White
Developmental Editor: Kim Fons
Publishing Services Manager: Pat Joiner
Project Manager: Karen M. Rehwinkel
Designer: Amy Buxton

Printed in the United States of America
Last digit is the print number: 9   8   7   6   5   4   3   2   1

WILBERT S. ARONOW, MD
Clinical Professor of Medicine,
New York Medical College;
Chief of Cardiology Clinic,
Westchester Medical Center,
Valhalla, New York
Spinal Cord Stimulation for the Treatment of Angina Pectoris

DONALD A. BISSON, MaR, RRP, CET, CCT
Dean and Chairman,
Ontario College of Reflexology,
New Liskeard, Ontario, Canada
Reflexology

ELAINE CALENDA, NCTMB
Academic Dean,
Boulder College of Massage Therapy,
Boulder, Colorado
Therapeutic Massage and Asian Bodywork

JOHN D. CAPOBIANCO, DO, FAAO
Acting Chair, Department of Osteopathic Medicine;
Clinical Associate Professor,
New York College of Osteopathic Medicine of the New York Institute of
Technology,
Old Westbury, New York
Osteopathic Manipulative Medicine in the Treatment of Hypertension

MICHAEL H. COHEN, JD, MBA
Assistant Professor of Medicine;
Director of Legal Programs,
Division for Research and Education in Complementary and Integrative
Medical Therapies,
Harvard Medical School,
Boston, Massachusetts
Legal Issues in Integration of Complementary Therapies Into Cardiology Practice

SUZANNE W. CRATER, RN, ANP-C
Duke Clinical Research Institute;
Director, Interventional Devices Clinical Trials,
Duke University Medical Center,
Durham, North Carolina
Prayer and Cardiovascular Disease

JEFFERY A. DUSEK, PhD
Associate Research Director,
Mind-Body Medical Institute;
Instructor of Medicine,
Harvard Medical School,
Boston, Massachusetts
Prayer and Cardiovascular Disease

ARTHUR E. FASS, MD, FACC, FACP
Chief of Cardiology,
Phelps Memorial Hospital,
Briarcliff Manor, New York;
Clinical Assistant Professor of Medicine,
New York Medical College,
Valhalla, New York
Hypnosis for the Relief of Cardiac Symptomatology

SUZAN FLECK, BA
Associate Faculty,
Boulder College of Massage Therapy,
Boulder, Colorado
Therapeutic Massage and Asian Bodywork

WILLIAM H. FRISHMAN, MD, FACC, FAHA, MACP
Rosenthal Professor and Chairman of Medicine,
Professor of Pharmacology,
New York Medical College;
Director of Medicine,
Westchester Medical Center,
Valhalla, New York
The Placebo Effect in Cardiovascular Disease
Nutriceuticals and Cardiovascular Illness
Herbal Approach to Cardiac Disease
Acupuncture in Cardiovascular Diseases
Chelation Therapy
Sauna as a Therapeutic Option for Cardiovascular Disease
Animal-Assisted Therapy and Cardiovascular Disease
Magnetic Biostimulation: Energy Therapy
Spinal Cord Stimulation for the Treatment of Angina Pectoris

STEPHEN P. GLASSER, MD
Professor of Epidemiology;
Director of Graduate Studies in Clinical Research,
University of Minnesota, School of Public Health,
Minneapolis, Minnesota
The Placebo Effect in Cardiovascular Disease

JAMES G. GRATTAN, MD, FACC
Clinical Assistant Professor,
Department of Internal Medicine,
Texas Tech University Health Sciences Center,
Lubbock, Texas
Mind-Body Approach to Cardiac Illness

SUZANNE B. HANSER, EdD, MT-BC
Chair, Music Therapy Department,
Berklee College of Music;
President, World Federation of Music Therapy,
Boston, Massachusetts
The Effects of Music Therapy in Cardiac Healthcare

ALAN R. HIRSCH, MD, FACP
Neurological Director,
Smell and Taste Treatment and Research Foundation,
Chicago, Illinois
Aromatherapy in Cardiac Conditions

LINDA C. NADIA HOLE, MD
Guest Faculty,
American Academy of Pain Management,
American Holistic Medical Association,
World Congress of Qigong;
Faculty, Traditional Chinese Medical College of Hawaii,
Pope Valley, California
Heart Qi and the Heart of Healing: Qigong for the Prevention and Treatment of Cardiac Disease

ROGER JAHNKE, OMD
Director, Institute of Integral Qigong and Tai Chi;
Chair, Qigong and Tai Chi Department,
Santa Barbara College of Oriental Medicine,
Santa Barbara, California
Qigong and Tai Chi: Traditional Chinese Health Promotion Practices in the Prevention and Treatment of Cardiovascular Disease

MITCHELL W. KRUCOFF, MD, FACC, FCCP
Associate Professor, Medicine/Cardiology,
Duke Clinical Research Institute;
Director, Interventional Devices Clinical Trials,
Duke University Medical Center;
Durham, North Carolina
Prayer and Cardiovascular Disease

NATHAN A. KRUGER, MD
Internal Medicine Resident,
Yale–New Haven Hospital,
New Haven, Connecticut
Nutriceuticals and Cardiovascular Illness

WEI-NCHIH LEE, MD
Assistant Professor of Medicine,
Section of General Internal Medicine,
New York Medical College,
Westchester Medical Center,
Valhalla, New York
The Placebo Effect in Cardiovascular Disease

RAVINDER MAMTANI, MD, MSc
Professor, Clinical Preventive Medicine;
New York Medical College;
Chief, Section of Complementary Medicine,
Department of Medicine,
Department of Community and Preventive Medicine,
Westchester Medical Center,
Valhalla, New York
Ayurveda and Yoga in Cardiovascular Diseases
Homeopathy With a Special Focus on Treatment of Cardiovascular Diseases
Acupuncture in Cardiovascular Diseases

RONAC MAMTANI, BS
Medical Student,
Stony Brook Medical School,
Port Jefferson, New York
Ayurveda and Yoga in Cardiovascular Diseases

SUSAN E. MANDEL, MEd, MT-BC
Music Therapy Consultant and Researcher,
Lake Hospital System Inc.,
Willoughby, Ohio;
Doctoral Student,
Union Institute and University,
Cincinnati, Ohio
The Effects of Music Therapy in Cardiac Healthcare

ANGELE MCGRADY, PhD
Professor, Department of Psychiatry,
Medical College of Ohio,
Toledo, Ohio
Biofeedback in Cardiovascular Disease

MOHAMMED MOIZUDDIN, MD
Medical Resident,
Department of Internal Medicine,
St. Barnabas Hospital,
Weill Medical College of Cornell University,
New York, New York
Herbal Approach to Cardiac Disease

NAUMAN NASEER, MD
Assistant Professor of Medicine,
New York Medical College,
Division of Cardiology,
Westchester Medical Center,
Valhalla, New York
Sauna as a Therapeutic Option for Cardiovascular Disease

YEN NGUYEN, MD
Medical Resident,
Santa Clara Valley Medical Center,
Stanford Medical School,
San Jose, California
Sauna as a Therapeutic Option for Cardiovascular Disease

TERRY OLESON, PhD
Doctoral Program Director,
Emperor's College of Traditional Oriental Medicine,
Santa Monica, California
Auriculotherapy for Cardiovascular Disorders

MEHMET OZ, MD
Professor;
Vice Chairman, Department of Surgery;
Director, Cardiovascular Institute,
Columbia University, College of Physicians and Surgeons,
New York, New York
Integrative Medicine in Cardiothoracic Surgery

STEPHEN J. PETERSON, MD, FACP
Vice Chairman, Department of Medicine;
Professor of Clinical Medicine;
Chief, Section of General Internal Medicine,
New York Medical College;
Director, Internal Medicine Residency Training Program,
Westchester Medical Center,
Valhalla, New York
The Placebo Effect in Cardiovascular Disease

JAMES ROSADO, PhD
Postdoctoral Psychology Fellow,
Harvard Medical School,
Spaulding Rehabilitation Hospital,
Massachusetts General Hospital,
Boston, Massachusetts
Cognitive-Behavioral Therapy in Cardiac Illness

RONALD SCHOUTEN, MD
Associate Professor of Psychiatry,
Harvard Medical School;
Director, Law and Psychiatry Services,
Massachusetts General Hospital,
Boston, Massachusetts
Legal Issues in Integration of Complementary Therapies Into Cardiology Practice

STEPHEN T. SINATRA, MD, FACC, CNS
Assistant Clinical Professor of Medicine,
University of Connecticut School of Medicine,
Farmington, Connecticut
Nutriceuticals and Cardiovascular Illness
Herbal Approach to Cardiac Disease

ADAM J. SPIEGEL, DO
Resident Physician,
Clinical Assistant Instructor,
Department of Medicine,
Stony Brook University Hospital,
Stony Brook, New York
Osteopathic Manipulative Medicine in the Treatment of Hypertension

TRACI R. STEIN, MPH
Director, Columbia Integrative Medicine Program,
Department of Surgery,
Columbia University, College of Physicians and Surgeons,
New York Presbyterian Hospital,
New York, New York
Integrative Medicine in Cardiothoracic Surgery

AI GVHDI WAYA (EILEEN NAUMAN), DHM (UK)
Desert Institute of Classical Homeopathy,
Phoenix, Arizona
Native American Healing for the Heart

MICHAEL I. WEINTRAUB, MD, FACP, FAAN
Clinical Professor of Neurology and Medicine,
Departments of Neurology and Internal Medicine,
New York Medical College,
Westchester Medical Center,
Valhalla, New York
Magnetic Biostimulation: Energy Therapy

RONALD D. WHITMONT, MD
President,
Homeopathic Medical Society of the State of New York,
Rhinebeck, New York
Homeopathy With a Special Focus on Treatment of Cardiovascular Diseases

ALAN WITKOWER, EdD, CGP
Instructor, Harvard Medical School;
Clinical Associate, Department of Psychiatry,
Massachusetts General Hospital;
Director of Psychology, Pain Program,
Spaulding Rehabilitation Hospital,
Boston, Massachusetts
Cognitive-Behavioral Therapy in Cardiac Illness

ANDREW I. WOLFF, MD
Resident, Internal Medicine,
Strong Memorial Hospital,
Rochester, New York
The Placebo Effect in Cardiovascular Disease
Chelation Therapy
Animal-Assisted Therapy and Cardiovascular Disease

JONATHAN E.E. YAGER, MD
Division of Cardiology,
Duke Clinical Research Institute,
Duke University Medical Center,
Durham, North Carolina
Prayer and Cardiovascular Disease

To all those health care providers who have preceded us,
who currently work with us,
and who will follow us

More and more individuals are looking outside the borders of conventional medicine for at least part of their health care needs. In the United States, more visits are being made to nonconventional healers than to physicians, at an annual cost of over $30 billion; most of this cost is out-of-pocket.

As a health care discipline, alternative medicine has been defined in recent years as medical approaches that were not traditionally addressed in allopathic medical schools. *Complementary medicine* is a term first used in Great Britain to describe the use of alternative medicine as an adjunct to, and not primarily a replacement for, conventional medical care. In the 21st century, there is an ongoing effort to integrate complementary and alternative medicine (CAM) into conventional medicine practice (Integrative Medicine). In 1998, the National Institutes of Health, recognizing the need to vigorously evaluate CAM therapies, created the National Center for Complementary and Alternative Medicine (NCCAM), which supports ongoing research. Multiple medical centers have formed Centers of Integrative Medicine, and most medical schools are now offering course work in complementary/alternative medicine.

Many of the complementary and alternative medicine modalities, as defined today, have been used for thousands of years as the mainstay of the healing arts in various cultures and societies. Chinese medicine has used bioenergy ("qi" manipulation [qi gong], insertion of needles [acupuncture] and ingestion [herbs and foods]) as part of a systematic approach to health care. Practitioners of Indian medicine (Ayurveda and Yoga) have used the combination of meditation and exercise as part of their healing approach. Native American medicine emphasizes "shamanism" and spiritualism. Recently, western medicine has included the development of allopathic medicine along with the CAM fields of homeopathy, vitamin therapy, osteopathic manual manipulation, chelation therapy, and talk therapies.

The scientific community no longer ignores the worldwide exponential surge in public enthusiasm for CAM therapies. This surge in interest relates to the chronicity of many illnesses, the information explosion on the Internet, and a more active participation of individuals in their own health care. At the same time, a large percentage of individuals who use CAM therapies do not even inform their personal physicians of this activity, making them vulnerable to the possible adverse effects from herb-drug interactions and other potential side effects of CAM treatments.

CAM therapies have also been used to treat cardiovascular disorders for thousands of years. However, the use of CAM for treating cardiovascular disease is a highly-charged subject, with both critics and proponents. Critics do not understand or accept anecdotal statements of benefit from CAM and demand rigorous placebo-controlled studies. These are essentially lacking in most situations. CAM therapies are a challenge to the scientific training of many cardiovascular physicians, with most positive observations being considered a placebo effect. However, physicians can no longer turn a deaf ear to the possibilities of CAM, and a growing number are already integrating CAM into their practices or are referring their patients to other CAM practitioners. The American College of Cardiology is sponsoring an annual course on CAM as part of its continuing medical education efforts. In a recent workshop, the NCCAM emphasized the need for an exchange of ideas between CAM practitioners and scientists, and for collaborative research efforts.

Complementary and Integrative Therapies for Cardiovascular Disease describes the major CAM therapies and approaches in chapters written by noted experts in their respective fields, with the overall text edited by a cardiovascular clinical researcher and two physician leaders in the field of CAM. Each chapter describes a specific CAM practice or approach, with its history, philosophy, and a discussion of the strengths and weaknesses of clinical studies regarding the prevention and treatment of cardiovascular disease. Chapters contain the most updated reference citations regarding the various CAM practices. The book recognizes the shortcoming of many of the CAM therapies regarding critical scientific scrutiny; however, it opens up the possibility for considering some of these approaches as part of an integrative approach to the management of cardiovascular disease, and also possible future clinical trial investigations.

The book is organized into six sections. The introductory section addresses the placebo effect in cardiovascular medicine, the minimum standard of efficacy by which all CAM therapies may be judged. A chapter that deals with the legal and ethical issues of CAM as part of a cardiovascular practice is also included.

The second section covers nutritional and herbal approaches to the treatment of cardiovascular disease and includes discussions of nutriceutical use (e.g. vitamins, enzymes, amino acids, carnitine, and antioxidants) and herbal botanical remedies, including their potential adverse effects and interactions with conventional drugs.

The third section deals with talk therapies and various cognitive approaches to the prevention and management of cardiovascular disease, including mind-body healing therapies, hypnosis, biofeedback, and cognitive behavior therapy.

The fourth section deals with regional CAM approaches to cardiovascular health care, including those coming from the Chinese tradition (Qigong and Tai Chi), Indian tradition (Ayurveda and Yoga), Native American tradition, and Western tradition (homeopathy and osteopathic manipulation).

The fifth section critically reviews specific CAM methodologies used in the prevention and treatment of heart disease and includes acupuncture, auriculotherapy, reflexology, chelation, aromatherapy, music therapy, sauna, meditation and prayer, pet therapy, Shiatsu and massage, magnetotherapy, and spinal cord stimulation. Some practices, such as art, horticultural, and humor therapies, are not included because there are no reported experiences with these approaches in cardiovascular medicine.

The final section consists of a chapter illustrating the function and design of a Center for Complementary and Alternative Medicine that is integrated into the workings of a conventional medical school and medical center (Columbia Presbyterian, New York City). Programs such as this are opening in medical centers across the country (e.g., Duke, Harvard, University of California at San Francisco, New York Medical College, Thomas Jefferson University), highlighting the growing desire to make available to patients, under one roof, both conventional and CAM therapies as part of an integrated approach to cardiovascular health care.

The editors are indebted to the many contributors of this book who come from various health care disciplines, and to our trainees and colleagues who have served as research collaborators and sources of intellectual stimulation. A special acknowledgement must be given to Joanne Cioffi-Pryor, who has served as the editorial assistant for this book and for other cardiovascular texts and journals we have published over a 25-year period. Her meticulous attention to detail and critical eye have contributed to the successful completion of this text.

We wish to acknowledge our editor Kellie White and the editorial staff at Elsevier, especially Kim Fons and Kendra Bailey, who have guided the book through the editorial process.

Finally, the most important contributors continue to be our families, who provide the ongoing support and love that have enabled our academic careers to flourish.

We are privileged to bring together this unique and timely book that we hope will increase the understanding of CAM and augment dialogue between traditional cardiovascular health care providers and the practitioners of CAM. Ultimately, it is the fusion of the best medical practices that will provide the most favorable clinical outcomes for cardiovascular patients in the years to come.

WILLIAM H. FRISHMAN, MD
MICHAEL I. WEINTRAUB, MD
MARC S. MICOZZI, MD

CONTENTS

COMPLEMENTARY AND INTEGRATIVE THERAPIES FOR CARDIOVASCULAR DISEASE

PART I

Introduction

CHAPTER I

The Placebo Effect in Cardiovascular Disease*

William H. Frishman, MD

Andrew I. Wolff, MD

Wei-Nchih Lee, MD, MPH

Stephen J. Peterson, MD

Stephen P. Glasser, MD

The three general reasons for clinical improvement in a patient's condition are the following: (1) natural history and regression to the mean; (2) the specific effects of the treatment; and (3) the nonspecific effects of the treatment attributable to factors other than the specific active components (this latter effect being included under the heading of "placebo effect").[1] Each time a physician recommends a diagnostic or therapeutic intervention for a patient, the possibility of a placebo effect, a clinical effect unrelated to the intervention itself, is built into this clinical decision.[2,3] Simple diagnostic procedures such as phlebotomy or more invasive procedures such as cardiac catheterization have been shown to have important associated placebo effects.[4,5] Indeed, Chalmers has stated that one only has to review the graveyard of therapies to realize how many patients would have benefited by being assigned to a placebo control group.[6] In fact, the first known clinical trial—attributed to Galen in 150 BC—may have reached erroneous conclusions because it lacked a placebo control group. Galen wrote that "some patients that have taken this herb have recovered, while some

*Modified with permission from Frishman WH, Lee W-N, Glasser SP, Bienenfeld L, Chien P, Peterson SJ: The placebo effect in cardiovascular disease. In Frishman WH, Sonnenblick EH, Sica DA, editors: Cardiovascular Pharmacotherapeutics, ed 2, New York, 2003, McGraw Hill. pp 15-25.

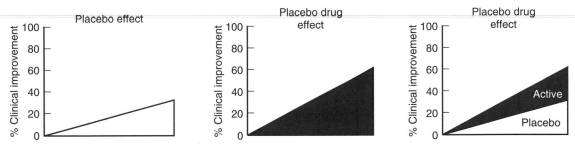

Fig 1-1. Any perceived total drug effect is likely to comprise an active drug effect component and a placebo effect component. *(From Archer TP, Leier CV: Placebo treatment in congestive heart failure, Cardiology 81:125-33, 1992.)*

have died; thus, it is obvious that this medicament fails only in incurable diseases."

Placebo effects are commonly observed in patients with cardiac disease who also receive drug and surgical therapies as treatments (Figure 1-1). In this chapter, the placebo effect in cardiovascular disease is reviewed, and the implications of this clinical phenomenon to the study of new treatments are discussed.

DEFINITION

Stedman's Medical Dictionary gives the following two meanings for the word *placebo*, which originates from a Latin phrase meaning "I shall please": (1) an inert substance prescribed for its suggestive value; and (2) an inert substance identical in appearance with the compound being tested in experimental research, which may or may not be known by the physician and/or the patient; and which is given to distinguish between a compound's action and the suggestive effect of the compound under study.[7]

The exact definition of *placebo* is debated today. Many recent articles on the subject include a broader definition, as described by Shapiro in 1961:

"....any therapeutic procedure (or that component of any therapeutic procedure) which is given deliberately to have an effect or unknowingly has an effect on a patient, symptom, syndrome, or disease, but which is objectively without specific activity for the condition being treated. The therapeutic procedure may be given with or without conscious knowledge that the procedure is a placebo, may be an active (non-inert) or nonactive (inert) procedure, and includes, therefore, all medical procedures no matter how specific—oral and parenteral medication, topical preparations, inhalants, and mechanical, surgical, and psychotherapeutic procedures. The placebo must be differentiated from the placebo effect which may or may not occur and which may be favorable or unfavorable. The placebo effect is defined as the changes produced by placebos. The placebo is also used to describe an adequate control in research".[8]

A further refinement of the definition was proposed by Byerly in 1975: "any change in a patient's symptoms that is the result of the therapeutic intent and not the specific physiochemical nature of a medical procedure."[9]

THE PLACEBO EFFECT IN CLINICAL TRIALS

Placebo controls in medical research date back to 1753, when Dr. James Lind advocated their use when he evaluated the effects of lime juice on scurvy.[10] After World War II, research protocols designed to assess the efficacy and safety of new pharmacologic therapies began to include the recognition of the placebo effect. Recognition of placebos and their role in controlled clinical trials occurred in 1946, when the Cornell Conference on therapy devoted a session to placebos and double-blind methodology. At that time, placebos were associated with increased heart rate, altered respiration patterns, dilated pupils, and increased blood pressure.[7] In 1951, Hill[11] concluded that for a specific treatment to be attributable to a change for better or worse in a patient, this result must be repeatable a significant number of times in similar patients. Otherwise, the result was merely due to the natural history of the disease or to the simple passage of time. He also proposed the inclusion of a control group that received identical treatment except for the inclusion of an "active ingredient." Thus the active ingredient was separated from the situation within which it was used. This control group, also known as a placebo group, would help in the investigations of new and promising pharmacologic therapies.[11]

Beecher was among the first investigators to promote the inclusion of placebo controls in clinical trials.[12] He emphasized the importance of ensuring that neither the patient nor the physician know what treatment the experimental subject was receiving and referred to this as the *double unknown technique*. Today, this term is called the *double-blind trial*. It ensures that the expectations and beliefs of the patient and physician are excluded from evaluation of new therapies. Beecher reviewed 15 studies that included 1082 patients and found that an average of 35% of these patients benefited from placebo therapy.[12] He also concluded that placebos can relieve pain from conditions in which either physiologic or psychologic etiologies were present. He described many diverse objective changes from placebo therapy. Some medical conditions—including severe postoperative wound pain, cough, drug-induced mood changes, pain from angina pectoris, headache, seasickness, anxiety, tension, and the common cold—improved with placebo therapy.

CHARACTERISTICS OF THE PLACEBO EFFECT

An inverse relationship seems to exist between the number of placebo doses that need to be administered and treatment outcomes. In a study of patients with postoperative wound pain, 53% of the subjects responded to one placebo dose, 40% to two or three doses, and 15% to four doses.[12] In analyzing the demographics of placebo responders and nonresponders, Beecher and his associates could find no differences in gender ratios or intelligence quotients between the two groups.[13] They did find significant differences in attitudes, habits, educational backgrounds, and personality structure between consistent responders and nonresponders. In attempting to understand the reproducibility of the placebo effect, they observed that there was no relationship between an initial placebo response and subsequent responses with repeated placebo doses of saline. Beecher and his colleagues concluded that placebos are most effective when stress, such as anxiety and pain, is greatest.

Patient adherence to placebo[14-17] has been shown to provide symptom relief and to affect discrete end points, such as survival. A patient's preference for a certain type of treatment has been shown to produce an enhanced placebo response as well. Kaptchuk examined the effect of placebo on patients receiving various types of alternative therapies.[17] Kaptchuk believed that patients who were more willing to use alternative medicines may be influenced by alternative medicine's "romantic vision," thus enhancing the placebo response to their medications.

A recent study of the effects of placebo on hypertension found that older white people are the predominant age-race subgroup that responds to placebo.[18] The subjects who were able to reach the goal blood pressure and maintain a diastolic blood pressure lower than 95 mm Hg for one year were broken down according to their age and race. Nine of 44 (20%) were African Americans; eight of 31 (26%) were younger whites; 12 of 44 (27%) were older African Americans; and 24 of 64 (38%) were older whites.

Placebos can produce both desirable and adverse reactions.[19,20] Beecher and his associates described over 35 different adverse reactions from placebo;[12,13] the most common are described in Box 1-1. These reactions were recorded without the patient's or physician's knowledge that a placebo had been administered. In one study in which lactose tablets were given as a placebo, major

Box **1-1** Most Common Adverse Reactions From Placebo Therapy	
Dry mouth	9%
Nausea	10%
Sensation of heaviness	18%
Headache	25%
Difficulty concentrating	15%
Drowsiness	50%
Warm glow	8%
Relaxation	9%
Fatigue	18%
Sleep disturbance	10%

From Frishman WH, Lee W-N, Glasser SP et al: The placebo effect in cardiovascular disease. In Frishman WH, Sonnenblick EH, Sica DA, editors: Cardiovascular Pharmacotherapeutics, ed 2, New York: McGraw Hill 2003: pp 15-25.

adverse reactions occurred in three patients.[21] The first patient experienced overwhelming weakness, palpitation, and nausea after taking placebo. The second patient experienced a diffuse rash that disappeared after discontinuing placebo administration. The third patient experienced epigastric pain that was followed by watery diarrhea, urticaria, and angioneurotic edema of the lips after receiving placebo.

In more general terms, Beecher went on to describe negative consequences of the use of placebo: "Placebos may divert patients from seeking more effective treatments, mask symptoms that may need attention, add to cost of treatment, and may have unexpected physiological effects."[12] Indeed, because of the substantial evidence of placebo "efficacy" and placebo "side effects," some have wittingly suggested that if placebo were submitted to the US Food and Drug Administration (FDA) for approval, the agency—although it might be impressed with the efficacy data—would probably recommend disapproval based on the high incidence of side effects. Some have questioned whether placebos are truly inert. Davis points out that "part of the problem with the placebo paradox is our failure to separate the use of an inert medication (if there is such a substance) from the phenomenon referred to as the placebo effect.[22] It might help us if we could rename the placebo effect the 'obscure therapeutic effect.'" That is, in lactase deficiency, could the amount of lactose in placebo tablets actually cause true side effects? Because of the small amount of lactose, this seems unlikely, but it is perhaps more likely that allergies to some of the so-called inert ingredients in placebos could cause reactions in predisposed individuals (although in the latter case it would seem unlikely that this could explain more than a small percentage of placebo side effects). The placebo effect has also been called the "meaning response." Moerman and Jonas[23] found that previous attempts to define the placebo effect were incorrect and argued that "placebos are inert and don't cause anything."[23] They went on to define the meaning response as the physiologic or psychologic effects of meaning in the origins or treatment of illness. The positive responses elicited should be termed "placebo effect" and when they are undesirable "nocebo effect".[24]

The most recent validation of the placebo effect occurred in 1962, when the United States enacted the Harris-Kefauver Amendments to the Food, Drug, and Cosmetic Act. These amendments require proof of efficacy as well as documentation of relative safety in terms of the risk-to-benefit ratio for the disease to be treated before an experimental agent can be approved for general use.[25] In 1970, the FDA published rules for "Adequate and Well-Controlled Clinical Evaluations." The federal regulations identified five types of controls (i.e., placebo, dose-comparison, active, historical, and no treatment) and identified use of the placebo control as an indispensable tool to achieve the standard.[26] However, one should remember that the FDA does not mandate placebo controls and in fact has stated that placebo groups are "desirable, but need not be interpreted as a strict requirement... the speed with which blind comparisons with placebo and/or positive controls can be fruitfully undertaken varies with the nature of the compound."[27] The FDA publication "General Considerations for the Clinical Evaluation of Drugs" further states that "it should be recognized that there are other methods of adequately controlling studies. In some studies, and in some diseases, the use of an active control drug rather than a placebo is desirable, primarily for ethical reasons."[27]

An important statistical concept that may mimic a placebo response is regression to the mean. Regression to the mean addresses the fact that in biologic systems most variables increase and decrease around a mean (one might conceptualize this idea by envisioning a sine wave). Thus any value measured at a specific point in time is likely—by chance—to be either above or below the mean and that a second measurement will be at a different point around the mean and therefore will be different from the first measurement. This change between measurements could then represent an improvement or worsening and thereby mimic a placebo response. The presumption is that this variability about the mean will be the same in the placebo group as the active treatment group (assuming adequate sample size and randomization), so that differences between the two groups relative to regression to the mean will "cancel out."

A recent meta-analysis of randomized clinical trials with three arms—a treatment arm, a placebo arm, and a nontreatment arm—demonstrated a clear placebo effect in its comparison of continuous variable outcomes among subjects in the placebo arm with subjects in the nontreatment arm.[28] The beneficial effect, however, decreased with increasing sample size. The authors suggest that although placebo should continue to play a role in future clinical trials, it should not be used as an actual treatment.

PLACEBO IN ISCHEMIC HEART DISEASE AND CHRONIC, STABLE EXERTIONAL ANGINA PECTORIS

The rate of improvement in the frequency of symptoms in patients with chronic, stable, exertional angina pectoris with placebo therapy has been assessed to be from 30% to 80%.[29] A summary of subjective and objective placebo effects in cardiovascular disease is provided in Tables 1-1 and 1-2. Because of the magnitude of the placebo effect, studies of new antianginal therapies had generally been performed with a placebo control.[30] However, the safety of this practice came under scrutiny in the late 1980s in response to concern that patients with coronary artery disease would have periods without drug treatment. Accordingly, Glasser et al explored the safety of exposing patients with chronic, stable exertional angina to placebos during short-term drug trials with an average double-blind period of 10 weeks.[31] The study samples were taken from new drug applications (NDAs) submitted to the FDA. The results of these drug trials

Table 1-1   SYMPTOMATIC PLACEBO EFFECTS IN CARDIOVASCULAR DISEASE

Chronic, stable angina pectoris improvement	30% to 80%[29]
Heart failure improvement	25% to 35%[45]

From Frishman WH, Lee W-N, Glasser SP et al: The placebo effect in cardiovascular disease. In Frishman WH, Sonnenblick EH, Sica DA, editors: Cardiovascular Pharmacotherapeutics, ed 2, New York: McGraw Hill 2003: pp 15-25.

Table 1-2   OBJECTIVE PLACEBO EFFECTS IN CARDIOVASCULAR DISEASE

Heart Failure	
Exercise tolerance testing	
with 1 to 2 baseline measurements	90 to 120 seconds[45]
with 3 to 10 baseline measurements	10 to 30 seconds[45]
Increase in ejection fraction of 5%	20% to 30% of patients[45]
Hypertension	
Measured by noninvasive, automatic, ambulatory 24-hour monitoring	0%[57]
Arrhythmias based on comparison of one control 24-hour monitoring period to one 24-hour treatment period (variability is so great that it may be inadvisable to pool individual patient data to detect trends in ectopic frequency in evaluating new potential antiarrhythmic agents in groups of patients)	
Mean hourly frequency of ventricular tachycardia	<65%[69]
Mean hourly frequency of couplets	<75%[69]
All ventricular ectopics, without regard for complexity	<83%[69]
When differentiating proarrhythmia in patients with mixed cardiac disease and chronic ventricular arrhythmias from spontaneous variability, with a false-positive rate of only 1%	
When baseline VPCs >100/h	<3 times baseline[70]
When baseline VPCs <100/h	<10 times baseline[70]
Silent Ischemic Coronary Disease	
Reduction in the frequency of ischemic events	44%[35]
Reduction of ST-segment integral	50%[35]
Reduction in duration of ST-segment depression	50%[35]
Reduction of total peak ST-segment depression	7%[35]
Other	
Compliance with treatment at a rate ≥ 75%	<3 times baseline[15,72]

were submitted regardless of whether they were favorable, and all adverse events were reported. Qualifying studies used symptom-limited exercise tolerance testing as an end point. No antianginal medication except sublingual nitroglycerin was taken after a placebo or drug-free washout period. The placebo-controlled samples consisted of 12 studies: six that used beta-adrenergic blockers and six that used calcium antagonists.[31] A total of 3161 patients entered the studies; 197 withdrew because of adverse cardiovascular events. Beta-blocker therapy was not significantly different than placebo therapy. Conversely, calcium antagonist therapy had a significantly higher cardiovascular event rate than placebo therapy had, thus leading to withdrawal from the trials. However, this significantly higher cardiovascular event rate was due to one calcium antagonist study that reported a disproportionately higher number of adverse events than the other five studies. This study found evidence that supported the safety of a placebo group in short-term drug trials for chronic, stable exertional angina.[31]

The safety of using placebo in longer-term drug trials for chronic, stable exertional angina has not been established. A placebo-controlled trial by a European group in 1986 enrolled 35 patients and followed them while administering placebo and short-acting nitroglycerin for 6 months.[32] This study of the long-term effects of placebo treatment in patients with moderately severe, stable angina pectoris found a shift toward the highest dosage during the titration period. Seven patients were kept on the lowest dosage. The average ending dosage was 65% more than the initial dose. The compliance, determined by pill count, for 27 patients was more than 80%. During the first 2.5 months of the trial, all the patients who were noncompliant or could not physically continue the study were determined. No patients died or experienced myocardial infarction.

Data regarding any gender differences in placebo response are sparse. Female patients represented 43% of the population in the aforementioned European study and were more likely to have angina despite normal coronary arteries.[32] Because the placebo effect may be more pronounced in patients with normal coronary arteries, data from male patients were analyzed separately to be compared with the overall results. However, the data from male patients were very similar to the overall results. In fact, the functional status of males showed more improvement due to placebo (61%) than overall (48%) at 8 weeks. The results of this study showed no adverse effects of long-term placebo therapy, with 65% of patients reporting subjective clinical improvement and 27% of patients reporting objective, clinical improvement on exercise performance.[32] Of note was the fact that improvement in exercise performance can occur when patients are repeatedly exposed to testing.[33]

Two problems inherent in all of the modern-day antianginal trials is that anginal patterns vary and modern-day treatments render attacks of angina rather infrequent. Therefore the FDA has adopted a surrogate measure of antianginal effect: treadmill walking time to the point of moderate angina. Just as anginal frequency responds to a placebo effect, a patient's treadmill walking time often (50% to 75%) improves with placebo therapy.

Other potential mechanisms partially explain the improvement but are unrelated to a treatment effect in exercise walking time in antianginal studies: the so-called learning phenomenon and the training effect. Patients often improve their walking times between the first and second treadmill test in the absence of any treatment. The anxiety and unfamiliarity of the first test are presumably reduced with the second test. Of greater importance is the training effect, in which the frequency of treadmill testing might result in a true improvement of exercise performance irrespective of treatment. The effect of placebo on exercise tolerance in patients with angina was demonstrated in the Transdermal

Nitrate Therapy Study, which compared various doses of nitroglycerin administered for 24-hour durations from transcutaneous patch formulations to placebo patch treatment.[34] This study was particularly important because it was the first large study to address the issue of nitrate tolerance with transcutaneous patch drug delivery in outpatient, ambulatory subjects. The study demonstrated tolerance in all treated groups in that the treated groups performed at the study's end no better than the placebo group did. However, the placebo and active treatment groups improved a striking 80 to 90 seconds in in the primary efficacy end point of exercise walking time on a treadmill. This improvement in placebo could have masked any active treatment effect, but it also demonstrated the importance of placebo control, since without such a control one could have deduced a significant improvement due to active therapy.

Myocardial ischemia was assessed via 48-hour ambulatory ECG monitoring for ST-segment analyses in 250 males with stable angina pectoris and coronary artery disease based on at least 70% stenosis of one major coronary artery, previous myocardial infarction at least 2 months before screening, coronary artery bypass surgery, angioplasty, or a positive exercise tolerance test within the last 12 months prior to screening.[35] These participants were reassessed after 7 weeks of therapy with amlodipine or placebo by repeating the 48-hour ambulatory ECG monitoring. The monitoring showed the well-known circadian pattern of ischemic activity with peaks in the morning and afternoon. Amlodipine significantly reduced ischemia in comparison to placebo. However, transient silent myocardial ischemia was less common in all groups, including the placebo group.

Internal mammary artery ligation was thought to improve angina pectoris until studies showed similar benefit in patients where a sham operation was performed—that is, skin incision with no ligation. Beecher tried to analyze the effect of doctors' personalities on clinical outcomes by comparing the results of the same placebo procedure performed by one of two groups, the "enthusiasts" or the "skeptics."[36] His analysis indicated that the enthusiasts achieved nearly four times more "complete relief" for patients than the skeptics, although the procedure has no known specific effects.[36] Five patients receiving the sham operation emphatically described marked improvement.[37] Objectively, a patient undergoing the sham operation had an increase in work tolerance from 4 to 10 minutes with no inversion of T waves on ECG and no pain. This procedure was used in the United States for 2 years before it was disproven by three small, well-planned, double-blind studies and thus discontinued.[38] Carver and Samuels also have addressed the issue of sham therapy in the treatment of coronary artery disease.[39] They point out that although the pathophysiology of coronary artery disease is well-known, many of the expressions of myocardial ischemia are subjective, thus rendering the placebo effect more important. This has resulted in a number of treatments that are based upon testimonials rather than on hard scientific evidence and have been touted as "miracle cures" and "breakthroughs." Among therapies cited by these authors are chelation therapy (see Chapter 17), various vitamin therapies, and mineral supplements (see Chapter 3). Chelation therapy—probably one of the most instructive examples of a sham—

is briefly discussed here. An estimated 500,000 patients per year are treated by this technique in the United States alone. Before 1995, the data to support claims regarding the effectiveness of chelation therapy were uncontrolled open-label studies. In 1994, van Rij and associates performed a double-blind, randomized, placebo-controlled study in patients with intermittent claudication and demonstrated no benefits of chelation over placebo.[40] A number of variables were evaluated, including both objective and subjective measures, with improvement in many of the measures of both therapies. Again, without the use of a placebo control, the results could have been interpreted as improvements related to chelation treatment. The National Institutes of Health has started a large multicenter, placebo-controlled trial to definitively assess whether chelation is of any clinical benefit in patients with coronary artery disease.

THE PLACEBO EFFECT IN HEART FAILURE

Until recently, the importance of the placebo effect in patients with congestive heart failure (CHF) had not been recognized. In the 1970s and early 1980s, vasodilator therapy was administered to patients in clinical trials without placebo control. Investigators believed that the cause of heart failure was predictable, so placebo-controlled trials were unnecessary. Another view of the unfavorable course of heart failure concluded that withholding a promising new agent was unethical. The ethical issues regarding placebo use in cardiovascular disease are discussed further in this chapter and elsewhere.[41-44]

Clinical trials with placebo controls documented a 25% to 35% improvement in patients' symptoms. This placebo response occurred in patients with mild to severe symptoms and did not depend on the size of the study. The assessment of left ventricular (LV) function can be determined by several methods, including noninvasive echocardiography, radionuclide ventriculography, and invasive pulmonary artery balloon-floatation catheterization. These methods measure the patient's response to therapy or the natural progression of the patient's heart failure.[45]

Noninvasive measurements of LV ejection fraction vary, especially when the ventricular function is poor and the time interval between tests is 3 to 6 months. Packer found that when a 5% increase in ejection fraction is used to determine a beneficial response to a new drug, 20% to 30% of patients show improvement with placebo therapy. Overall, changes in noninvasive measures of LV function have not been shown to correlate closely with observed changes in clinical status of patients with CHF. Most vasodilator and inotropic drugs can produce clinical benefit without a change in LV ejection fraction. Conversely, LV ejection fraction may increase significantly in heart failure patients with worsening clinical status.[45]

Because spontaneous fluctuations in hemodynamic variables are possible in the absence of drug therapy, one must carefully interpret the results of studies that use invasive catheterization to evaluate the efficacy of a new drug. To avoid recognition of spontaneous variability attributable to drug therapy, the researcher should assess postdrug effects at fixed times; threshold values should eliminate changes due to spontaneous variability. Another factor that can mimic a beneficial drug response by favorably affecting hemodynamic measurements is measurement performed immediately after catheterization of the right side of the heart or after ingestion of a meal. Systemic vasoconstriction occurs after intravascular instrumentation and resolves in 12 to 24 hours. When predrug measurements are done during the postcatheterization period, any subsequent measurements will show beneficial effects because the original measurements were done during the vasoconstricted state. Thus comparative data must be acquired after the postcatheterization vasoconstricted state has resolved.[45]

The most common test for evaluating drug efficacy for heart failure is the exercise tolerance test (ETT). An increased duration of ET represents a beneficial therapy. However, this increased duration is also recorded during placebo therapy, possibly because of the patient's familiarity with the test and the physician's increased willingness to encourage the patient to exercise to exhaustion. Placebo response to repeated ETT can be an increase in duration of 90 to 120 seconds when only one or two baseline measurements are done. This response can be reduced to 10 to 30 seconds when 3 to 10 baseline measurements are performed. The placebo response cannot be explained by changes in gas-exchange measurements during the ETT; presumably, it relates to an improvement in subjects' mechanical efficiency of walking during the ETT.[45,46]

Because all methods used to measure efficacy of a treatment for heart failure include placebo effects, studies must include placebo controls to prove efficacy of a new drug therapy. Statistical analysis of placebo-controlled studies must compare between groups for statistical significance. "Between groups" refers to comparison of the change in one group, such as a new drug therapy, with the change in another group, such as a placebo.[45]

In 1992, Archer and Leier reported on placebo therapy for 8 weeks in 15 patients with CHF, which resulted in a mean improvement in exercise duration of 81 seconds, or 30% above baseline.[47] This result was statistically significant in comparison to the 12-second improvement by the 9 patients in the non–placebo control group. Between-group statistical analysis revealed no statistically significant differences between the placebo and nonplacebo groups at baseline nor at week 8 of treatment. Echocardiography studies showed no significant improvement in either group and no significant differences between the two groups at baseline or during the treatment period. To prove the existence of the therapeutic power of placebo treatment in CHF and to quantify it, the same principal investigator performed all studies with identical study methods and conditions. Moreover, all patients were similarly familiarized with the treadmill testing procedure before baseline measurements. Also, the study used a well-matched, non–placebo control group and illustrated the spontaneous variability of congestive heart failure.

The Placebo Effect in Hypertension

Some studies of placebo response in hypertensive patients have shown a lowering of blood pressure;[18,48–50] others have not.[51–53] In the Medical Research Council study, no treatment that was compared to placebo therapy in patients with mild hypertension for several months found similar results in both groups, an initial fall in blood pressure followed by stabilization.[53] Of historical note is a study by Goldring and associates published in 1956.[54] These authors fabricated an "electron gun" designed to be as "dramatic as possible, but without any known physiologic action other than a psychogenic one." Initial exposure to the gun was 1 to 3 minutes; the length was increased to 5 minutes three times per day. The investigators noticed a substantially lower pressure during therapy than before therapy. In six of nine hospitalized patients, blood pressure dropped 39/28 mm Hg.

An important factor to consider is the method of measuring blood pressure. With standard sphygmomanometry, blood pressure falls initially. During placebo therapy, intraarterial pressures and circadian curves measured over 24 hours did not show a decline in blood pressure or heart rate. Intraarterial blood pressure was lower at home than at the hospital. The circadian curves from intraarterial ambulatory blood pressure monitoring were reproducible on separate days several weeks apart.[50,55] Like 24-hour invasive intraarterial monitoring, 24-hour noninvasive automatic monitoring of ambulatory blood pressure also has been reported to lack a placebo effect. Upon the initial application of the blood pressure device, a small reduction of ambulatory blood pressure values in the first 8 hours occurred with placebo therapy. This effect, however, did not change the mean 24-hour value. The home monitoring values were lower than the office measurements. Heart rate was also measured, with no variance in either setting. The office measurement of blood pressure—but not the 24-hour blood pressure—was lower after 4 weeks of placebo therapy.[56] This study confirms the absence of a placebo effect in 24-hour noninvasive ambulatory blood pressure monitoring as suggested by several specific studies on large numbers of patients.[57-59] The 24-hour monitoring was measured by the noninvasive automatic Spacelabs 5300 device (Spacelabs Inc., Redmond, Washington).[60] Another important factor in 24-hour noninvasive monitoring is that the intervals of measurement were less than 60 minutes.[61]

In a study of the influence of observer's expectation on the placebo effect in blood pressure, 100 patients were followed for a 2-week single-blind period and for a 2-week double-blind period.[62] During this time, the patients' blood pressures were measured by two methods: a 30-minute recording with an automatic oscillometric device and a standard sphygmomanometric measurement performed by a physician. All patients were seen in the same examining room, monitored by the same automatic oscillometric device, and seen by the same physician. The results during the single-blind period showed a slight but statistically significant decline in diastolic blood pressure detected by the automatic oscillometric device but no decline measured by the physician. During the double-blind period, the oscillometric device measured no additional decline in diastolic blood pressure, but the physician measured significant decreases in both systolic and diastolic blood pressures. Overall, the blood pressures measured by the automatic oscillometric device in the absence of the physician were lower than those measured by the physician. However, there was significant correlation of the two methods. The investigators concluded that correcting for the placebo effect in clinical trials that use ambulatory monitoring to study hypertension requires the same design standards as those in using conventional sphygmomanometry.[63]

A randomized double-blind comparison of placebo and active treatment for elderly patients with isolated systolic hypertension showed a small effect of placebo on BP.[64] Patients older than 60 years old were randomly assigned to the administration of nitrendipine 10 to 40 mg daily with the possible addition of enalapril 5 to 20 mg daily and hydrochlorothiazide 12.5-25 mg daily or matching placebos. After a 2-year follow-up period, the sitting systolic BP fell by 13 mm Hg in the placebo and by 23 mm Hg in the active treatment group.

Although a placebo effect on blood pressure was measured with auscultatory technique in the Systolic Hypertension in the Elderly Program (SHEP), it was less significant than the reduction of blood pressure produced by active therapy in patients 60 years of age and older with isolated systolic hypertension.[65,66] In a subsequent study of patients with isolated systolic hypertension, a substantial portion of the long-term blood pressure change observed during active treatment was attributed to a placebo effect. Twenty-four–hour blood-pressure monitoring was no more reliable than conventional sphygmomanometry in correcting for the actions of placebo.

The use of placebo control in mild disease states such as stage 1 and 2 hypertension has undergone much debate. Although the ethical considerations will be discussed later in this article, placebo treatment has been shown to be effective for such conditions. Preston et al compared the rates of blood pressure control and adverse effects of placebo and active treatment in stage 1 and 2 hypertension.[18] The randomized controlled trial performed at 15 Veterans Affairs hypertension centers consisted of 1292 subjects who were randomly allocated to receive treatment with one of six active drugs or placebo. Of those patients given placebo, 30% achieved a goal diastolic blood pressure lower than 90 mm Hg 1 year after treatment. Patients whose blood pressure was nonresponsive and became too high were discontinued from the study. This consisted of 14% in the placebo arm and only 7% in the active treatment arm. Preston et al concluded that placebo does have a place in trials of treatments for stage 1 and 2 hypertension.

Placebo in long-term trials has been associated with an increased risk. The Syst-Eur Study showed 8.7% of 2297 patients given placebo had a serious adverse event, as opposed to 5.8% of 2398 patients given active treatment.[63] A similar study of the effects of enalapril in patients with renal impairment found an adverse event rate of 13% in the placebo arm and 3% in the active arm.[67]

THE PLACEBO EFFECT IN ARRHYTHMIA

Spontaneous variability in the natural history of disease or in its signs and/or symptoms is another reason that placebo controls are necessary. In a study of ventricular arrhythmias, Michelson and Morganroth found marked spontaneous variability of complex ventricular arrhythmias such as ventricular tachycardia and couplets.[68] Their study followed 20 patients for 4-day periods of continuous ECG monitoring. They recommended that statistically significant therapeutic efficacy in evaluation requires a comparison of one 24-hour control period to four 24-hour test periods that shows a 41% reduction in the mean hourly frequency of ventricular tachycardia and a 50% reduction in the mean hourly frequency of couplets. They also suggested that individual patient data not be pooled to detect trends because individual variability is so great.

A study by Morganroth et al provides an algorithm to differentiate spontaneous variability from proarrhythmia in patients with benign or potentially lethal ventricular arrhythmias.[69] A total of 495 patients were evaluated with two or more Holter tracings during placebo therapy. The algorithm defines proarrhythmia as an increase of more than three times when the hourly frequency of baseline ventricular premature complexes (VPCs) is greater than 100 and greater than 10 times when it is less than 100. The false-positive rate is 1% with this algorithm.

The Cardiac Arrhythmia Suppression Trial (CAST) evaluated the effect of antiarrhythmic therapy in patients with asymptomatic or mildly symptomatic ventricular arrhythmia.[70,71] Response to drug therapy was determined by a greater than or equal to 80% reduction of ventricular premature depolarizations or a greater than or equal to 90% reduction of runs of unsustained ventricular tachycardia as measured by 24-hour Holter monitoring 4 to 10 days after the initiation of pharmacologic treatment; this response previously had been considered an important surrogate measure of antiarrhythmic drug efficacy. Ambulatory ECG (Holter) recording screened for arrhythmias. The CAST Data and Safety Monitoring Board recommended that encainide and flecainide therapy be discontinued based on the increased number of deaths from arrhythmia, cardiac arrest, or any cause in comparison the placebo group (1455 patient were assigned to drug regimens). The CAST investigators' conclusion emphasized the need for more placebo-controlled clinical trials of antiarrhythmic drugs with a mortality end point.[70]

THE RELATIONSHIP OF TREATMENT ADHERENCE TO SURVIVAL IN PATIENTS WITH AND WITHOUT HISTORY OF MYOCARDIAL INFARCTION

One important consideration in determining study results is adherence to therapy and the assumption that any differences in adherence rates are equal in the active and the placebo treatment groups. The Coronary Drug Project planned to evaluate the efficacy and safety of several lipid-influencing drugs in the long-term treatment of coronary heart disease.[14] This randomized double-blind placebo-controlled multicenter clinical trial found no significant difference in the 5-year mortality of 1103 men treated with the fibric acid derivative clofibrate in comparison to 2789 men given placebo. However, good adherers—patients who took 80% or more of the protocol drug—had lower mortality than poor adherers in both the clofibrate and placebo groups.[14]

A similar association between adherence and mortality was found in patients after myocardial infarction in the Beta-Blocker Heart Attack Trial (BHAT) data.[15] The same phenomenon was extended to women after myocardial infarction. On analysis of the BHAT data for 505 women randomized to both beta-blocker therapy and placebo therapy, mortality increased two-and-a-half– to three-fold within the first 2 years in patients who took less than 75% of their prescribed medication. Adherence among men and women was similar, at about 90%. However, the cause of the increased survival resulting from good adherence is not known. Good adherence has been speculated to reflect a favorable psychological profile—an individual's ability to make lifestyle adjustments that limit disease progression. Alternatively, adherence may be associated with other advantageous health practices or social circumstances not measured. Another possible explanation is that improved health status may facilitate good adherence.[16]

The Lipid Research Clinics Coronary Primary Prevention Trial did not find a correlation between compliance and mortality.[72] The trial randomized 3806 asymptomatic hypercholesterolemic men to cholestyramine or placebo. Over 7 years, the main effects of the drug on cholesterol, death, and nonfatal myocardial infarction were compared to placebo. In the active drug group, a relationship between compliance and outcome existed and was mediated by lowering cholesterol. However, no effect of compliance on cholesterol or outcome was observed in the placebo group.[72]

The Physicians' Health Study randomized 22,000 American male physicians between the ages of 40 and 84 years who were free of myocardial infarction and cerebral vascular disease.[73] This study analyzed the benefit of differing frequencies of aspirin consumption on the prevention of myocardial infarction. The study also identified factors associated with adherence and analyzed the relationship of adherence with cardiovascular outcomes in the placebo group. In this study, an average compliance of 80% in the aspirin and placebo groups over the 60 months of follow-up was observed.[73] Adherence during the trial was associated with several baseline characteristics in the aspirin and placebo groups. Trial participants with poor adherence (<50% compliance with pill consumption) were more likely than those with good adherence to be younger than 50 years at randomization, to smoke cigarettes, to be overweight, to not exercise regularly, to have a parental history of myocardial infarction, and to have angina. These associations were statistically significant. In a multivariant logistic regression model, cigarette smoking, being overweight, and angina remained significant predictors of poor compliance. The strongest predictor of adherence during the trial was adherence during the run-in period. Baseline characteristics with little relationship to adherence included regular alcohol consumption and a history of diabetes and hypertension.[73]

According to an intention-to-treat analysis, the aspirin group had a 41% lower risk of myocardial infarction than the placebo group had. On subgroup analysis, participants who reported excellent (95%) adherence in the aspirin group had a significant (51%) reduction in risk of first myocardial infarction relative to those with similar adherence in the placebo group. Lower adherence in the aspirin group did not produce a statistically significant reduction of first myocardial infarction in comparison to the placebo group with excellent adherence. Excellent adherence in the aspirin group was associated with a 41% lower relative risk of myocardial infarction than in those with lower adherence in the aspirin group. Excellent adherence in the placebo group did not show a reduction of relative risk.

The rate of stroke was different from myocardial infarction. In the intention-to-treat analysis, the aspirin group had an insignificant (22%) increased rate of stroke than the placebo group. Excellent adherence in the placebo group produced a lower rate of strokes than among participants in the aspirin and placebo groups with poor (<50%) adherence. Excellent adherence in the placebo group was associated with a 29% lower risk of stroke than among those with excellent adherence in the aspirin group.

The overall relationship of adherence to aspirin therapy with cardiovascular risk examined a combined end point of all important cardiovascular events—including first fatal or nonfatal myocardial infarction or stroke or death from cardiovascular disease with no prior myocardial infarction or stroke. In an intention-to-treat analysis, risk of all important cardiovascular events was decreased by 18% in the aspirin group in comparison to the placebo group. Participants with excellent adherence in the aspirin group had a 26% reduction of risk of a first major cardiovascular event in comparison to those with excellent adherence in the placebo group. However, those participants in the aspirin group with poor compliance had a 31% increased risk of a first cardiovascular event in comparison to those in the placebo group with excellent adherence. Within the placebo group, level of adherence and risk of first cardiovascular event were not associated.

In analysis of death from any cause with no prior nonfatal myocardial infarction or stroke, poor adherence in both the aspirin and placebo groups was associated with a four-fold increase in the risk of death. In analysis of the 91 deaths due to cardiovascular causes, similar risks were found to be associated with poor adherence in both the aspirin and placebo groups relative to excellent adherence in the placebo group.

The Physicians' Health Study found similar results to the Coronary Drug Project, in which all-cause mortality and cardiovascular mortality were considered.[14,73] These relationships remained strong when adjusted for potential confounding variables at baseline. The strong trend for higher death rates among participants with poor adherence in both the aspirin and placebo groups may be due to the tendency for individuals to lessen or discontinue study participation as their health declines with serious illness. Acute events such as myocardial infarction did not accompany an increased risk associated with poor adherence in the placebo group. Thus placebo effects seem to vary according to the outcome considered.

A systematic review of trials using placebo as a treatment for disease showed little evidence of placebo having powerful clinical effects.[28] The only place placebo was shown to have a small effect was in conditions with continuous subjective outcomes and for pain. Therefore placebo has no place in treating disease outside the realm of clinical trials.

CLINICAL TRIALS AND THE ETHICS OF USING PLACEBO CONTROLS

Since the 1962 amendments to the Food, Drug and Cosmetic Act, the FDA has had to rely on the results of "adequate and well-controlled" clinical trials to determine the efficacy of new pharmacologic therapies. Regulations governing pharmacologic testing recognize several types of controls that may be used in clinical trials to assess the efficacy of new pharmacologic therapies. These include the following: 1) placebo concurrent control; 2) dose-comparison concurrent control; 3) no-treatment concurrent control; 4) active-treatment concurrent control; and 5) historical control. However, regulations do not specify the circumstances for the use of these controls because any number of study designs could be adequate in a given set of circumstances.[74,75]

Vickers et al[76] suggests that choosing a research design depends upon the particular question being asked and must be considered in terms of the distinction between internal and external validity. Among the several advantages of using the placebo, according to Vickers et al, is that the placebo group controls for placebo effect, natural remission, and nontrial interventions. It also facilitates outcome blinding and promotes subject and physician compliance via double-blinding.[77] Furthermore, placebo control is advantageous because without it the researcher cannot discern whether the effects of control therapy are greater than those achieved with the placebo effect. However, placebo-controlled trials do not give clinically useful information such as the effect size or the comparative effectiveness of real-world choices. The studies do not reveal how drugs A and B compare to each other but rather how each compares to placebo. Therefore the trial has "high internal validity, or rigor, and low external validity, or generalizability."[76]

The debate concerning the ethics of using placebo controls in clinical trials of cardiac medications is ongoing.[41,42,78] The issue revolves around administration of placebo in lieu of a proven therapy. Rothman and Michels[43] argue that the common practice in clinical trials of administering placebo therapy instead of a proven therapy for the patient's medical condition directly violates the Nuremberg Code and the World Medical Association's adaptation of this code in the Helsinki Declaration. The fifth revision of the Helsinki Declaration drafted in 2000 states, "The benefits, risks, burdens and effectiveness of a new method should be tested against those of the best current prophylactic, diagnostic, and therapeutic method. This does not exclude the use of placebo or no treatment in studies where no proven prophylactic, diagnostic, or therapeutic method exists."[79] The Nuremberg Code, a 10-point ethical code for experimentation in human beings, was formulated in response to the human experimentation atrocities recorded during the post–World War II trial of Nazi physicians in Nuremberg, Germany. According to Rothman and Michels, placebo-controlled studies violate these principles because the use of placebo as control denies the patient the best proven therapeutic treatment.[43] They argue that the practice occurs despite the establishment of regulatory agencies and institutional review boards yet seem to ignore the fact that informed consent is part of the current practice, as certainly was not the case with the Nazi atrocities. One reason that placebo-controlled trials are approved by institutional review boards is that they are part of the FDA's general recommendation for demonstrating therapeutic efficacy before an investigational drug can be approved. When the investigational drug is found to be more beneficial than placebo, therapeutic efficacy is proven.[80] As more drugs are found to be more effective than placebo in treating disease, inclusion of a placebo group is often questioned. However, this objection ignores the fact that, in many cases, drug efficacy had been established by surrogate measures and—as new and better measures of efficacy become available—additional study becomes warranted. For instance, the suppression of ventricular arrhythmia by antiarrhythmic therapy was later proven to be unrelated to survival; in fact, results with this therapy were worse than those with placebo. Likewise, in studies of inotropic therapy for heart failure, exercise performance rather than survival was used as the measure of efficacy, and in fact a presumed efficacious therapy performed worse than placebo. In the use of immediate short-acting dihydropyridine calcium antagonist therapy for the relief of symptoms of chronic stable angina pectoris, again, a subject might have fared better had he or she been randomly assigned to placebo therapy.

Also important to the concept that established beneficial therapy should not necessarily prohibit use of placebo for evaluating new therapies is that the natural history of a disease may change and thus the effectiveness of the so-called established therapy (e.g., antibiotic agent for treatment of infection) may diminish. The prevailing standard for choosing to use an investigational drug in a clinical trial is that confidence in the new drug should be high enough to risk patient exposure to it yet enough doubt about the drug to risk exposure to placebos. A placebo control is thus warranted, particularly when other life-saving therapy is not discontinued.

Placebo-controlled trials may be advocated on the basis of a scientific argument. When pharmacologic therapy has been shown effective in previous placebo-controlled clinical trials, conclusions drawn from trials without placebo controls may be misleading because the previous placebo-controlled trial becomes a historical control. These historical controls are the least reliable for demonstrating efficacy. In active-controlled clinical trials, one assumes that the active control treatment is as effective under the new experimental conditions as it was in the previous placebo-controlled trial. This assumption can result in misleading conclusions when results with an experimental therapy are found to be equivalent to those with active, proven therapy. This conclusion of equivalence can be magnified by conservative statistical methods, such as the "intent to treat" approach, analysis of all randomized patients regardless of protocol deviations, and attempts to minimize the potential for introduction of bias into the study. Concurrent placebo controls account for factors other than drug-effect differences between study groups. When an untreated control group is used instead of a placebo-control group, blinding is lost, and treatment-related bias may occur.[17,23,26,81]

Clark and Leaverton[26] and Rothman and Michel[43] agree that the placebo controls are ethical when no existing treatment favorably affects morbidity and mortality or survival. Furthermore, some treatment for chronic diseases exists but does not favorably alter morbidity and mortality or survival. For example, no clinical trial has found the treatment of angina to increase a patient's survival. In contrast, treatment after a myocardial infarction with beta-blocking agents has been convincingly proven to increase a patient's survival.[26] However, Clark and Leaverton[26] disagree with Rothman and Michels[43] by asserting that a placebo-controlled clinical trial of short duration is ethical for chronic disease because no alteration in long-term outcome for the patient usually occurs. The short duration of the trial represents a small segment of the lifetime management of a chronic disease. For instance, treatment of chronic symptomatic congestive heart failure (CHF) and a low ejection fraction (<40%) with enalapril was shown to decrease mortality by 16%. This decrease in mortality was most marked in the first 24 months of an average 40 months of follow-up. Therefore only long-term compliance with pharmacologic therapy resulted in some decrease in mortality. Another example of a chronic medical condition that requires long-term treatment and in which short-term placebo is probably not harmful is hypertension.[82] Halpern & Karlawish, however, believe that there is no longer any scientific or clinical value of placebo therapy and that it is unethical, even in the setting of short term trials of stage 1 and 2 hypertension.[42] They believe that many patients receive placebo therapy that exceeds blood-pressure limits, possibly causing problems with the long-term consequences of uncontrolled blood pressure. Furthermore, an extraordinary number of efficacious antihypertensive medications are available; the value of knowing that another one exists is not beneficial or worth the risk.

In some studies, men and women with a history of myocardial infarction and at least 80% compliance with treatment, including placebo therapy, had an increased survival. This increased survival was also described in patients in a 5-year study of the effect of lipid-influencing drugs on coronary heart disease.[14-16]

Therefore Rothman and Michels[43] and Clark and Leaverton[26] agree that a placebo should not be included in a trial when a proven therapy that favorably affects morbidity and mortality exists, but they disagree with regard to chronic cardiovascular diseases and short-term trials. Brief interruption of effective therapy has not been found to alter long-term outcome when the effective treatment is a long-term therapy. The claim that the use of placebos in clinical trials violates the Nuremberg Code and the Helsinki Declaration if a proven therapy exists does not account for all of the information currently available. The proven therapies for chronic congestive heart failure and hypertension are long-term therapies. The belief that patients receiving placebo are being harmed is inaccurate because no adverse effect on morbidity and mortality or survival results from short-term withholding of proven long-term therapy.

Temple and Ellenberg state that not all placebo-controlled trials are unethical if a proven efficacious therapy exists.[83,84] Active controlled trials cannot definitively prove therapeutic efficacy without comparing it to placebo or to no treatment. Furthermore, if the Declaration of Helsinki is followed closely, no clinical trial could be considered ethical because every patient fails to receive the most proven efficacious therapy. The American Medical Association,[85] the World Health Organization,[86] and the Council for International Organizations of Medical Sciences[87] have rejected the Declaration of Helsinki's position on barring all trials in which a proven therapy is available; therefore a revision of the Declaration is of interest.

Treating serious medical conditions in placebo-controlled trials unanimously is considered unethical. To estimate how a new drug would compare to placebo in this instance, one must extend from an active control trial. This requires a significant amount of scientific judgment and expertise, because of the significant uncertainty associated with historical data. Over time, changes occur in patients, their surroundings, and other factors that may affect the comparability with historical trial data. Therefore differences in opinion will exist in various clinical settings.[78]

Many have argued for placebo-controlled trials on the grounds that the smaller sample size required to demonstrate statistical significance exposes fewer people to the potentially risky therapy and makes the study quicker and less expensive.[81] Another way in which placebo controls are considered ethical is the existence of the informed consent process. A patient is asked to participate before the trial begins, and the informed consent process describes use of placebo and other aspects of the trial. In this written agreement the patient is responsible for notifying the physician of any medical problems and is informed of his or her right to withdraw from the study at any time, as described in the Nuremberg Code and Helsinki Declaration. During this disclosure, patients are presented with some new concepts and with risks and benefits to understand. On the basis of this information, a patient voluntarily decides whether to participate, knowing that he or she may receive a placebo or investigational medication.

However, despite physicians' efforts to inform the patient of research methods and the risk and benefits of trial participation, some patients agree to participate simply because of their trust in their physicians. This situation may produce conflict between the physician-patient relationship and the physician's role as investigator. A partial resolution of this conflict is the double-blind technique, in which neither the patient nor the investigator knows which therapy a patient is receiving. This technique allows the doctor and patient to make medical decisions on the basis of clinical signs and symptoms. Moreover, because of the informed consent requirement, participation in a clinical trial is the patient's rather than the physician's sole decision. However, the patient's physician evaluates the suitability of the patient for a particular trial before asking him or her to participate.

For every pharmacologic therapy, patient compliance with the regimen is an assumption. In clinical trials, investigators try to monitor compliance by having patients bring their pill bottles to their appointments and counting the pills. Ultimately, the patient decides whether the beneficial effects of therapy outweigh the adverse effects. If a medication produces annoying and adverse side effects, the patient may not continue to take the medication. Other factors that affect compliance are the number of pills taken daily and the frequency of dosing. For instance, taking a medication once a day is easier than three times a day. Furthermore, studies of patient compliance have found increased survival in patients with at least an 80% rate of compliance with therapy, including placebo therapy.[14-16] All parties should be responsible for their research and accountable for the ethical conduct of their research. Clinical trials that violate the Nuremberg Code and the Helsinki Declaration should not be conducted nor accepted for publication. However, determining which research methods are in compliance with the Nuremberg Code and Helsinki Declaration is controversial. Scientific needs should not override ethical needs. Clinical trials must be carefully designed to produce a high-quality trial performance, and experimentation with human subjects must abide by the universal standards of the Nuremberg Code and Helsinki Declaration.

Until the mechanism of the placebo action is understood and controlled, data from clinical trials that lack a placebo group should be interpreted cautiously. Assessing efficacy of a therapy is difficult without a placebo group to which to compare it because clinical improvement attributed to drug therapy might have occurred as well in a control group. As was found in studies of heart failure, chronic diseases have variable courses; until those courses are understood, placebo controls must help explain it. Furthermore, because each clinical trial has a different setting and study design within the context of the physician-patient relationship, a placebo group helps the investigator distinguish true drug effects from placebo effects.

Patients who receive placebo may report subjective, clinical improvements and show objective, clinical improvements—for instance, on ETT or Holter monitoring of ischemic events. Findings such as these dispel the implication that placebo therapy is the same as no therapy. The factors that influence these findings include elements of the physician-patient relationship, such as the psychological state of the patient; the patient's expectations and conviction regarding the efficacy of the method of treatment; and the physician's biases, attitudes, expectations, and methods of communication.[88] Close attention from investigators explains some patients' improvement during trials. Baseline laboratory values are checked to ensure the patient's safety and compliance with the study protocol. This positive response by the patient is called a *positive placebo effect* when it is found in control groups of patients who receive placebo therapy.[*]

Conversely, placebos have worsened patient response in some cases.[†] Every drug has side effects. These side effects are also found with placebo therapy and can be so great that they preclude the patient's continuation with the therapy. Finally, placebos can act synergistically and antagonistically with other specific and nonspecific therapies. Therefore much remains to be discovered about the effects of placebo in cardiovascular medicine.

CONCLUSION

The effect of placebo on the clinical course of systemic hypertension, angina pectoris, silent myocardial ischemia, CHF, and ventricular tachyarrhythmias is well described and continues to be the focus of many investigative interests. A direct relation seems to exist between compliance with placebo treatment and favorable clinical outcomes for prevention of myocardial infarction. The safety of short-term placebo-controlled trials has now been well documented in stud-

---

[*]References 29, 33, 36, 38, 45, 62, and 69.
[†]References 21, 32, 45, 62, 89, and 90.

ies of drug treatment of angina pectoris. The ethical basis for performing placebo-controlled trials continues to be challenged in the evaluation of drugs and alternative therapies for treating cardiovascular diseases.[41,43,91] However, as long as life-saving treatment is not being denied, placebo-controlled studies remain a prudent approach for obtaining reliable scientific information regarding the efficacy and safety of new treatments.[92,93]

REFERENCES

1. Turner JA, Deyo RA, Loeser JD et al: The importance of placebo effects in pain treatment and research, JAMA 271:1609-14, 1994.
2. Talbot M: The placebo prescription, New York Times Magazine January 9, 2000.
3. Weiner M, Weiner GJ: The kinetics and dynamics of responses to placebo, Clin Pharmacol Ther 60:247-54, 1996.
4. Packer M, Medina N, Yushak M: Hemodynamic changes mimicking a vasodilator drug response in the absence of drug therapy after right heart catheterization in patients with chronic heart failure, Circulation 71: 761-66, 1985.
5. Carruthers SG, et al editors: Melmon and Morrelli's clinical pharmacology: basic principles in therapeutics, ed 4, New York, 2000, McGraw-Hill.
6. Chalmers TC: Prophylactic treatment of Wilson's disease, N Engl J Med 278:910-11, 1968.
7. Stedman's Medical Dictionary, ed 26, Baltimore, 1995, Williams & Wilkins.
8. Shapiro AK: Factors contributing to the placebo effect: their implications for psychotherapy, Am J Psychother 18:73, 1961.
9. Byerly H: Explaining and exploiting placebo effects, Perspect Biol Med 19:423-36, 1976.
10. Lind JA: A treatise of the scurvy, Edinburgh, 1753.
11. Hill AB: The clinical trial, Br Med Bull 7:278, 1951.
12. Beecher HK: The powerful placebo, JAMA 159:1602, 1955.
13. Lasagna L, Masteller F, von Felsinger JM, Beecher HK: A study of the placebo response, Am J Med 16:770, 1954.
14. The Coronary Drug Project Research Group: Influence of adherence to treatment and response to cholesterol on mortality in the Coronary Drug Project, N Engl J Med 303:1038-41, 1980.
15. Horwitz RI, Viscoli CM, Berkman L et al: Treatment adherence and risk of death after a myocardial infarction, Lancet 336:542-45, 1990.
16. Gallagher EJ, Viscoli CM, Horwitz RI: The relationship of treatment adherence to the risk of death after myocardial infarction in women, JAMA 270:742-44, 1993.
17. Kaptchuk TJ: The placebo effect in alternative medicine: Can the performance of a healing ritual have clinical significance? Ann Intern Med 136:817-25, 2002.

18. Preston, RA, Materson BJ, Reda DJ, Williams DW. Placebo-associated blood pressure response and adverse effects in the treatment of hypertension: observations from a Department of Veterans Affairs Cooperative Study, Arch Intern Med 160:1449-54, 2000.

19. Barsky AJ, Saintfort R, Rogers MP, Borus JF: Nonspecific medication side effects and the nocebo phenomenon. JAMA 287:622-27, 2002.

20. Feinstein AR: The placebo effect. In Education of Health Professionals in Complementary/Alternative Medicine. Conference sponsored by Josiah Macy Jr. Foundation, Phoenix, AZ, November 2-5, 2000. Published by Josiah Macy Jr. Foundation, New York, New York, 2001.

21. Wolf S, Pinsky RH: Effects of placebo administration and occurrence of toxic reactions. JAMA 155:339, 1954.

22. Davis JM: Don't let placebos fool you, Postgrad Med 88:21-24, 1990.

23. Moerman DE, Jonas WB: Deconstructing the placebo effect and finding the meaning response, Ann Intern Med 136:471-76, 2002.

24. Hahn RA: The nocebo phenomenon: concept, evidence, and implications for public health, Prev Med 26:607-11, 1997.

25. Nies AS: Principles of therapeutics. In Hardman JG, Limbird LE, editors: Goodman and Gilman's Pharmacological Basis of Therapeutics, ed 10, New York, 2001, McGraw Hill: 45-66.

26. Clark PI, Leaverton PE: Scientific and ethical issues in the use of placebo controls in clinical trials, Annu Rev Public Health 15:19-38, 1994.

27. FDA Draft: Guidelines for the Clinical Evaluation of Anti-anginal Drugs, January 10, 1989.

28. Hrobjartsson A, Gotzsche PC: Is the placebo powerless? An analysis of clinical trials comparing placebo with no treatment, N Engl J Med 344:1594-1602, 2001.

29. Amsterdam EA, Wolfson S, Gorlin R: New aspects of the placebo response in angina pectoris, Am J Cardiol 24:305-06, 1969.

30. Kim MC, Kini A, Sharma SK: Refractory angina pectoris: mMechanism and therapeutic options, J Am Coll Cardiol 39:923-34, 2002.

31. Glasser SP, Clark PI, Lipicky RJ et al: Exposing patients with chronic, stable, exertional angina to placebo periods in drug trials, JAMA 265:1550-54, 1991.

32. Boissel JP, Philippon AM, Gauthier E et al: Time course of long-term placebo therapy effects in angina pectoris, Eur Heart J 7:1030-36, 1986.

33. McGraw BF, Hemberger JA, Smith AL, Schroeder JS: Variability of exercise performance during long-term placebo treatment, Clin Pharmacol Ther 30:321-27, 1981.

34. Transdermal Nitroglycerin Cooperative Study Group Steering Committee: Acute and chronic antianginal efficacy and continuous 24-hour application of transdermal nitroglycerin, Am J Cardiol 68:1263-73, 1991.

35. Deanfield JE, Detry JRG, Lichen PR et al for the CAPE Study Group: Amlodipine reduces transient myocardial ischemia in patients with coronary artery disease: double-blind circadian anti-ischemia program in Europe (CAPE Trial), J Am Coll Cardiol 24:1460-67, 1994.

36.   Beecher HK: Surgery as a placebo: a quantitative study in bias, JAMA 176:1102, 1961.

37.   Dimond EG, Kittle CF, Crockett JE: Comparison of internal mammary artery ligation and sham operation for angina pectoris, Am J Cardiol 5:484, 1960.

38.   Cobb LA: Evaluation of internal mammary artery ligation by double-blind technique, N Engl J Med 260:1115, 1959.

39.   Carver JR, Samuels F: Sham therapy in coronary artery disease and atherosclerosis, Pract Cardiol 14:81, 1988.

40.   van Rij AM, Solomon C, Packer SGK, Hopkins WG: Chelation therapy for intermittent claudication, Circulation 90:1194-99, 1994.

41.   Enserink M: Psychiatry: Are placebo-controlled drug trials ethical? Science 288:416, 2000.

42.   Halpern SD, Karlawish JHT: Placebo-controlled trials are unethical in clinical hypertension research, Arch Intern Med 160: 3167-69, 2000.

43.   Rothman KJ, Michels KB: The continuing unethical use of placebo controls, N Engl J Med 331:394-98, 1994.

44.   Frishman WH, Lee W-N, Glasser SP et al: The placebo effect in cardiovascular disease. In Frishman WH, Sonnenblick EH, Sica DA, editors: Cardiovascular Pharmacotherapeutics, ed 2, New York: McGraw Hill 2003: 15-25.

45.   Packer M: The placebo effect in heart failure, Am Heart J 120:1579-82, 1990.

46.   Russell SD, McNeer FR, Beere PA et al: Improvement in the mechanical efficiency of walking: An explanation for the "placebo effect" seen during repeated exercise testing of patients with heart failure. Duke University Clinical Cardiology Studies (DUCCS) Exercise Group, Am Heart J 135:107-14, 1998.

47.   Archer TP, Leier CV: Placebo treatment in congestive heart failure, Cardiology 81:125-33, 1992.

48.   Pugsley DJ, Nassim M, Armstrong BK, Beilin L: A controlled trial of labetalol (Trandate), propranolol and placebo in the management of mild to moderate hypertension, Br J Clin Pharmacol 7:63-68, 1979.

49.   Martin MA, Phillips CA, Smith AJ: Acebutolol in hypertension: a double-blind trial against placebo, Br J Clin Pharmacol 6: 351-56, 1978.

50.   Report of Medical Research Council Working Party on Mild to Moderate Hypertension: Randomized controlled trial of treatment for mild hypertension: design and pilot trial, Br Med J 1:1437-40, 1977.

51.   Wilkinson PR, Raftery EB: A comparative trial of clonidine, propranolol and placebo in the treatment of moderate hypertension, Br J Clin Pharmacol 4:289-94, 1977.

52.   Veterans Administration Cooperative Study Group on Antihypertensive Agents: Effects of treatment on morbidity in hypertension: results in patients with diastolic blood pressures averaging 115 through 129 mm Hg, JAMA 202:1028-34, 1967.

53. Veterans Administration Cooperative Study Group on Antihypertensive Agents: Effects of treatment on morbidity in hypertension: results in patients with diastolic blood pressures averaging 90 through 114 mm Hg, JAMA 213:1143-52, 1970.

54. Goldring W, Chasis H, Schreiner GE, Smith HW: Reassurance in the management of benign hypertensive disease, Circulation 14:260, 1956.

55. Raftery EB, Gould BA: The effect of placebo on indirect and direct blood pressure measurements, J Hypertens 8(Suppl 6):S93-100, 1990.

56. Mutti E, Trazzi S, Omboni S et al: Effect of placebo on 24-h non-invasive ambulatory blood pressure, J Hypertens 9:361-64, 1991.

57. O'Brien E, Cox GP, O'Malley K: Ambulatory blood pressure measurements in the evaluation of blood pressure lowering drugs, J Hypertens 7:243-47, 1989.

58. Coats AJS, Conway J, Somers VK et al: Ambulatory blood pressure monitoring in the assessment of antihypertensive therapy, Cardiovasc Drugs Ther 3 (Suppl 1):303-11, 1989.

59. Parati G, Pomidossi G, Casadei R et al: Evaluation of the antihypertensive effect of celiprolol by ambulatory blood pressure monitoring. Am J Cardiol 61:27C-33C, 1988.

60. Casadei R, Parati G, Pomidossi G et al: Twenty-four hour blood pressure monitoring: Evaluation of Spacelabs 5300 monitor by comparison with intra-arterial blood pressure recording in ambulant subjects. J Hypertens 6:797-803, 1988.

61. Portaluppi F, Strozzi C, degli Uberti E et al: Does placebo lower blood pressure in hypertensive patients? A noninvasive chronobiological study, Jpn Heart J 29: 189-97, 1988.

62. Sassano P, Chatellier G, Corvol P, Menard J: Influence of observer's expectation on the placebo effect in blood pressure trials, Curr Ther Res 41:304, 1987.

63. Staessen JA, Thijs L, Bieniaszewski L et al: On behalf of the Systolic Hypertension in Europe (SYST-EUR) Trial Investigators: ambulatory monitoring uncorrected for placebo overestimates long-term antihypertensive action, Hypertension 27(3 Pt 1):414-20, 1996.

64. Staessen JA, Fagard R, Thijis H. Randomised double-blind comparison of placebo and active treatment for older patients with isolated systolic hypertension, The Lancet 350:757-63, 1997.

65. SHEP Cooperative Research Group: Prevention of stroke by anti-hypertensive drug treatment in older persons with isolated systolic hypertension: final results of the Systolic Hypertension in the Elderly Program (SHEP), JAMA 265:3255-64, 1991.

66. Davis BR, Wittes J, Pressel S et al: Statistical considerations in monitoring the Systolic Hypertension in the Elderly Program (SHEP), Control Clin Trials 14:350-61, 1993.

67. Keane WF, Polis A, Wolf D et al. The long-term tolerability of enalapril in hypertensive patients with renal impairment, Nephrol Dial Transplant 12 (Suppl 2):75-81, 1997.

68. Michelson EL, Morganroth J: Spontaneous variability of complex ventricular arrhythmias detected by long-term electrocardiographic recording, Circulation 61:690-95, 1980.

69. Morganroth J, Borland M, Chao G: Application of a frequency definition of ventricular proarrhythmia, Am J Cardiol 59:97-99, 1987.

70. The CAST Investigators: Preliminary report: Effect of encainide and flecainide on mortality in a randomized trial of arrhythmia suppression after myocardial infarction, N Engl J Med 321:406-12, 1989.

71. Capone RJ, Pawitan Y, El-Sherif N et al and the CAST Investigators: Events in the Cardiac Arrhythmia Suppression Trial: baseline predictors of mortality in placebo-treated patients, J Am Coll Cardiol 18:1434-38, 1991.

72. Lipid Research Clinics Program: The Lipid Research Clinics Coronary Primary Prevention Trial Results, II: the relationship of reduction in incidence of coronary heart disease to cholesterol lowering, JAMA 251:365-74, 1984.

73. Glynn RJ, Buring JE, Manson JE et al: Adherence to aspirin in the prevention of myocardial infarction: the Physicians' Heart Study, Arch Intern Med 154:2649-57, 1994.

74. Cleophas TJM: Clinical trials: design flaws associated with use of a placebo, Am J Ther 3:529, 1996.

75. Emanuel EJ, Miller F: The ethics of placebo-controlled trial: a middle ground, N Engl J Med 345: 915-19, 2001.

76. Vickers AJ, Craen A. Why use placebo in clinical trials? A narrative review of the methodological literature, J Clin Epidemiol 53:157-61, 2000.

77. Pledger GW, Hall D. Active control trials: do they address the efficacy issue? Proc Am Stat Soc 1-10, 1986.

78. Fisher LD, Gent M, Büller HR: Active control trials: how would a new agent compare with placebo? A method illustrated with clopidogrel, aspirin, and placebo, Am Heart J 141:26-32, 2001.

79. World Medical Association Declaration of Helsinki: Ethical principles for medical research involving human subjects, JAMA 284: 3043-46, 2000.

80. Cagliano S, Traversa G: The use of placebo controls (correspondence), N Engl J Med 332:60, 1995.

81. AI-Khatib SM, Califf RM, Hasselblad V et al: Placebo-controls in short-term clinical trials of hypertension, Science 292: 2013-15, 2001.

82. Alderman MH: Blood pressure management: individualized treatment based on absolute risk and the potential for benefit, Ann Intern Med 119:329-35, 1993.

83. Temple R, Ellenberg SS. Placebo controlled trials and active controlled trials in the evaluation of new treatments, part 1: ethical and scientific issues, Ann Intern Med 133:455-63, 2000.

84. Ellenberg SS, Temple R. Placebo controlled trials and active-control trials in the evaluation of new treatments, part 2: practical issues and specific cases, Ann Intern Med 133:464-70, 2000.

85. American Medical Association Council on Ethical and Judicial Affairs. The use of placebo controls in clinical trials: report 2-A-1996. Chicago, 1996, American Medical Association.
86. Grof P, Akhter MI, Campbell M et al: Clinical evaluation of psychotropic drugs for psychiatric disorders: principles and proposed guidelines, WHO Expert Series on Biological Psychiatry, Volume 2, Seattle, 1993, Hogrefe & Huber, 28-29.
87. Council for International Organizations of Medical Sciences: International ethical guidelines for biomedical research involving human subjects, Geneva: Council for International Organization of Medical Sciences, 1993.
88. Benson H, Epstein MD: The placebo effect, a neglected asset in the care of patients, JAMA 232:1225-27, 1975.
89. Roberts AH: The powerful placebo revisited: magnitude of non specific effects, Mind/Body Med 1:35, 1995.
90. Drici MD, Raybaud F, DeLunardo C et al: Influence of the behavior pattern on the nocebo response of healthy volunteers, Br J Clin Pharmacol 39:204, 1995.
91. Flynn JT: Ethics of placebo use in pediatric clinical trials. The case of antihypertensive drug studies. *Hypertension* 42:865-869, 2003.
92. Miller FG, Emanuel EJ, Rosenstein DL, Straus SE: Ethical issues concerning research in complementary and alternative medicine. *JAMA* 291; 599-604, 2004.
93. Arnstein P: The placebo effect. *Sem Integr Med* 1:125-135, 2003.

CHAPTER 2

Legal Issues in Integration of Complementary Therapies Into Cardiology Practice

Ronald Schouten, MD, JD
Michael H. Cohen, JD

Complementary and alternative medical (CAM) therapies are moving into the mainstream of American medicine.[1,2] Indeed, for some conditions, physicians may resort to CAM therapies more than conventional treatments.[3] However, the innovative nature of these treatments does not free them from the medical-legal issues that affect conventional medical practice. As CAM providers venture into traditional areas of medicine, they may expose themselves to liability issues previously limited to practitioners of standard forms of Western medicine.[4,5] In this chapter, we review basic medical-legal issues as they apply to the application of CAM therapies by physicians in cardiology, as well as steps that might be taken to reduce potential liability risk.

MEDICAL MALPRACTICE

MALPRACTICE GENERALLY

The threat of being sued for malpractice poses an ongoing general concern for healthcare professionals. Approximately once a decade a "crisis" in medical malpractice occurs and is marked either by skyrocketing malpractice insurance premiums, increased incidence of claims, large damage awards, or some combination of these.[3] In the 1990s, increasing damage awards and declining investment income for insurers set the stage for increasingly burdensome malpractice insurance premiums.[4]

Physicians have been the traditional objects of malpractice claims. The reasons for this are numerous and include the relatively high-risk conditions that they address and the more invasive treatments that they provide.

Because of the increased risk of suit, physicians have carried substantial insurance coverage, providing "deep pockets" that likely have the double effect of encouraging litigation. Malpractice insurance serves dual purposes: it protects the practitioner from personal liability for acts of negligence and ensures that compensation is available for patients injured by negligent acts of physicians. Whether malpractice insurance should be regarded as personal protection for practitioners or as a fund to compensate injured patients is the subject of lengthy debate that is outside the scope of this chapter.[5] States vary in their requirements regarding malpractice coverage. In some states, specific amounts of coverage are mandated, whereas other states do not require any coverage.[6] Regardless, it is a risky matter for a physician to practice without malpractice insurance, or "go bare", and the decision to do so must be made carefully.

Malpractice is a subset of personal injury or tort law. A tort is defined as a civil (as opposed to criminal) wrong that gives rise to a right to sue for damages. The purpose of awarding damages is twofold. First, it provides compensation to those injured by the acts of others. Second, the imposition of liability for negligent behavior serves as a disincentive for negligence and an inducement to exercise reasonable care.[7,8]

There are two basic types of torts: intentional and unintentional. Intentional torts arise when one person purposefully engages in an act that is likely to cause harm to another person. Unintentional torts arise when an injury results from negligence in the pursuit of an activity that is not intended to cause harm, such as medical treatment.[3,9]

Malpractice insurance is intended to protect practitioners from liability for medical negligence and not for liability from intentional acts.[5,8] Certain intentional torts are covered by malpractice policies, however. Battery (the intentional touching of another person without consent or justification) is an intentional tort that may fall within the realm of malpractice coverage if the touching occurred in the course of medical treatment, such as a case in which a patient is injured after a treatment for which full informed consent was not obtained. This scenario is battery because battery was a theory of recovery that later morphed, in many states, into treatment with inadequate informed consent (see Informed Consent, p. 40); furthermore, the nonconsensual touching itself may be the negligent act. A battery by a practitioner that is unrelated to treatment would not fall within malpractice coverage, however. For example, injury to a patient in the course of spinal manipulation by a chiropractor might be covered—because the battery, negligence, and failed informed consent are related—whereas injury to a patient in the course of an altercation in the waiting area would not be. In addition to battery, malpractice coverage may be afforded in some cases for certain intentional acts such as abandonment and, on a limited basis, for inappropriate sexual involvement with a patient.[10,11] These two areas will be discussed specifically below. It should be noted that although malpractice insurance may cover these arenas, courts are reluctant to allow physicians to disclaim liability or to have patients waive their right to sue for damages, in these arenas.

ELEMENTS OF A MALPRACTICE CLAIM

For a claim of malpractice to succeed, the plaintiff (the injured party making the claim) must establish four elements: that the defendant had a duty toward the plaintiff to use reasonable care, that the defendant was derelict in that duty, that dereliction directly led to harm, and that harm can be measured in the form of damages that are provable.[12]

Duty

Every practitioner has a duty to possess the skills and knowledge of the average, reasonable practitioner in his or her field of practice. Pursuant to the "school rule," each practitioner is judged according to the standards of practice of his or her field.[13] Thus physicians generally are held to a medical standard of practice, but CAM providers are each held to the standard of care in their own professions (e.g., acupuncture, chiropractic, massage therapy, etc.)[14] However, a general standard of practice is applied to all those who present themselves to the public as being able to diagnose and treat illness.[15] Thus when CAM providers offer treatment that overlaps with medical diagnosis and treatment (e.g., a chiropractor ordering an X-ray), that provider could be held to a medical standard.[14] Similarly, when a physician incorporates CAM therapies, it is unclear whether that physician will be held to a "mixed" standard of care that includes medical and CAM practice standards—that is, the physician might be compared to that of similarly situated physicians incorporating CAM therapies in like fashion; physicians in this situation may, however, be able to use as a potential defense to malpractice the "respectable minority" argument, which suggests that practice is legitimate if it is followed by a significant number of similarly situated clinicians.[14]

The locality rule, which calls for practitioners to be judged according to the standard of practice in their communities, has been in decline with the wide availability of medical information in publications, at conferences, and online.[15,16] Instead, courts tend to judge practitioners according to national standards of care. In addition, those who represent that they have specific expertise in a given area are held to a higher standard of knowledge and skill. Thus a primary care physician who represents having special expertise in treating heart ailments will be judged according to the standard of practice of cardiologists, not of other primary care physicians or CAM practitioners who treat general ailments.

The number of schools of CAM poses a challenge in terms of identifying specific schools of practice and determining what standards of practice might apply to CAM practices that are not clearly defined by any one profession. Statutory recognition, specialized education, and distinctive treatment can all be considered in determining whether a type of practice represents a distinct school.[15] In any event, practitioners of all types—licensed or unlicensed—have a duty to refer when the condition to be treated is outside the range of their knowledge and experience.[17,18] CAM providers therefore have a duty to refer the patient to a physician when the condition exceeds the CAM provider's knowledge, skill, and expertise, although no court yet has found such a reverse duty back from the physician to the CAM provider.[14]

Dereliction (Breach of Duty)

Dereliction (or breach of duty) refers to negligent failure to comply with the standard of care. This may occur when the practitioner fails to take routine steps in the course of evaluation and treatment—for example, treating chest pain with spinal manipulation without taking a thorough history and obtaining appropriate testing, such as an ECG. It can also arise when an appropriate workup is done but the information is handled negligently (e.g., ignoring key elements of the history or misinterpreting the ECG).

Direct Causation

The negligent departure from the standard of care must have a direct connection with some injury to the plaintiff.[19] This has two aspects to it. The first is direct causation in the mechanical sense, as measured by the "but for" rule: but for the negligent behavior, the injury would not have occurred. The second aspect is proximate or legal cause. This refers to the principle that liability will only be imposed for harm that was reasonably foreseeable from any negligent action.[20] Foreseeability is broadly interpreted, and physical injury after medical treatment is easy to establish through the testimony of a medical expert that—to a "reasonable degree of medical certainty"—the alleged negligence caused the harm in question.[21]

Damages

Finally, to recover on a claim of negligence, the plaintiff must prove that damages have been suffered. Damages can be financial (e.g., lost earning capacity, medical costs), physical (e.g., loss of a body part or function), or emotional (e.g., depression or anxiety after an injury).[19,20] Damages, like the other elements of a malpractice claim, are established through the testimony of expert witnesses. For example, an economist is typically called to testify about the lost value of future earnings and a psychiatrist or psychologist to testify about emotional damages.

Where the negligent behavior results in a missed opportunity to prevent harm, a plaintiff may recover under the "loss of chance" doctrine. For example, a physician who does not perform a physical examination on his patient and thus misses a cancerous breast lump that ultimately leads to the patient's death may be held liable for wrongful death under the loss of chance rule. Clearly, the lack of examination did not cause the cancer, but it represented a lost opportunity for the cancer to be detected.[22,23] Loss of chance is a potent legal theory with regard to negligence in the field of CAM. Failure to diagnose or treat, or prescription of ineffective treatment techniques in the absence of full informed consent (see Case G below), or use of the wrong treatment could all serve as bases for such claims.

BURDEN OF PROOF

In any personal injury litigation, the plaintiff has the burden of establishing his or her case by a preponderance of the evidence (i.e., it is more likely than not that the facts are as the plaintiff alleges and so the plaintiff is entitled to judgment).

This should be contrasted with the burden of proof in criminal cases, which is "beyond a reasonable doubt." Thus the plaintiff must present testimony that establishes each of the elements of a malpractice claim outlined above. The testimony of an expert witness must be introduced on the subjects of standard of care and proximate cause.[12]

Under the doctrine of *res ipsa loquitur* ("the thing speaks for itself"), the burden of proof shifts to the defendant, who then has to prove compliance with the standard of care or lack of proximate cause. This doctrine applies where the procedure, instrument, or medication was under the sole control of the defendant and the defendant alone has knowledge of the events leading up to the injury. For example, if a patient has complications from a surgical sponge discovered in the abdomen, the surgeon who performed the prior surgery has the burden of proving compliance with the standard of care, a lack of relationship between the sponge and the new injury, or that the sponge got there by some other means.[12]

SELECTED MALPRACTICE ISSUES IN CAM

To date, CAM has been light on malpractice claims relative to medicine. Studdert et al found that from 1990 to 1996, malpractice claims against chiropractors, acupuncturists, and massage therapists were fewer in number and involved less serious injuries than those against traditional practitioners.[24] This situation is likely to change, however. As the field grows, expands the range of conditions it treats and makes greater claims for efficacy, it will come to the attention of the plaintiff's personal injury bar and be subjected to the same malpractice rules as other areas of medicine.[24-27]

This section reviews some of the specific areas of CAM in which claims for malpractice may arise. Consider the following case and its variations[*]:

C is a board-certified cardiologist who is well versed in mind-body therapies and in herbal medicine and nutrition and has taken sufficient weekend courses in acupuncture and traditional oriental medicine to receive certification appropriate to the state law requirements. C also has a referral network consisting of a licensed chiropractor, a licensed naturopathic physician, and a clinical psychologist who have staff privileges at the same hospital as C. P, the patient, visits C and complains of chest pain. C takes a medical history and learns that P is 2 weeks away from taking a state exam to become a licensed stockbroker.

Case A

C determines that P is suffering from anxiety over the coming exam and refers P to the clinical psychologist for a mental health check-up and some relaxation techniques. On the drive to the clinical psychologist, P suffers a heart attack. An autopsy reveals that the heart attack easily could have been prevented had C, instead of referring P, simply followed conventional diagnostic and monitoring techniques.

[*]Copyright Ronald Schouten MD, JD and Michael Cohen JD, reprinted with permission.

Case B

Part 1. C summarily concludes that P is simply suffering from anxiety, fails to treat P with necessary medication for P's heart condition, and does not refer him to anyone. The next day, P has a heart attack that could have been prevented by conventional diagnosis and treatment.

Part 2. C applies regular diagnostic methods and concludes that P is at risk of a heart attack if P continues to neglect diet and exercise and pile up stressors. C recommends the Ornish diet, a regimen of light yoga and various stress reduction methods. "I want you to come back in 2 weeks and let's test you again," C says, "In the meanwhile, try these methods and call me if your chest pain worsens or you feel any other symptoms. And try to ease off on your hours at the firm."

Case C

C applies regular diagnostic methods and concludes that P is at risk of an impending heart attack. C applies magnets to P's chest wall, telling P, "This treatment will reverse your cardiovascular disease." The next day, P has a heart attack that could have been prevented by conventional diagnosis and treatment.

Case D

C tells P: "With your lifestyle and emotional constitution, your heart's in danger." C recommends that P adopt a nutritional protocol and seek counseling for anger management. P yells back, "But I love my salami for breakfast, lunch, and dinner and I refuse to change. Stop trying to control me!" C replies, "You're a lost cause. I refuse to see you anymore. Good luck finding someone who can handle your temper tantrums." The next day, P has a heart attack that could have been prevented by conventional diagnosis and treatment.

Case E

Part 1. In Case D above, C goes to the chief of cardiology and reports the stormy encounter with P. The chief replies: "That's okay; our patient volume is up, and your research grant just came through. You don't have to deal with an obstreperous personality like that; why get yourself all stressed out? Walk the talk and take some deep breaths, and let that one go." C goes for a long walk and determines never to speak to P again.

Part 2. Assume instead that after speaking with the chief, C goes for a walk; takes some deep breaths; and, feeling responsible for P, calls and suggests that P make an appointment with the clinical psychologist affiliated with the hospital. P does so. C fails to mention P's angry blow-ups, and, during P's visit, P is in a mild and charming state. The psychologist fails to do an adequate assessment. The next day, P is involved in a minor traffic accident but in an act of road rage severely injures the other driver in a physical confrontation. P is arrested and is prevented from getting his broker's license.

Case F

C describes P's case (and discloses P's name) to the licensed chiropractor, a licensed naturopathic physician, and a clinical psychologist without receiving an appropriate, signed consent form from P. P receives a phone call from one of these providers, who offers services. P is embarrassed and irate.

Case G

C diagnoses P conventionally and determines that P must schedule bypass surgery to avoid a possible myocardial infarction. P has the bypass surgery and later learns that there is some evidence in the medical literature, albeit conflicting, that chelation therapy might have been a preferred alternative. P is angry at C for not disclosing the possibility of chelation therapy and claims that if he had been properly informed, he would have elected to try this treatment instead of bypass surgery.

Case H

C diagnoses P conventionally and determines that P might have to schedule bypass surgery to avoid a possible myocardial infarction; C also discloses to P that some evidence, albeit conflicting, in the medical literature suggests that chelation therapy might be a preferred alternative. P wants to try the therapy. "We'll schedule you for follow-up," C tells P. "If chelation therapy doesn't work, we'll have to do the bypass surgery." P receives chelation therapy and, delighted by the results, tells his clinical psychologist, who promptly reports C to the state medical board for engaging in professional misconduct by using an off-label therapy that is not supported by medical evidence.

Case I

C continues to treat P over a number of years and during one visit attempts to console P for a family tragedy by giving him a hug. P mistakes the gesture for an uninvited sexual intimacy.

MISDIAGNOSIS

Misdiagnosis refers to both a failure to diagnose a condition as well as inaccurate diagnosis. It is important to emphasize the fact that an error alone is not sufficient to establish negligence. The error must result from a departure from the standard of care in order to provide a basis for a successful claim.[28,29] For CAM practitioners, misdiagnosis may be an issue with which adherence to a particular school of practice leads to a failure to detect a condition. Thus both the physician who fails to diagnose ischemic cardiovascular disease and the chiropractor who misdiagnoses intermittent chest pain as the product of subluxation of the thoracic spine, rather than angina, could be held liable for misdiagnosis.

In Case A, the cardiologist misdiagnosed the patient's impending heart attack by failing to implement standard conventional diagnostic techniques. C's referral without conventional diagnosis is inexcusable, as is the diagnosis of P as simply a case of "anxiety." C's inclusion of CAM therapies does not relieve the obligation to practice in accordance with the standard of care as regards conventional medical diagnosis.

FAILURE TO TREAT

Most malpractice cases arise from an act of misfeasance—that is, failure to act in an appropriate manner. Generally speaking, there is no obligation to act to help another person in distress. However, once a person undertakes to provide such assistance, a duty arises to exercise reasonable care. Once a condition is diagnosed—or should have been diagnosed by the reasonable practitioner practicing in accordance with the standard of care—the clinician is obligated to offer treatment or to transfer care to another clinician. Claims that a necessary treatment is not offered by the practitioner do not alleviate the duty to treat or refer for treatment. This can be an issue when newer treatments with demonstrated efficacy have not been adopted by a particular practitioner who continues to offer treatments that were previously state-of-the-art but no longer retain that status.[30,31]

In case B, Part 1, the cardiologist compounds the initial misdiagnosis with failure to treat, thus presenting an additional and alternate theory of malpractice liability. Case B is egregious and represents one end of a possible spectrum, in which overreliance on CAM therapies or on the mind-body connection leads to ignoring tested, conventional methods of diagnosis and treatment.

In Part 2, the cardiologist is offering some CAM therapies that have some reasonable evidence of safety and efficacy in the medical literature, without neglecting conventional monitoring and diagnosis.[32,33] In such a scenario, malpractice liability is unlikely. When a CAM therapy has significant evidence of safety and efficacy, physicians should recommend that therapy to patients, and know that liability is highly unlikely; when a CAM therapy has significant evidence of safety but not efficacy—or vice versa—physicians should allow fully informed and consenting patients to try such a therapy, while continuing to monitor conventionally and intervening conventionally when necessary because liability is possible but again unlikely. In cases in which CAM therapy has significant evidence of either serious danger or inefficacy, physicians should avoid and actively discourage patients from using such a therapy because liability would be highly likely.[25]

FRAUD AND MISREPRESENTATION

The tort of fraud and misrepresentation is defined as the knowing inducement of reliance on inaccurate or false information for the benefit of the person committing the fraud and to the detriment of the victim. The following elements must be established to prove fraud and misrepresentation by any type of practitioner:

1. A false representation by the practitioner
2. Knowledge or belief on the part of the practitioner that the representation is false or insufficient basis in fact to make the representation
3. Intent to induce the patient to rely upon the false representation either by accepting the offered treatment or foregoing other treatment
4. Reliance upon the representation by the patient that is reasonable and justified under the circumstances. The reasonableness of the reliance is determined by a number of factors, including the credentials of the person recommending the treatment, the sophistication and educational level of the patient, and the nature of the representation. The more outlandish the claim of efficacy, the more persuasive the misrepresentation must be in order to establish reasonable reliance.
5. Damage to the patient as a result of relying upon the false representation.[12] As mentioned previously, this damage may take the form of injury that

results from the patient being induced to rely on a fraudulent treatment, thus preventing the patient from pursuing care that is more likely to have a positive result.

In case C, all five elements are present: the cardiologist falsely represented to the patient that applying magnets to the chest wall would reverse the patient's cardiovascular condition; the cardiologist knew this representation was false (or recklessly believed it to be true); it would be sufficient if the cardiologist either knew the claim is false or lacked a scientific basis for making the claim. The cardiologist induced the patient to rely on the magnet claim and thereby forego necessary, conventional care; the patient reasonably relied on the cardiologist's advice and thereby was injured. This cardiologist therefore would be liable for fraud, a higher level of culpability than negligence—one that would likely trigger punitive (as well as compensatory) damages.

ABANDONMENT

Abandonment in the context of malpractice liability is defined as the unilateral and unjustified termination of the treatment relationship by the treater that results in damage to the patient. As the term *unjustified* indicates, in some situations it is reasonable and appropriate for treaters to unilaterally terminate the treatment relationship. These include threatening or violent patients, patients who repeatedly fail to keep appointments, and patients who are noncompliant to the point where the clinician can no longer justify seeing them.[34-36]

Even when termination of the relationship may seem justified to the clinician, however, it is advisable (1) to consult with one or more colleagues to see how they assess the situation, (2) make arrangements for emergency coverage until the patient can find another caregiver, and (3) wherever possible, help facilitate the identification of a new treater and transfer of patient care. When the treater needs to withdraw, for whatever reason, reasonable time must be allowed to enable the patient to obtain substitute treatment.[37]

Case D certainly presents a patient who may be difficult to manage. The patient's anger, refusal to comply with medical advice—and even, one might argue—tendency to lash out against the provider may (in the physician's mind) justify terminating treatment. As mentioned, however, the physician has a legal and ethical duty not to abandon the patient who needs conventional medical care. C in this hypothetical situation would be wise to refer the patient to a provider who is a better match, where P can receive the necessary conventional care, augmented by any psychological intervention that may be necessary.

VICARIOUS LIABILITY/REFERRAL

Clinicians may be held liable for the harm caused by employees or others under their direction (as may institutions in which those clinicians are employed) under the doctrine of vicarious liability or *Respondeat superior* ("Let the master answer").[38] This legal principle holds that an employer may be vicariously liable for acts performed by his or her employees within the scope of their duties in cases when the employer has the right to control the employee in the performance of those duties.[12] The liability may arise as a result of negligent hiring (i.e., employment of someone who is known—or should be known—to pose a risk of negligent or inappropriate behavior). For example, a clinician who hires an assistant with a history of sexual misconduct with patients may be held liable for such misconduct if it is again repeated with the employing clinician's patients.[39]

Vicarious liability may be imposed on physicians who supervise residents and other trainees or on nonphysicians who treat the physician's patients. Whether liability will be imposed in these situations is determined by the degree to which the defendant has actual or potential control over the supervisee's clinical decision-making and performance of other duties. Liability is unlikely to be imposed if it is primarily a consulting relationship, in which the defendant provides recommendations but does not control whether or not those recommendations are accepted.[40-42]

Vicarious liability may be imposed in CAM in connection with employees, cotreaters, and clinicians to whom patients are referred.[43-44] An arm's-length referral to a specialist, without more, however, rarely generates liability. In integrative care—in which conventional providers closely collaborate with CAM providers to comanage patient diagnosis, monitoring, and treatment—shared liability is more likely.[45]

In Case E, Part 1, the hospital would be vicariously liable under *respondeat superior* for any negligence on C's part. In addition, the chief cardiologist may be directly negligent for failing to properly supervise C and for encouraging C to engage in patient abandonment.

In Part 2, C would not necessarily be liable simply for referring P to the clinical psychologist. If, however, the cardiologist and clinical psychologist were actively working together and thus engaged in joint treatment of the patient, each may have liability for the other's negligent acts.[45] When referring to a CAM provider, the physician should take reasonable care to ensure that the CAM provider does not have a significant history of malpractice liability or professional discipline and does not include practices that are marginal to or outside the CAM profession itself.[25] These reasonable steps will help protect against a claim of negligent referral and/or vicarious liability for the CAM provider's negligence. Some basic information is available to help physicians reasonably assess a CAM provider's credentials and qualifications.[46]

CONFIDENTIALITY

Medical information is highly personal. Society, through case law and statutes, recognizes that the privacy of that information is entitled to protection. This is true regardless of the discipline of the person providing the treatment. Unauthorized breach of that privacy can cause personal embarrassment and have implications for personal and professional relationships. For those reasons, the decision to disclose personal medical information is left to the patient, except under limited circumstances. The law protects the privacy of medical information by imposing a duty of confidentiality on clinicians.[47,48] Confidentiality is the ongoing obligation of physicians and other clinicians to keep private the information shared with them by patients in the course of treatment. It is an obligation that exists until the patient grants permission for confidentiality to be breached or a situation arises that falls within one of the exceptions to confidentiality. Signed release of information forms, which grants the clinician permission to release information to a specific party or parties, have become routine, although many clinicians traditionally have felt comfortable obtaining verbal permission and recording it in the patient's record. State and Federal statutes, including the Health Insurance Portability and Accountability Act (HIPAA), have increased the requirements for signed releases. HIPAA formalizes many of the preexisting protections of medical information, which it calls *Protected Health Information* (PHI).[49,50] It is important to note, however, that HIPAA is aimed in part at facilitating the disclosure of information to increase the efficiency of health care. For example, HIPAA would allow the sharing of information between cotreaters without the patient's permission. Physicians should be aware that HIPAA regulations set the minimum standard for protection of confidentiality. If state law provides greater protection for confidentiality, the state law governs.[51]

The duty of confidentiality imposed by case law and statutes applies to all medical information, including that related to CAM. Although it is an evolving field, these obligations will be applied to nonphysician practitioners who treat various ailments because the focus of confidentiality is the privacy of the information and not the discipline of the practitioner. Thus a physician who offers chelation therapy and discloses the identity of a patient at a conference or in an article will be as subject to liability for breach of confidentiality as a physician who offers more widely-accepted treatments.[25,50,52] In case F, disclosure of P's confidential health information to the licensed chiropractor, a licensed naturopathic physician, and a clinical psychologist without receiving an appropriate, signed consent form likely would result in liability.

Certain exceptions to the duty of confidentiality allow information to be disclosed without a patient's express permission. The exceptions to confidentiality include emergency, implied or express waiver, incompetence, and imminent danger to self or others. Even under these exceptions, however, confidentiality should be breached to the least extent necessary to accomplish the necessary goal. For example, under the emergency exception, the identity of a patient brought unconscious to the emergency room could be revealed in the course of telephone calls to numbers found in the patient's address book. Such calls are permissible because they have the goal of gathering medical information necessary to provide emergency care, and the potential risk of harm from releasing the patient's identity is outweighed by the risk of having inadequate information. In a nonemergency situation, with a stable patient, such a call without the patient's permission would not be considered permissible and might lead to a legitimate complaint of breach of confidentiality.

Clinicians may also have a duty to breach confidentiality when it is necessary to protect third parties from potential violence, other risks posed by a patient (such as infection), or genetic predisposition to serious diseases. A detailed discussion of this exception is beyond the scope of this chapter, but readers are advised to familiarize themselves with the law on this topic in their jurisdictions.[53-55]

INFORMED CONSENT

The doctrine of informed consent is one of the most important developments in law, medicine, and ethics of the 20th century. It is grounded in the fundamental ethical and legal notions that "every human being of adult years and sound mind has a right to determine what shall be done with his body."[56] Informed consent has evolved from an ethical to a medical-legal construct, with an unfortunate focus on the latter. Freed from such legalistic thinking, informed consent is an essential element of good patient care, improved compliance, and risk management. As a matter of medical ethics, it promotes the autonomy of individuals with regard to making individual medical decisions.[57] In CAM, informed consent issues are of utmost importance because patients must be given an opportunity to weigh the risks and benefits of choosing a CAM approach rather than a more conventional approach.[58] While the doctrine of informed consent emphasizes that the choice belongs to the patient, it in no way discourages the age-old practice of the patient looking to the physician for advice and the physician providing it.[59]

Informed consent is the process through which a clinician proposing treatment provides information to a current or prospective patient, who then voluntarily consents to the treatment. It is this process of exchanging information that constitutes informed consent. The signing of a form, as required by various hospital, administrative, and governmental regulations, is merely evidence that the informed consent process has taken place.[60]

All three elements of informed consent—information, voluntariness, and competence—must be present for consent to be valid. Informed consent, standing alone, is infrequently the subject of malpractice claims. The proximate cause element of malpractice, discussed previously, requires that "but for" the failure to obtain proper informed consent, that harm would not have occurred (i.e., the patient would not have accepted the treatment).[12] As a result, a patient from whom proper informed consent was not obtained would have to argue that he or she would have foregone the treatment in question. This is potentially a greater risk issue for CAM than for traditional medical treatments because the patient could more easily argue that, had he known that more widely accepted treatments with established efficacy were available, he would have chosen one of those as opposed to the CAM treatment offered.

Information

Questions are often raised about the amount of information that needs to be provided in order for consent to be valid. Does every risk and side effect have to be described? As a rule of thumb, patients should be advised of risks and side effects along a continuum, from those that are common but not very serious to those that are infrequent but are potentially significant. It is the materiality of risks that govern whether they need to be discussed specifically.[60,61]

As a legal requirement, the amount and type of information that must be provided depends upon the jurisdiction in which the physician is practicing. In jurisdictions that apply a physician-oriented or community standard, the physician must provide the information that the average, respectable physician in the community would provide under similar circumstances. The patient-oriented or materiality standard applied in other jurisdictions requires that all the information that an average patient (or in some states, the specific patient) would find material in making a decision.[62]

In *Harnish* v. *Children's Hospital Medical Center*,[63] the Massachusetts Supreme Judicial Court set out requirements for information sharing that satisfy legal and ethical requirements in virtually all jurisdictions. They include the following:

- The diagnosis and nature of the condition being treated
- The benefits the patient can reasonably expect from the proposed treatment
- The nature and probability of material risks
- The inability to predict results
- The potential irreversibility of the procedure
- The likely results, risks, and benefits associated with CAM treatments and no treatment.

The last element of the *Harnish* requirements is of particular relevance in CAM. Clinicians need not inform their patients of all available CAM therapies—only of those that would be offered by the average, reasonable physician in the community. Thus in *Moore* v. *Baker*, a Federal Court held that a physician had not breached a statutory duty to obtain informed consent by failing to inform a patient of chelation therapy as an alternative to carotid endarterectomy. The court held that the physician was obligated to inform the patient only about those treatments that are practical and "generally recognized and accepted by reasonably prudent physicians."[64]

Although such an approach does not help promote CAM therapies, it does not prevent them from being offered. Rather, it remains true to the reasonableness standard with regard to the imposition of duties on physicians. If, over time, chelation therapy were to be established as an accepted and reasonable treatment option, the court noted, the same case might be decided differently. On the other hand, the CAM practitioner who fails to advise the patient of more widely accepted treatment as another option to CAM therapies, may be breaching the duty to provide adequate information. In Case G, P would not likely succeed without offering convincing evidence of general medical acceptance of the CAM therapy proposed.

Voluntariness

The consent to treatment must be voluntary, meaning that it cannot be the result of coercion by the person offering the treatment. The largely elective nature of CAM treatments and the conditions treated make it unlikely that overt coercion would be used. More subtle forms of coercion, such as denying access to requested treatment unless other treatments or supplements are also accepted, can also render consent invalid.

Although the voluntariness requirement speaks to coercion by the clinician, questions sometimes arise about coercion by family members. This could arise, for example, with an elderly parent whose child insists that she accept alternative treatment modalities that are the preference of the child but not the parent, on pain of losing a place to live or other support. While such coercion does not

automatically violate the legal acceptability of the consent, it does raise significant ethical and clinical compliance issues. In such situations, it is advisable for
the treating clinician to focus the consent process on the patient while including
concerned family members, in order to reach a clinical resolution. Similar problems arise in the treatment of children and adolescents.[65]

Competence

This is the threshold element of informed consent; only a competent person can
give valid consent to treatment or treatment refusal. The law presumes that all
adults are legally competent to make their own medical treatment decisions.
That legal status remains intact until a court declares the person legally incompetent. In medical care, questions often arise about an individual patient's
capacity to make treatment decisions. Although a clinical determination of lack
of decision making capacity does not strip the patient of competency in the eyes
of the law, clinicians are obligated to take note of this potential lack of capacity
before accepting a patient's consent (or refusal) as being informed.[64,66] The fact
that a patient disagrees with the physician's recommendations—or even
chooses a course of treatment that most others would reject—does not mean
that he or she lacks capacity. Competent individuals are well within their rights
to make decisions that are incompetent in the eyes of others.[67,68]

As with other rules, exceptions to informed consent exist. Full informed consent does not need to be obtained in emergencies or in cases in which the patient
waives the consent process, is incompetent, or—in very limited cases—the
informed consent process would worsen the patient's condition.[69-71]

If the emergency exception is to be invoked, the patient's capacity to participate in the decision making process must be assessed first. If the patient lacks
capacity, the physician acting in an emergency should turn to a family member
for consent, if time and circumstances permit. The emergency exception does
not allow the treating physician to override the patient's refusal of care
expressed before the emergency.[72]

Just as patients have the right to make their own decisions, they have the right to
leave the decision making to others, including their physicians. The key inquiry
here, as with other aspects of informed consent, is whether the decision to waive is
being made by someone who has the capacity to do so. If the patient from whom
consent is sought lacks the capacity to engage in the decision-making process, then
an alternate decisionmaker should be sought. The decision to seek a substitute
decisionmaker turns on the degree of impairment and the risk-benefit balance of
the proposed treatment. A sliding scale approach—with less capacity required for
consent to low-risk/high-benefit treatments and refusal of high-risk/low-benefit
treatments and more capacity required for consent to high-risk/low-benefit treatments and refusal of low-risk/high-benefit treatments—is widely endorsed as an
acceptable and practical approach to the competency issue.[73,74]

In many jurisdictions, judicial involvement is required for treatments that are
considered to be extraordinarily intrusive or dangerous.[75]

The doctrine of therapeutic privilege allows informed consent from the
patient to be deferred and consent to be obtained from another decisionmaker

in cases in which the consent process itself would have a deleterious effect on the patient's condition. Such situations are rare, and this exception must be invoked only with great care. Even when it may be justified, one is obligated to seek an alternate decisionmaker.[76,77]

OFF-LABEL USE OF FDA-APPROVED MEDICATIONS

The Food and Drug Act of 1936 was enacted to protect public health and safety by ensuring that food and medications offered to the public would not pose inherent risks. It was not intended to interfere with the doctor-patient relationship or the ability of physicians to exercise clinical judgment in treating patients. Once a medication receives FDA approval, physicians are free to use it for any treatment purpose based on their clinical judgment. Use of medications for nonapproved or off-label purposes exposes the physician to potential liability if an injury results. Although the lack of FDA approval may not be considered a material risk for informed consent purposes, discussing the lack of FDA approval and its implications along with other information as part of the informed consent process is advisable.[78-80]

Although the FDA cannot regulate the practice of medicine, state licensing boards can discipline physicians for professional misconduct. Most state statutes contain a number of defined categories for such misconduct, including such matters as practicing while under the influence of alcohol or drugs, sexual misconduct (see next section), and malpractice liability. In addition, most state medical boards can discipline physicians for using therapies that are not generally medically accepted.[14] Unfortunately, such a broad mandate leaves medical boards free to discipline physicians who include CAM therapies because many such therapies may not be medically accepted. In response to this conundrum, many states have enacted medical freedom laws, which provide that medical boards may not discipline physicians *solely* based on inclusion of CAM therapies.[14] The Federation of State Medical Boards recently has issued Model Guidelines on Physician Use of Complementary and Alternative Therapies in Medical Practice that reiterate this principle.[81] In Case H, C may or may not be subject to discipline, depending on the medical board's view of chelation therapy and the applicable state licensing rules; cardiologists should investigate the law in the state in which they practice.

SEXUAL INVOLVEMENT WITH PATIENTS

In the 1980s and 1990s, sexual contact between physicians and therapists and their patients came to be recognized as a significant problem. It has been the basis for numerous ethics complaints against physicians and nonphysician treaters alike and has been addressed by the American Medical Association [82] and specialty societies.[83]

Sexual involvement with patients, also known as sexual misconduct and boundary violations, has been the subject of malpractice suits.[84,85] These suits have a number of bases, depending upon the specialty of the clinician and the nature of the relationship. Among the allegations are negligent handling of the doctor-patient relationship, fraud and misrepresentation, breach of fiduciary duty, undue influence, and lack of valid consent because of disparity in the levels of power within the relationship.[86] In addition, a number of states have made sexual contact with a current patient a criminal offense, with physicians being sentenced to prison time for such activity.[87]

The issue of sexual involvement with patients traditionally has been viewed as a problem for mental health professionals. This relates, in part, to the level of emotional intimacy that occurs in the course of psychotherapy and the emotional vulnerability of many patients (often because of previous sexual abuse or exploitation). Similar problems are encountered in obstetrics and gynecology and parishioner-clergy relationships.[88] The sexual relationships between attorneys and clients have also received increasing criticism.[89] The basis for recovery in psychotherapy cases has been on negligent handling of the transference (the emotional reaction of the patient to the therapist) and countertransference (the emotional reaction of the therapist to the patient).

It should be expected that a similar analysis would apply to other treaters who endeavor to treat the emotional problems of their patients and have close physical and emotional contact with them. For example, those who practice in the field of mind-body medicine, which acknowledges the essential interplay between psychological and physical states, would be expected to understand and properly handle the emotional and physical feelings that arise in the course of the treatment.

In Case I, the issue of physical touch has always been a hot button for mental health professions, but supportive gestures such as this are rarely problematic, even in mental health. As hands-on treatments such as chiropractic and massage therapy enter conventional settings, the boundaries around physical contact with patients will change, and new emphasis is being given to how psychic boundaries are defined.[90] If C had treated P for many years, it is possible that a sensitive and engaged relationship in which such a gesture would be well within professional boundaries would have arisen. Indeed, integrative care emphasizes the power of the therapeutic relationship, including the closeness of provider and patient in the shared aligning of therapeutic intentionality.[91] In the absence of such a relationship, a gesture like this could be misinterpreted as being unduly familiar and experienced by the patient as inappropriate. Crossing of those boundaries, either in the form of treatment using physical contact or a supportive hug, needs to be done with consideration and with the patient's consent. Boundary violations, such as sex with patients, is outside the realm of treatment and, as noted previously, may be considered inherently nonconsensual.

LIABILITY RISK MANAGEMENT

The experience of being sued for malpractice, charged with regulatory violations, or being brought up on ethics charges are universally acknowledged to be unpleasant. Such allegations disrupt the defendant's relationships with friends, family, patients, and colleagues. They cause tremendous personal sadness, often accompanied by anger and self-doubt.[47,92] The goal, then, is liability risk management: taking steps to decrease the likelihood of becoming the subject of malpractice or other litigation.

RELATIONSHIP MATTERS

Liability risk management efforts often focus on the technical aspect of medicine. Only a small percentage of medical errors lead to allegations of malpractice, however, thus suggesting that other factors usually account for the decision of a patient or family member to pursue a malpractice claim.[93,94]

The prevailing view is that the relationship between the caregiver and the patient and his or her family plays the greatest role in determining whether a given adverse event will give rise to litigation. It has been widely suggested that malpractice cases arise from the combination of bad outcomes plus bad feelings.[95] A more sophisticated but less widely publicized formulation hones in on how some physicians may behave or be regarded by their patients. This formulation, known as Russell's Rule of Risk (after its creator, statistician A. Russell Localio) posits that the probability of a malpractice suit is directly proportional to a physician's arrogance (real or perceived) divided by physician's competence.[96]

Much can be done to improve the doctor-patient relationship, including the perception of arrogance. Good communication with patients, which includes tailoring the communication content and style to the needs of the individual patient, has been shown to enhance the perception of the physician's competence and decrease the risk of malpractice.[97,98] Scheduling enough time to talk with patients, answering telephone calls directly (rather than having a staff member return them), being aware of one's own stress level, and achieving general satisfaction with one's own professional practice all seem to be associated with decreased risk.[99] One study suggested that characteristics of the relationship had a greater effect for primary care physicians than for surgeons.[100]

These communication skills—along with respect for patients' time, appreciation of the validity of their concerns, and honest sharing of what we know and do not know—humanize the doctor-patient relationship. By disabusing patients and their families of the myths that physicians know and can control everything and that outcomes are guaranteed, we can manage expectations in a way that limits the risk of unnecessary disappointments and surprises. That, in turn, can decrease the risk of litigation.[101]

If this prevailing view of the role of relationships in risk management is valid, it may explain why CAM practitioners have experienced fewer malpractice claims. It may also bode well for the future. Attention to the whole patient, a focus on the person rather than the procedure, and a willingness to listen to patient concerns should all have a positive impact on risk reduction. It is the context and not the substance of the treatment that is protective, however. As CAM becomes part of mainstream medicine and as the treatments are offered during rushed office visits with little time for communication, we should expect the risk of litigation to approach that of conventional treatment.

An often-overlooked risk-reduction measure is the practice of apologizing for adverse or unexpected outcomes. This does not mean that the clinician should engage in self-blame and assume all fault for every adverse event; no guarantees exist in any field of medicine, and the ultimate adverse outcome is preordained for every human being. Rather, this is the very simple practice of saying "I'm sorry" and offering support when things go badly. Genuine sympathy can do much to decrease the anger, frustration, and perception of indifference that may lead to litigation.[102] Beyond risk management, acknowledgment of errors and apology may be seen as ethical obligations.[95,103]

GOOD CLINICAL CARE

Beyond attention to the doctor-patient relationship, a number of steps can be taken to decrease the likelihood of suit and increase the chances of prevailing, should one occur.[104] First among these is consistently good clinical care, which includes ongoing education and management of clinical information.[105] Good clinical care includes monitoring for potential adverse reactions between conventional and CAM therapies—such as, for example, monitoring for adverse herb-drug interactions. Recent literature has suggested that not all herbal products are safe (or natural, for that matter) and that significant adverse interactions can result from their use.[106]

The case examples have emphasized the importance of conventional diagnosis and monitoring when CAM therapies are recommended or allowed. This is probably the most important means of ensuring that patients do not receive substandard care.[25] Continuing to monitor conventionally and intervene conventionally when medically necessary means that the standard of care will have been met and the possibility of patient injury minimized. For example, the cardiologist and patient may wish to try a CAM therapy for a predefined period of time instead of conventional care (e.g., a combination of lifestyle changes) and return to conventional care (e.g., surgery) when it becomes necessary.

Another risk-reduction measure is the practice of obtaining consultation. Ongoing supervision as well as occasional "curbside" consultations regarding a specific case should be documented in the patient's record. These serve to establish the standard of care in the community, can provide valuable input into clinical decision-making, and show that the clinician is willing to take extra steps for the benefit of the patient.[95]

DOCUMENTATION

Good clinical care is not sufficient if the medical record does not adequately document that care. The record should reflect the diagnosis and the proposed treatment, the bases for them, the informed consent process, and the treatment plan, including follow-up.[107,108] In the absence of documentation, the litigation may come down to the word of the injured patient versus the memory and reputation of the defendant clinician. Poor medical records can suggest negligence to a jury. In general, keeping complete and accurate medical records that include documentation of the patient's medical history concerning use of CAM therapies and of conversations with patients concerning potential inclusion of such therapies is advisable. Such thorough documentation can help physicians prove that informed consent requirements were satisfied and also may help protect against undue disciplinary action by state medical boards concerned with use of CAM therapies.[25]

If the physician recommends or allows use of a CAM therapy based on the medical literature, it is a good idea to keep a back-up file of the medical literature supporting the specific medical recommendation.[25] On the other hand, if the physician believes that, based on the medical literature, the patient's continued use of one or more CAM therapies is medically inadvisable and if the patient insists on using such therapies against medical advice, this event should be documented in the medical record. Such a record may help show the patient's involvement in selection and use of such therapies (see below). Physicians should familiarize themselves with documentation standards suggested by the Federation of State Medical Board Guidelines and know whether these are applicable in their state or home institution.

ASSUMPTION OF RISK

As noted previously, competent patients have the right to make decisions that others consider ill advised. Under the doctrine of voluntary assumption of risk, a patient who requests or consents to a novel or high risk procedure may do so, so long as the decision is voluntary and is based on adequate information. For assumption of risk to apply as a defense to a malpractice claim, it must be shown that the injured party knew that there was a risk, understood the nature of the risk, and voluntarily agreed to undertake it.[12]

Assumption of risk has been allowed in at least one case involving patient election of a CAM therapy instead of conventional care (i.e., of a nutritional protocol in lieu of conventional oncology care).[109] In this case, the court allowed the patient's signing of an appropriate consent form to serve as an "express" assumption of risk and therefore a complete defense to the claim of medical malpractice. In another case, a New York court found that the patient had "impliedly" assumed the risk because she was aware of and voluntarily chose a CAM protocol for cancer care, even without signing the requisite form.[110] Most courts, however, disfavor waivers of negligence,[111] and many might not allow either express or implied assumption of risk as a defense to a malpractice claim involving CAM therapies. Physicians should nonetheless engage in clear conversations with patients concerning options involving CAM therapies because such an approach is likely to satisfy informed consent concerns, respects an ideal of shared decision-making, and encourages positive relationships that can help mitigate the prospect of litigation.

ETHICAL ISSUES IN CAM

The dominant ethical principles in medicine are nonmaleficence (doing no harm), beneficence (acting for the good of the patient), and autonomy (promoting the patient's independence and freedom of choice regarding treatment).[112-115] Conventional medicine and CAM share these same ethical principles and the same clinical goals of curing disease, relieving suffering, and promoting the quality of life.

Ethical issues in CAM may arise when a patient requests an alternative treatment that the physician does not endorse or when the patient refuses a treatment that the physician feels is best. Others relate to the dissemination of information (i.e., does a conventional physician have an obligation to inform a patient with back pain that chiropractic or acupuncture may help the condition?). Courts by and large have not explicitly imposed a legal obligation on conventional physicians to provide information about CAM therapies, but as individual CAM therapies become more widely used and accepted, such an obligation may be imposed.[116]

Although the legal obligation to provide such information is not well established, one should keep in mind that legal and ethical obligations are not always the same. Patient autonomy and risk-management arguments can be made for providing that information. As discussed in the section on informed consent, patients have a right to information as to the risks and benefits of proposed treatments, CAM therapies, and no treatment. That includes treatments that the clinician does not offer or even fully endorse. An important part of this obligation is the provision of information about the risks of CAM therapies,[117,118] the extent to which their efficacy has been demonstrated,[119] and their risks and benefits relative to conventional treatments.[116] Clinical experience and research evidence show that patients want to hear the options, but they also want to hear what their physician recommends and usually base their decisions upon it.[120] The sharing of information about CAM therapies strengthens, rather than dilutes, the physician-patient relationship. Physicians who disagree with patient choices may choose not to treat those patients but preferably will see whether they can engage their patients in shared decision making while continuing to monitor and treat conventionally when necessary. If this fails, referral can be made to a provider who can fulfill these functions.[121]

Finally, as a matter of nonmaleficence and beneficence, as well as good clinical practice, physicians should maintain an ongoing record of what medications, herbal and mineral supplements, and other treatments a patient may be using. This provides an opportunity to review and discuss the relative risks and benefits of these treatments and, as suggested earlier, to assess for possible drug interactions.[122]

CONCLUSION

Generally, cardiologists should inform and engage patients in shared decision making about the option of trying CAM therapies that have reasonable support in the medical literature concerning safety and efficacy. Nutritional, exercise and lifestyle, and mind-body approaches may be viable ways to help patients empower themselves and augment conventional medical care with self-care.

At the same time, cardiologists should monitor patients conventionally and be prepared to intervene conventionally when medically necessary. On the other hand, cardiologists should discourage patients from CAM therapies that the literature suggests may be unsafe or inefficacious. Such an approach respects patient interest in autonomy and choice, expands the repertoire of medical alternatives, incorporates health and wellness concepts, yet preserves the duty to do no harm. The suggested approach also makes sense from the standpoint of trying to minimize risk of potential malpractice liability.

REFERENCES

1. Eisenberg DM, Davis RB, Ettner SL et al. Trends in alternative medicine use in the United States, 1990-1997: results of a follow-up national survey, JAMA 280:1569-1575, 1998.
2. Kessler RC, Soukup J, Davis RB et al. The use of complementary and alternative therapies to treat anxiety and depression in the United States. Am J Psychiatry 158:289-294, 2001.
3. Studdert DM, Mello MM, Brennan TA. Medical malpractice, N Engl J Med 350:283-292, 2004.
4. Government Accounting Office. Medical malpractice insurance: multiple factors have contributed to increased premium rates. Washington, DC, 2003.
5. Schwartz GT. The ethics and economics of tort liability insurance, Cornell Law Rev 75:313-365, 1990.
6. American Medical Association. Liability insurance requirements. Available at http://www.ama-assn.org/ama/pub/category/print/4544.html. Accessed March 9, 2004.
7. Rakatansky H. Medical malpractice tort actions provide two benefits: compensation for the victim of medical malpractice, and a reminder to the health care profession of the legal consequences of negligence, Med Health R I 83(11):368, 2000.
8. Schwartz WB, Komesar NK. Doctors, damages, and deterrence: an economic view of medical malpractice, N Engl J Med 298:1282-1289, 1978.
9. Gittler GJ, Goldstein EJ. The elements of medical malpractice: an overview, Clin Infect Dis 23:1152-1155, 1996.
10. Lang DM. Sexual malpractice and professional liability: some things they don't teach in medical school—a critical examination of the formative case law, Conn Ins Law J 6:151-186, 1999.
11. Rice WE. Insurance contracts and judicial discord over whether liability insurers must defend insureds' allegedly intentional and immoral conduct: a historical and empirical review of federal and state courts' declaratory judgments—1900-1997, Am Univ Law Rev 47:1131-1219, 1998.
12. Keeton WP. Prosser and Keeton on the law of torts, St. Paul, Minnesota, 1984, West Publishing.

13. *Dolan v. Galluzo*, 379 N.E. 2d 795 (Ill. Ct. App. 1978)., aff'd 396 N.E. 2d 13 (Ill. 1979).
14. Cohen MH. Complementary and alternative medicine: legal boundaries and regulatory perspectives, Baltimore, 1998, Johns Hopkins University Press.
15. Feasby C. Determining standard of care in alternative contexts, Health Law J 5:45-65, 1997.
16. Karlson HC, Erwin RD. Medical malpractice: informed consent to the locality rule, Indiana Law Rev 12:653-685, 1979.
17. *Mackey v. Greenview Hospital, Inc.*, 587 S.W.2d 249, (Ky. Ct. App. 1979).
18. *Keir v. United States*, 853 F.2d 398 (6th Cir. 1988).
19. *Monahan v. Weichert* 82 A.D. 2d 102, 442 N.Y.S. 2d. 295, 298 (1981)
20. Wright RW. Causation, responsibility, risk, probability, naked statistics, and proof: Pruning the bramble bush by clarifying the concepts, Iowa Law Rev 73:1001-1077, 1988.
21. Lewin JL. The genesis and evolution of legal uncertainty about "reasonable medical certainty," Univ Maryland Law Rev 57:380-502, 1998.
22. Garwin MJ. Risk creation, loss of chance, and legal liability, Hematol Oncol Clin North Am 16(6):1351-1363, 2002.
23. Negligence—Failure to carry out physical examination and biopsy—Damages for loss of chance of extended lifespan, J Law Med 9:397-398, 2002.
24. Studdert D, Eisenberg D, Miller F et al. Medical malpractice implications of alternative medicine. JAMA 280:1620-1625, 1998.
25. Cohen MH, Eisenberg DM. Potential physician malpractice liability associated with complementary and integrative medical therapies, Ann Intern Med 136:596-603, 2002.
26. Doyle A. Alternative medicine and medical malpractice: emerging issues, J Leg Med 22:533-552, 2001.
27. Silverstein D, Spiegel A. Are physicians aware of the risks of alternative medicine? J Community Health 26:159-174, 2001.
28. Tracy TF, Jr., Crawford LS, Krizek TJ, Kern KA. When medical error becomes medical malpractice: the victims and the circumstances, Arch Surg 138:447-454, 2003.
29. *Vergara v. Doan* 593 N.E. 2d 185 (Ind. 1992).
30. Klerman GL. The psychiatric patient's right to effective treatment: implications of *Osheroff v. Chestnut Lodge*, Am J Psychiatry 147:409-418, 1990.
31. Stone AA. Law, science, and psychiatric malpractice: a response to Klerman's indictment of psychoanalytic psychiatry, Am J Psychiatry 147:419-427, 1990.
32. Koertge J, Weidner G, Elliott-Eller M et al. Improvement in medical risk factors and quality of life in women and men with coronary artery disease in the Multicenter Lifestyle Demonstration Project, Am J Cardiol 91:1316-1322, 2003.

33. Ornish D, Scherwitz LW, Billings JH et al. Intensive lifestyle changes for reversal of coronary heart disease, JAMA 280:2001-2007, 1998.

34. Fentiman LC, Kaufman G, Merton V et al. Current issues in the psychiatrist-patient relationship: outpatient civil commitment, psychiatric abandonment and the duty to continue treatment of potentially dangerous patients: balancing duties to patients and the public, Pace Law Rev 20:231-262, 2000.

35. Gerber PC. Abandonment and the nonpaying patient, Physicians Manage 24:86-93, 96, 1984.

36. Gutheil TG, Simon RI. Abandonment of patients in split treatment, Harv Rev Psychiatry 11:175-179, 2003.

37. *Hongsathavij v. Queen of Angels/Hollywood Presbyterian Medical Center* 62 Cal. App. 4th 1123, 1138 73 Cal. Rptr. 2d 695 (Ct.App. Cal.1998).

38. Black's Law Dictionary. 1990: 1311.

39. Jorgenson LM, Sutherland PK, Bisbing SB. Transference of liability: employer liability for sexual misconduct by therapists, Brooklyn Law Review 60:1421-1481, 1995.

40. Schouten R. Legal aspects of consultation. In Cassem NH, Stern TA, Rosenbaum JF, Jellinek MS, editors: Massachusetts General Hospital Handbook of general hospital psychiatry, St Louis, 1997, Mosby-Year Book, 415-436.

41. Fox BC, Siegel ML, Weinstein RA. "Curbside" consultation and informal communication in medical practice: a medicolegal perspective, Clin Infect Dis 23:616-622, 1996.

42. Sederer L, Ellison J, Keyes C. Guidelines for prescribing psychiatrists in consultative, collaborative, and supervisory relationships, Psychiatric Svcs 49:1197-1202, 1998.

43. Cohen MH. Malpractice and vicarious liability for providers of complementary and alternative medicine, Benders Health Care Law Mon 3-13, 1996.

44. Josefek K. Alternative medicine's roadmap to mainstream, Am J Law Med 26:295, 2000.

45. Cohen MH. Beyond complementary medicine: legal and ethical perspectives on health care and human evolution. Ann Arbor, 2000, University of Michigan Press.

46. Eisenberg DM, Cohen MH, Hrbek A et al: Credentialing complementary and alternative medical providers, Ann Intern Med 137:965-973, 2002.

47. Ryan M. Medical malpractice: a review of issues for providers, Hematol Oncol Clin North Am 16:1331-1350, 2002.

48. Torres A, Proper S. Medicolegal developments and the dermatologist, Adv Dermatol 12:299-322, 1997.

49. Health Insurance Portability and Accountability Act of 1996. Public Law 104-191. 1996.

50. Office of the Secretary DoHaHS. Standards for privacy of individually identifiable health information, Federal Register 67:53182-53273, 2002.

51. Brendel RW, Bryan E. HIPAA for psychiatrists, Harv Rev Psychiatry. In press.

52. Stone J. Ethical issues in complementary and alternative medicine, Complement Ther Med 8:207-213, 2000.

53. Beck JC. Legal and ethical duties of the clinician treating a patient who is liable to be impulsively violent, Behav Sci and the Law 16(3):375-389, 1998.

54. Kennedy I. Duty to warn third parties: *Bradshaw v. Daniel.* Med Law Rev 2(2):237-239, 1994.

55. McAbee GNSJaD-FB. Physician's duty to warn third parties about the risk of genetic diseases, Pediatrics 102:140-142, 1998.

56. *Schloendorff v. Society of New York Hospital*, 92 N.E. 105 (NY 1914).

57. Schouten R. Informed consent: resistance and reappraisal. Crit Care Med 17:1359-1361, 20

58. Monaco GP, Smith G. Informed consent in complementary and alternative medicine: current status and future needs, Semin Oncol 29:601-608, 2002.

59. Ubel PA. "What should I do, Doc?": some psychologic benefits of physician recommendations, Arch Intern Med 162:977-980, 2002.

60. English DC. Valid informed consent: a process, not a signature, Amer Surgeon 68:45-48, 2002

61. *Precourt v. Frederick*, 481 N.E. 2d 1144 (Mass. 1985).

62. Appelbaum PS, Lidz CW, Meisel A. Informed consent: legal theory and clinical practice, New York, 1987, Oxford University Press.

63. *Harnish v. Children's Hospital Medical Center*, 439 NE 2d 240 (Mass. 1982).

64. *Moore v. Baker*, 98 F.2d 1129 (11th Cir. 1993).

65. Schouten R, Duckworth KS. Medical-legal and ethical issues in the pharmacological treatment of children. In Werry JS, Aman MG, editors: Practitioner's guide to psychoactive drugs in children and adolescents, New York, 1993, Plenum Publishing, 161-178.

66. Grisso T, Appelbaum PS. Assessing competence to consent to treatment: a guide for physicians and other health professionals. New York, 1998, Oxford University Press.

67. Brock DW, Wartman SA. When competent patients make irrational choices, N Engl J Med 322:1595-1599, 1990.

68. Kerridge I, Lowe M, Mitchell K. Competent patients, incompetent decisions. Ann Intern Med 123:878-881, 1995.

69. Moskop JC. Informed consent in the emergency department. Emerg Med Clin North Am 17:327-329, 1999.

70. Nora LM, Benvenuti RJ, III. Medicolegal aspects of informed consent. Neurol Clin 16(1.:207-216, 1998.

71. Sprung CL, Winick BJ. Informed consent in theory and practice: legal and medical perspectives on the informed consent doctrine and a proposed reconceptualization. Crit Care Med 17:1346-1354, 1989.

72. *Shine v. Vega*, 58 N.E. 2d 709 (Mass.1999).

73. Roth LH, Meisel A, Lidz CW. Tests of competency to consent to treatment. Am J Psychiatry 134:279-284, 1977.
74. President's Commission for the Study of Ethical Problems in Medicine and Biomedical and Behavioral Research. Making Health Care Decisions: A Report on the Ethical and Legal implications of Informed Consent in the Patient-Practitioner relationship. 1982. Washington, DC: US Government printing Office.
75. *Rogers v. Commissioner of Department of Mental Health*, 458 N.E.2d 308 (Mass. 1983).
76. *Canterbury v. Spence*, 464 F.2d 772 (D.C. Cir.1972)., *cert. denied*, 409 U.S. 1064.
77. Dickerson DA. A doctor's duty to disclose life expectancy information to terminally ill patients. Cleveland State Law Review 43:319-350, 1995.
78. Beck JM, Azari ED. FDA, off-label use, and informed consent: debunking myths and misconceptions. Food Drug Law J 53:71-104, 1998.
79. Choonara I, Conroy S. Unlicensed and off-label drug use in children: implications for safety. Drug Safety 25:1-5, 2002.
80. Smith JJ, Berlin L. Off-label use of interventional medical devices. Am J Roentgenol 173:539-542, 1999.
81. Federation of State Medical Boards. Model Guidelines for the Use of Complementary and Alternative Therapies in Medical Practice. 2002. Available at *www.fsmb.org* Last accessed 3-4-2004.
82. Sexual misconduct in the practice of medicine. Council on Ethical and Judicial Affairs, American Medical Association. JAMA 266:2741-2745, 1991.
83. Sexual misconduct in the practice of obstetrics and gynecology: ethical considerations. ACOG Committee Opinion No. 144. ACOG Comm Opin 1994; No. 144:3.
84. Schouten R. Maintaining boundaries in the doctor-patient relationship. In: Stern TA, Herman JB, Slavin PL (eds).. The MGH Guide to Psychiatry in Primary Care. New York: McGraw Hill, 2004: 743-747.
85. Simon R. Therapist-patient sex: from boundary violations to sexual misconduct. Psychiatr Clin North Am 22:31-47, 1999.
86. Bisbing SB, Jorgenson LM, Sutherland PK. Causes of Action. Sexual Abuse by Professionals: A Legal Guide. Charlottesville: The Michie Company 1995:121-154.
87. Bemmann KC, Goodwin J. New laws about sexual misconduct by therapists: knowledge and attitudes among Wisconsin psychiatrists. Wis Med J 88:11-16, 1989.
88. Young JL, Griffith EE. Developments in clergy malpractice: the case of Sanders v. Casa View Baptist Church. J Am Acad Psychiatry Law 27:143-147, 1999.
89. Gutheil T, Jorgenson L, Sutherland P. Prohibiting lawyer-client sex. Bull Am Acad Psychiatry Law 20:365-382, 1992.

90. Cohen MH. Future Medicine: Ethical Dilemmas, Regulatory Challenges, and Therapeutic Pathways to Health and Healing in Human Transformation. Ann Arbor: University of Michigan Press 2003.

91. Snyderman R, Weil AT. Integrative medicine: bringing medicine back to its roots. Arch Intern Med 162:395-397, 2002.

92. Charles SC. Coping with a medical malpractice suit. West J Med 174:55-58, 2001.

93. Localio AR, Lawthers AG, Brennan TA et al. Relation between malpractice claims and adverse events due to negligence. Results of the Harvard Medical Practice Study III. N Engl J Med 325:245-251, 1991.

94. Brennan TA, Hebert LE, Laird NM et al. Hospital characteristics associated with adverse events and substandard care. JAMA 265:3265-3269, 1991.

95. Gutheil TG, Appelbaum PS. Malpractice and Other Forms of Liability. Clinical Handbook of Psychiatry and the Law. Philadelphia: 2000, Lippincott Williams & Wilkins : 135-214.

96. Localio AR. Medical malpractice American style: Lies, damned lies, and statistics. Presented at the University of Pennsylvania, May 15, 2003.

97. Adamson TE, Tschann JM, Gullion DS, Oppenberg AA. Physician communication skills and malpractice claims. A complex relationship. West J Med 150:356-360, 1989.

98. Moore PJ, Adler NE, Robertson PA. Medical malpractice: the effect of doctor-patient relations on medical patient perceptions and malpractice intentions. West J Med 173:244-250, 2000.

99. Charles SC, Gibbons RD, Frisch PR et al. Predicting risk for medical malpractice claims using quality-of-care characteristics. West J Med 157:433-439, 1992.

100. Levinson W, Roter DL, Mullooly JP et al: Physician-patient communication: The relationship with mal-practice claims among primary care physicians and surgeons. JAMA 227:553-559, 1997.

101. Gutheil T, Bursztajn H, Brodsky A. Malpractice prevention through the sharing of uncertainty. N Engl J Med 311:49-51, 1984.

102. Kellett AJ. Healing angry wounds: the roles of apology and mediation in disputes between physicians and patients. Spec Law Dig Health Care 10:7-27, 1989.

103. Finkelstein D, Wu AW, Holtzman NA, Smith MK. When a physician harms a patient by a medical error: ethical, legal, and risk-management considerations. J Clin Ethics 8:330-335, 1997.

104. Blackston JW, Bouldin MJ, Brown CA et al. Malpractice risk prevention for primary care physicians. Am J Med Sci 324:212-219, 2002.

105. Frank-Stromborg M, Bailey LJ. Cancer screening and early detection: managing malpractice risk. Cancer Pract 6:206-216, 1998.

106. Ernst E. Second thoughts about safety of St John's wort. Lancet 354:2014-2016, 1999.

107. Alford DM. The clinical record: recognizing its value in litigation. Geriatr Nurs 24:228-230, 2003.

108. Weintraub MI. Documentation and informed consent. Neurol Clin 17:371-381, 1999.
109. *Schneider v. Revici*, 987 F.2d 817 (2nd Cir. 1987).
110. *Charell v. Gonzales*, 660 N.Y.Supp.2d 665 (S.Ct. N.Y.Cty.1997). affirmed and modified to vacate punitive damages award, 673 N.Y.Supp.2d 685 (App Div., 1st Dept., 1998)., reargument denied, appeal denied, 1998 New York Appellate Division LEXIS 10711 (App. Div., 1st Dept., 1998)., appeal denied, 706 N.E. Rptr 2d 1211 (1998).
111. *Tunkl v. Regents of the Univ. of California* . 383P 2d. 441 (Calif. 1963).
112. Sade RM. Autonomy and beneficence in an information age, Health Care Anal 9:247-254, 2001.
113. Ethics Committee, Society for Academic Emergency Medicine. An ethical foundation for health care: an emergency medicine perspective, Ann Emerg Med 21:1381-1387, 1992.
114. Ethical decision-making in obstetrics and gynecology. ACOG Tech Bull 1989; No. 136:1-7.
115. Blustein J. Doing what the patient orders: maintaining integrity in the doctor-patient relationship, Bioethics 7:290-314, 1993.
116. Ernst E, Cohen MH. Informed consent in complementary and alternative medicine, Arch Intern Med 161:2288-2292, 2001.
117. Ernst E. The risk-benefit profile of commonly used herbal therapies: ginkgo, St. John's Wort, Ginseng, Echinacea, Saw Palmetto, and Kava, Ann Intern Med 136:42-53, 2002.
118. Ernst E. Complementary medicine: where is the evidence? J Fam Pract 52:630-634, 2003.
119. Thompson Coon JS, Ernst E. Herbs for serum cholesterol reduction: a systematic view, J Fam Pract 52:468-478, 2003.
120. Ende J, Kazis L, Ash A, Moskowitz MA. Measuring patients' desire for autonomy: decision making and information-seeking preferences among medical patients. J Gen Intern Med 4:23-30, 1989.
121. Adams KE, Cohen MH, Jonsen AR, Eisenberg DM. Ethical considerations of complementary and alternative medical therapies in conventional medical settings, Ann Intern Med 37:660-664, 2002.
122. Sugarman J, Burk L. Physicians' ethical obligations regarding alternative medicine, JAMA 280:1623-1625, 1998.

PART II

Nutritional and Herbal Approaches

CHAPTER 3

Nutriceuticals and Cardiovascular Illness

William H. Frishman, MD

Stephen T. Sinatra, MD

Nathan Kruger, MD

V itamins and minerals are required in trace amounts for normal bodily functioning. A number of people have subscribed to the notion that "more is better." Ingestion of micronutrient supplements (vitamins and minerals) beyond the recommended daily allowances (RDAs) is beneficial in certain deficiency states resulting from inadequate intake, disturbed absorption, or increased tissue requirements; however, routine dietary supplementation of micronutrients in the absence of deficiency states and beyond what one can usually obtain from consumption of a well-balanced diet has been shown to be questionably beneficial; indeed, in some cases it may be harmful.[1,2] Of course, exceptions exist. This chapter reviews those micronutrient supplements with beneficial and harmful effects on the cardiovascular system.

In 1994 the US Congress passed the Dietary Supplement Health and Education Act, which prevents the FDA from regulating vitamins, minerals, and herbal products as drugs. The law permits the continued marketing of dietary supplements sold before October 15, 1994 (defined as vitamins, minerals, botanicals, amino acids, enzymes) without the review or approval of any government agency. To market a new ingredient, a manufacturer must notify the FDA and demonstrate that it is reasonably expected to be safe. Health claims can be made on the label if they are accompanied with a disclaimer saying that the product is not intended to diagnose, treat, cure, or prevent any disease.[3]

THE RATIONALE FOR TARGETED NUTRITIONAL SUPPLEMENTS FOR CARDIOVASCULAR HEALTH

The heart, which has approximately 5000 mitochondria per cell and functions in a high-oxygen environment, is one of the most susceptible of all organs to free-radical oxidative stress. Fortunately, it is also highly responsive to the benefits of targeted nutritional agents, such as phytonutrients, antioxidants, and nutriceuticals. The term *nutriceutical* includes a wide variety of nonprescription nutritional supplements normally found in the body or in natural sources (such as vitamins, amino acids, and herbals). Strong scientific evidence from large and repeated clinical trials have confirmed their efficacy and safety as well as guidelines for patient selection, dosage, and potential medication interactions. For example, fat-soluble vitamins (K, E, D, and A) are stored to a variable extent in the body and are more likely to cause adverse reactions than water-soluble vitamins, which are readily excreted in the urine. Excessive vitamin K can cause hemolysis in persons with glucose-6-phosphate dehydrogenase (G6PD) deficiency and anemia (with Heinz bodies), hyperbilirubinemia, and kernicterus in newborns; moreover, vitamin K can counter the effects of oral anticoagulants by conferring biologic activity on prothrombin and factors VII, IX, and X. In contrast, high doses of vitamin E may potentiate the effects of oral anticoagulants by antagonizing vitamin K and prolonging prothrombin time.

MEGAVITAMINS AND MINERALS

VITAMIN E

Vitamin E's antioxidant and anticoagulant properties are thought to protect against myocardial infarction and thrombotic strokes.[3a] A recent extensive review article assessed the preventive effects of vitamin E on the development of atherosclerosis.[4] α-Tocopherols are the key lipid-soluble, chain-breaking antioxidants found in tissues and plasma. Oxidation of unsaturated fatty acids in low-density lipoprotein (LDL) particles, as a pivotal factor in atherogenesis, is widely recognized. Vitamin E, a predominant antioxidant present in the LDL particle, blocks the chain reaction of lipid peroxidation by scavenging intermediate peroxyl radicals.[4] Vitamin E supplementation can reduce lipid peroxidation by as much as 40%. Stabilizing plaque, reducing inflammation, decreasing thrombolytic aggregation, reducing the expression of adhesion molecules on the arterial wall, and enhancing vasodilation are key cardioprotective effects of vitamin E.[4] However, prospective controlled clinical trials have presented a confusing picture.

The Alpha Tocopherol, Beta Carotene (ATBC) Cancer Prevention Study,[5] a randomized double-blind, placebo-controlled trial of 29,133 male smokers ages 50 to 69 with a median follow-up of 4.7 years, showed a minor but statistically significant decrease in angina pectoris with vitamin E supplementation of 50 mg per day [relative risk (RR) = 0.91]. A nonsignificant (8%) reduction in mortality rate from coronary artery disease (CAD) was also realized.

In the Cambridge Heart Antioxidant Study (CHAOS), patients with atherosclerosis who received 400 to 800 U of vitamin E daily appreciated a 77% decrease in the relative risk of nonfatal MI; however, there was a nonsignificant increase in death from cardiovascular disease.[6] The Heart Outcomes Prevention Evaluation (HOPE)[7] and the initial GISSI Prevenzioni data[8] failed to establish a clear benefit; however, one researcher's reevaluation of GISSI showed a 20% reduced risk of cardiovascular death.[9]

On the other hand, in one of the investigations of patients with a history of myocardial infarction (MI), mortality was higher when vitamin E was combined with β carotene.[10] In the most recent review of the major human trials on vitamin E supplementation—including the ATBC, CHAOS, GISSI, SPACE, and HOPE trials—a statistical reanalysis of the data, including the totality of the evidence, suggests that α-tocopherol supplementation does not have a place in treating patients with preexisting cardiovascular disease.[9,11] In addition, the results of the MRC/BHF Heart Protection Study[12] in 20,536 high risk individuals showed no benefit from Vitamin E supplementation (600 mg daily) on morbidity and mortality. However, it is important to keep in mind that the oxidative modification of LDL-cholesterol is only a hypothesis and has yet to be proven, which raises the question of whether or not cardiologists should routinely recommend vitamin E to their patients. In two large prospective Harvard studies (Nurses' Health Study[13] and the Health Professional Study[14]) of approximately 87,000 women and 40,000 men, investigators attributed reductions in heart disease and stroke to vitamin E rather than other unidentified factors. In another investigation of men with documented coronary heart disease,[15] 100 U or more of vitamin E per day was correlated with decreased progression of coronary artery lesions compared to untreated counterparts. In this study of 156 men 40 to 59 years old with a history of coronary artery bypass surgery, supplemental vitamin E intake was associated with angiographically proven reduction in progression of coronary artery lesions.

Given the many longitudinal epidemiologic studies and prospective randomized trials in which vitamin E consumption was associated with decreased cardiac risk, it is probably safe to say that some vitamin E supplementation could be considered for those individuals at high risk for coronary artery disease (CAD) or with documented CAD, however, no definitive data support such an approach. In addition, the rationale for vitamin E supplementation in healthy individuals is still open to question.[15a] In one investigation into the effects of vitamin E on lipid peroxidation in healthy individuals,[16] vitamin E was supplied as d-α-tocopherol capsules. Increased circulating vitamin E levels were not associated with any change in three urinary indices of lipid peroxidation. It would be interesting to note whether administration of a combination of mixed tocopherols and gamma tocopherols would have made any difference in the analysis of lipid peroxidation.

Whenever vitamin E supplements are being considered, gamma tocopherol should be included in the basic formula. α-Tocopherol in the absence of a gamma tocopherol may be ineffective in inhibiting the oxidative damage caused by the reactive peroxynitrite radicals and, in larger doses, α-tocopherol can displace gamma tocopherol in plasma.[17] Gamma tocopherol can also be obtained in the diet in the form of healthy nuts, such as almonds, sunflower seeds, wheat germ, and wheat germ oil. Vitamin E (α-tocopherol) and mixed tocopherols, including tocotrienols (other derivatives of vitamin E), may be the best combination of tocopherol biochemistry and may play an even greater role in modifying the oxidation of LDL.[17]

Natural—but not synthetic—forms of vitamin E also help to reduce platelet aggregability. In studies looking at healthy volunteers, researchers measured how well platelet cells absorb d-α-tocopherol, d-α-tocopherol acetate (both natural forms), and d-l-α-tocopherol (synthetic form). The research showed that platelets effectively absorbed d-α-tocopherol acetate and d-α-tocopherol but not synthetic vitamin E. Both forms of natural vitamin E reduced platelet aggregation by more than 50%, whereas no significant change was associated with synthetic vitamin E. The researchers determined that vitamin E's anticoagulant effect was unrelated to its antioxidant properties but appears to result from its inhibition of protein kinase C, an enzyme that facilitates blood clotting.[18]

Vitamin E has also been shown to significantly lower levels of C-reactive protein and monocyte interleukin-6, markers of atherogenesis.[19] Vitamin E is the least toxic of the fat-soluble vitamins; it rarely causes adverse reactions even at doses 20 to 80 times the recommended daily requirement taken for extended periods of time. However, malaise, gastrointestinal (GI) complaints, headache, and even hypertension have been reported, and parenteral vitamin E, which has been withdrawn from the market, has been shown to cause pulmonary deterioration, thrombocytopenia, and liver and renal failure in several premature infants.

Previous investigations also suggest that plasma levels of antioxidants like vitamins E and C are a more sensitive predictor of unstable angina than severity of atheroslcerosis is.[20] The fact that free-radical activity has been noted to influence the degree of coronary ischemia and spasm suggests that the beneficial effects of antioxidants in patients with CAD may result in part from a favorable influence on vascular reactivity rather than a reduction in atherosclerotic plaque. Results of randomized double-blind, placebo-controlled clinical trials have also indicated that vitamins E and C can prevent nitrate intolerance,[21,22] a major problem for patients who require long-term treatment with high-dose oral nitrates for relief of anginal symptoms.

Investigational research suggests that nitrate intolerance is associated with increased vascular production of superoxides.[23] When nitric oxide is released during metabolism of nitroglycerin, it reacts with superoxide anions, thus resulting in lower levels of cyclic guanosine monophosphate, an important intracellular intermediary that promotes vasorelaxation. There are key vitamins that warrant attention for the prevention of nitrate intolerance, including vitamin E, the main lipid-phase antioxidant, and vitamin C, the main aqueous-phase antioxidant. Supplementation with these nutrients boosts the free-radical scavenging ability of the superoxide radical, thus promoting the prevention of nitrate intolerance. As the primary aqueous antioxidant, vitamin C—the major antioxidant in the aqueous phase—acts as the first line of defense against oxidative stress.

VITAMIN C

Vitamin C is not only a scavenger antioxidant but also acts synergistically with vitamin E to reduce the peroxyl radical. In addition to blocking lipid peroxidation by trapping peroxyl radicals in the aqueous phase, vitamin C helps normalize endothelial vasodilative function in patients with heart failure by increasing the availability of nitric oxide. Although the evidence linking vitamin C to human cardiovascular disease is still being evaluated, one study did report that vitamin C slowed the progression of atherosclerosis in men and women older than 55 years.[24] It is also well known that many groups known to be at an increased risk for CAD have lower blood levels of vitamin C, such as men, the elderly, smokers, patients with diabetes, patients with hypertension, and possibly women who take oral estrogen contraceptives. Female users of vitamin C supplement in the Nurse's Health Study were shown to be at lower risk for CAD.[25] In a recent large, prospective population study, British researchers evaluated the health of almost 20,000 people ages 45 to 79 over 4 years.[26] They found that men and women who consumed about 109 to 113 mg of vitamin C daily had about half the risk of death of those who consumed only 51 to 57 mg of vitamin C per day. Higher blood levels of vitamin C were directly and inversely related to death from all causes and specifically death from ischemic heart disease in both men and women. The researchers strongly advocated modest consumption of fruits and vegetables because their results suggested that the equivalent of one extra serving of vitamin C–rich food reduced the risk of death by 20%. However, the consumption of carotenoids, flavonoids, magnesium, and other health-promoting nutrients affected these data. Improved endothelial function has been observed with the administration of vitamin C in patients with hypertension, hypercholesterolemia, and diabetes mellitus, suggesting that some vitamin C supplementation may be warranted.[27] Vitamin C at daily doses of 500 mg has been shown to increase red cell glutathione by 50%. Glutathione is not only the major antioxidant responsible for inhibiting lipid peroxidation but also a key contributing agent in stabilizing immune function. However, the results of the MRC/BHF Heart Protection Study showed no benefit from vitamin C supplementation (250 mg daily) on morbidity and mortality in high-risk patients with cardiovascular disease.[12] In addition both vitamin C and E were recently shown not to improve key mechanisms in the biology of atherosclerosis or endothelial dysfunction or to reduce LDL oxidation in vivo.[28]

Megadose vitamin C (>500 mg a day) in patients who are vulnerable to iron overload states should be avoided. Vitamin C supplements may exacerbate iron toxicity by mobilizing iron reserves. Such patients may accumulate harmful excess iron with higher doses of vitamin C, so caution must be employed for those with genetic diseases such as hereditary hemochromatosis, thalassemia major, or other diseases that promote iron overload.

B VITAMINS

Clinical cardiologists must be familiar with B vitamin support for their patients. B vitamin (thiamine) depletion commonly occurs as a result of high-dose diuretic therapy used in the treatment of congestive heart failure (CHF) and should be considered in any patient with refractory CHF that is unresponsive to high-dose diuretic therapy.[29] The nocturnal leg cramps associated with diuretic therapy are a hallmark symptom of B vitamin depletion. The involuntary, painful contraction of the calf muscles and other areas of the leg can be alleviated with B vitamin support, resulting in an improved quality of life. A randomized placebo-controlled double-blind study[30] validated the efficacy of B complex supplementation in the treatment of nocturnal cramps. Of 28 elderly patients, 86% taking vitamin B complex reported remission of prominent symptoms, compared to no benefit in the placebo group.

Most cardiologists are now familiar with the clinical significance of providing B vitamin supplementation to treat hyperhomocysteinemia.[29] In 1969, Kilmer McCully[31] first proposed the homocysteine hypothesis, thus identifying accelerated vascular pathology as a sequela to homocysteinuria, a rare autosomal recessive disease caused by a deficiency in cystathione B-synthetase. Several investigations have confirmed his proposed connection between high plasma homocysteine levels and occlusive arterial disease, including atherosclerosis, peripheral vascular disease, CAD, and CHF.[32-37]

Hyperhomocysteinemia may be even more detrimental in women. In one study, women with coronary disease had higher homocysteine levels than matched control subjects.[38] In a study comparing men and women with high homocysteine levels, women demonstrated greater carotid thickening ratios than their male counterparts did.[37] In another study involving postmenopausal women, high homocysteine levels in combination with hypertension resulted in an alarming 25 times higher incidence of stroke.[39]

The actual mechanism of action in homocysteine-associated endothelial damage remains unclear.[40] The fact that the injury may be inhibited by the addition of catalase suggests that the process may be the result of free-radical oxidative stress. This theory is strengthened by the fact that free-radical hydrogen peroxide is generated during the oxidation of homocysteine. Homocysteine also enhances thromboxane A_2 and platelet aggregation and increases the binding of lipoprotein(a) and fibrin. Because the association between homocysteine and atherothrombotic vascular events has been shown to be consistent regardless of other factors, high levels of homocysteine are a significant marker for atherothrombotic vascular disease. The relationship between high homocysteine and degree of myocardial injury was studied in 390 consecutive patients who presented with acute coronary syndromes: 205 with MI and 185 with unstable angina. In a multivariate analysis, a homocysteine level in the top quintile (>15.7 µg/L) was an excellent predictor of possible peak cardiac protein troponin T level in patients with acute coronary syndromes and an even stronger predictor in those with unstable angina.[41] The researchers suggest that homocysteine has a causal prothrombotic effect and indicate that further study is needed to assess homocysteine-lowering therapy. Because enzymatic deficiencies occur in as many as 5% of the population and because 28% of patients with premature vascular disease have high blood levels of homocysteine, screening for this lethal risk factor should be considered. Should future randomized trials correlate homocysteine lowering with a significant reduction in vascular events, supplementation with B complex therapy would then be strongly considered for patients with elevated homocysteine levels.

With the evidence in hand, trying to lower plasma homocysteine concentrations to prevent coronary disease seems premature.[42] No convincing evidence that such treatment in practice is helpful exists, and it may not be harmless. The results of the placebo-controlled Vitamin Intervention for Stroke Prevention Study (VISP), which used high daily doses of folic acid (2.5 mg), vitamin B_6 (25 mg), and vitamin B_{12} (0.4 mg) in stroke survivors, showed no benefit on vascular outcomes during 2 years of follow-up. However, an association of baseline homocysteine level with vascular risk was demonstrated.[43]

Certainly, administration of B vitamins at the recommended daily allowance levels (folic acid = 400 μg; B_6 = 2 mg; B_{12} = 6 μg) appears to be safe. Research shows a dose-dependent relationship between higher homocysteine levels and lower serum levels of B vitamins, so much higher doses must be administered to those patients with severe hyperhomocysteinemia and documented CAD.[44,45] It is also encouraging to note that the US FDA has required that enriched grains be fortified with folic acid at a concentration that provides the average individual with an extra 100 μg of folic acid per day.

A potential hazard of folic acid therapy is subacute degeneration of the spinal cord with a subclinical vitamin B_{12} deficiency; folic acid may mask the development of hematologic manifestations in these patients. This situation can be avoided by either ruling out B_{12} deficiency before initiating folic acid therapy or by supplementing folic acid with vitamin B_{12}.[44]

High-dose niacin (vitamin B_3) is used in the treatment of hyperlipidemia and hypercholesterolemia and helps curb the development of atherosclerosis and its complications. Over-the-counter niacin preparations are marketed under different names and some have no free nicotinic acid which is the cholesterol lowering component of niacin.[46] Side effects of niacin include cutaneous flushing, pruritus, GI disturbances, exacerbation of asthma, and even acanthosis nigricans. Very high doses can cause liver toxicity. Vasodilation and flushing, the most common side effect of niacin, may help patients who suffer from Raynaud's phenomenon.

In an attempt to find a safer form of niacin with fewer side effects, investigators have developed a new, extended-release, once-daily formulation of niacin (Niaspan). This slowly metabolized form of niacin does not reach maximum serum levels for several hours after ingestion, thus resulting in fewer and less severe side effects.[47,48] Randomized, double-blind, placebo-controlled investigations showed that sustained-released niacin had an impact in decreasing LDL-cholesterol, total cholesterol, and triglycerides while raising HDL-cholesterol.[47-49]

Niaspan and niacin also play a significant role in reducing lipoprotein Lp(a), a serious risk factor in atherogenesis. In one small study of patients with lipoprotein Lp(a) concentrations greater than 30 mg/dL, the ingestion of 1 g of niacin three times daily demonstrated reduction in lipid levels, with the level of lipoprotein Lp(a) showing the greatest reduction (36.4%).[50]

CAROTENOIDS

Serum carotenoids have been extensively studied in the prevention of CAD. Approximately 600 carotenoids are found in nature, predominantly in fresh fruits and vegetables. Carrots are the primary source of β carotene and tomatoes being the best source of lycopene. Although lycopene has twice the antioxidant activity of β carotene, the latter has been the primary focus of study because of its activity as a precursor to vitamin A.

Elevated levels of serum β carotene have been associated with a lower risk of cancer and overall mortality.[51] However, inconsistent data from randomized clinical trials regarding both β carotene's antioxidant properties on LDL in vitro and its preventive actions on cardiovascular disease cast doubt on the beneficial effects of β carotene supplementation.[52-54]

Research studies have shown an association between a high dietary intake of β carotene with a reduction in the incidence of cardiovascular disease.[55] One study reported that increased β carotene stores in subcutaneous fat were correlated with a decreased risk of MI.[56] However, controlled studies have found that excessive supplemental β carotene failed to lead to a reduction in rates of lung cancer or cardiovascular disease among heavy smokers.[57] An increased incidence of lung cancer was found in the β carotene and retinal efficacy trial, halting the study 21 months early when this alarming cancer rate was observed among smokers and workers exposed to asbestos.[58] Similarly, after the first Physician's Health Trial demonstrated that alternate-day administration of 50 mg of β carotene for 12 years showed no positive effects on coronary heart disease events, the enthusiasm for β carotene as a preventive intervention for cardiovascular disease declined.[59] The results of the MRC/BHF Heart Protection Study showed no benefit from β carotene 20 mg daily on morbidity and mortality in high-risk individuals.[12] Recently, the second Physician's Health Trial showed no beneficial effects of β carotene on cardiovascular outcomes in healthy individuals; results are not published to date.

The use of excess synthetic β carotene, as done in the ATBC and the β carotene and retinal efficacy trials,[57,58] should be avoided in any high-risk populations because of yet unidentified elements that may somehow affect cancer growth in vulnerable individuals. It is safer and more efficacious to take a natural supplement combination of mixed carotenoids including β carotene, lutein, lycopene, α carotene, and β cryptoxanthin. β carotene is responsible for only an estimated 25% of total serum carotenoid activity. Perhaps the lower mortality associated with higher levels of baseline serum β carotene had more to do with long-term dietary habits of individuals who eat more fruits and vegetables containing multiple carotenoids than with artificial elevation of serum β carotenes with supplementation. Excessive carotene ingestion is relatively innocuous and results in yellowing of the skin, particularly on the palms and soles but sparing the sclerae. Hypothyroid patients are more susceptible to carotenemia.

The other carotenoids, such as lutein, that enter the LDL and high-density lipoprotein (HDL) particles may retard CAD by their favorable effects on LDL oxidation. In the Toulouse Study, those participants with greater lutein activity in their blood had a lower incidence of CAD.[60] Some researchers consider the lutein found in a diet rich in green and yellow fruits and vegetables to be more responsible for the inhibition of CAD than the red wine benefit called "French paradox."

FLAVONOIDS (RED WINE)

Residents of France, whose diet is steeped in high-fat cheeses, rich sauces, gravies, patès, and other highly-saturated fats, have a lower incidence of CAD than their American counterparts. This paradoxical situation challenges the belief that a low-fat diet protects against heart disease. Offsetting the "risk" that we see in the typical French diet is the routine consumption of fresh fruits and vegetables that contain vital phytonutrients, including tocopherols, carotenoids (especially lutein), flavonoids (quercetin), phenols, catechins, and other phytonutrients that may effectively reduce peroxidative tendencies and retard the varied interactions involved in atherogenesis and thrombosis. Red wine consumption could be another factor.

The serum antioxidant activity of red wine was addressed in a small study of volunteers, the results indicating that two glasses of red wine consumed before a meal offered considerable antioxidant protection for at least 4 hours.[61] Red wine increased antioxidant activity through a flavonoid-polyphenol effect. In another small investigation performed in the Netherlands, the use of dietary bioflavonoids, phenolic acids, and quercetin showed a reduction in the incidence of heart attack and sudden death.[62] The findings in 64- to 85-year-old men showed an inverse relationship between the amount of quercetin ingested and mortality. Quercetin-rich black tea, apples, and onions were the best foods evaluated because they contain polyphenols in amounts similar to those found in the red grapes used in making wine and grape juice.

A recent study with grape juice in normal volunteers demonstrated favorable effects on platelet aggregation, platelet-derived nitric oxide release, and free oxygen-derived free radical production.[63] Short- and long-term consumption of black tea was shown to reverse endothelial vasomotor dysfunction in patients with CAD.[64]

Oligomeric proanthocyanidins, like carotenoids, are found predominantly in brightly colored fruits and vegetables and represent a safe source of polyphenols and quercetin, which are believed to be the most active protective ingredients in preventing the oxidation of LDL. Oligomeric proanthocyanidins are significant free-radical scavengers that inhibit lipid peroxidation and contain antiinflammatory and antiallergenic properties as well. A recent study by Plotnick et al demonstrated the benefit of flavonoid supplementation in reversing brachial artery reactivity seen with a high-fat meal.[65]

Data on the absorption and metabolism of flavonoids are lacking. Natural flavonoids are glycosylated, which plays an uncertain role in influencing absorption. Once absorbed, glucuronide conjugation commonly occurs—but at varying sites, which may affect the biological activity of the compounds. It is not known if all flavonoids are beneficial, with evidence to suggest that some may increase cholesterol uptake in LDL. Furthermore, as would be expected in a heterogeneous group of compounds, both antitumor and mutagenic properties have been described, and concerns have been raised that excess intake may be toxic. As such, the optimal amount of flavonoids in the diet, form or method of supplementation, and dose are uncertain. Nonetheless, many flavonoids are available as food supplements in doses as high as 500 and 1000 mg, an amount that may be 10 to 20 times the daily intake in a typical vegetarian diet. An epidemiologic report from the Physician's Health Study did not show a strong inverse association between intake of flavonoids and total CAD.[66] Until these issues are resolved in prospective controlled studies, patients may be encouraged to consume a diet that includes tea, apples, and onions in generous amounts. Current research does not support the benefits of supplemental flavonoid intake, but further research is needed.

MAGNESIUM

Magnesium has a profound influence on coronary vascular tone and reactivity; deficiencies have been shown to produce spasm of the coronary vasculature, thus pointing to the low-magnesium state as a possible risk factor in nonocclusive MI.[67] Hypomagnesemia can result in progressive vasoconstriction, coronary spasm, and even sudden death. In anginal episodes due to coronary artery spasm, treatment with magnesium has been shown to be considerably efficacious.[68]

Magnesium deficiency, which is better detected by mononuclear blood cell magnesium than the standard serum level performed at most hospitals, predisposes to excessive mortality and morbidity in patients with acute myocardial infarction. Several studies have shown an association between intravenous magnesium supplementation during the first hour of admission for myocardial infarction and reductions in both morbidity and mortality. Although other trials of magnesium therapy in patients with acute myocardial infarction have produced inconsistent results, the most efficacious use of magnesium, like thrombolytics, occurs with the earliest administration.[69] Multiple cardioprotective and physiologic activities of magnesium include antiarrhythmic effects, calcium channel–blocking effects, improvement in nitric oxide release from coronary endothelium, and the ability to help prevent serum coagulation, to name a few.[69]

Research into the inhibition of platelet-dependent thrombosis indicates that magnesium may have a positive preventive role for patients with CAD. In one double-blind, placebo-controlled study of 42 patients, median platelet-dependent thrombosis was reduced by 35% in 75% of patients receiving oral administration of magnesium oxide tablets (800-1200 mg daily) for 3 months.[70] This antithrombotic effect occurred despite the use of aspirin therapy in the study population.

Magnesium has also shown considerable efficacy in relieving symptoms of mitral valve prolapse (MVP). In a double-blind study of 181 participants, serum magnesium levels were assessed in 141 patients with symptomatic MVP and compared to those of 40 healthy control subjects; decreased serum magnesium levels were identified in 60% of the patients with MVP, whereas only 5% of control subjects showed similar decreases.[71] The second leg of the study investigated response to treatment. Subjective results in the magnesium group were dramatic, with significant reductions noted in weakness, chest pain, shortness of breath, palpitations, and even anxiety. Lower levels of epinephrine metabolites were also found in the urine. For patients with MVP, magnesium supplementation offers a reduction in symptomatology and improvement in quality of life. Blood-pressure lowering with magnesium, especially when combined with calcium and potassium, has also been reported.[72] Supplemental magnesium and potassium should be avoided in patients with renal insufficiency.

Magnesium has been shown to be neuroprotective in animal models of stroke. However, the results of the placebo-controlled Intravenous Magnesium in Stroke Trial did not show a benefit of intravenous magnesium sulfate on death or disability when given within 12 hours of stroke.[73]

TRACE MINERALS

Cobaltous chloride is sometimes used in the treatment of iron deficiency and chronic renal failure. Excessive cobalt intake may cause cardiomyopathy and CHF, with pericardial effusions due to deposition of cobalt-lipoic acid complexes in the heart. High cobalt consumption has also been implicated in thyroid enlargement, polycythemia, neurologic abnormalities, and interference with pyruvate and fatty acid metabolism. Rarely, excessive iron ingestion may cause cardiomyopathy, CHF, and cardiac arrhythmias from hemochromatosis.

Chromium assists in glucose and lipid metabolism. It may bring about regression of cholesterol-induced atherosclerosis.[74] In a double-blind study involving 34 male athletes with elevated cholesterol levels,[75] supplementation with 200 µg of elemental chromium (chromium as niacin-bound chromium complex) significantly lowered serum cholesterol by an average of 14%. In a more recent study of 40 hypercholesterolemic patients (total cholesterol 210 to 300 mg/dL), a combination of 200 µg of chromium polynicotinate (Cr) and (proanthocyanidin) grape-seed extract (GSE) 100 mg twice daily resulted in profound lowering of LDL and total cholesterol.[76] However, no significant change in either HDL or triglyceride level in either the treatment or the placebo group was found. Because insulin resistance may be the major factor in disturbed lipid metabolism, chromium's favorable action on glucose/-insulin metabolism may be the key factor in lowering cholesterol.[77] Although no significant adverse reactions from Cr have been observed at the dose of 400 µg per day, massive ingestion of chromium has been associated with renal failure.[78]

Selenium is an antioxidant and an essential mineral with immune-enhancing and cancer-fighting properties. The metabolic relationships between the mineral selenium and vitamin E are very close. Selenium is a cofactor of the enzyme glutathione peroxidase, which serves as an antioxidant and is found in the platelets and the arterial walls. In contrast to vitamin E, which prevents formation of lipid hydroperoxides in cell membranes and LDL by acting as a biological free-radical trap, selenium and glutathione peroxidase help destroy lipid hydroperoxides already formed by peroxidation of polyunsaturated fatty acids. Selenium thereby defends against the free-radical oxidative stress that escapes the protection of vitamin E.

In some areas of the world, soil deficiencies in selenium have produced Keshan disease, a disorder of cardiac muscle characterized by multifocal myocardial necrosis that causes cardiomyopathy, CHF, and cardiac arrhythmias. Men with low levels of serum selenium (<1.4 µmol/L) demonstrated increased thickness in the intima and media of the common carotid arteries. Selenium, when combined with coenzyme Q10, may also offer cardioprotective benefits in patients after myocardial infarction. In one study of 61 patients admitted for an acute myocardial infarction,[79] 32 subjects in the experimental group received 100 mg of coenzyme Q10 with 500 µg of selenium in the first 24 h of hospitalization followed by daily doses of 100 mg of coenzyme Q10, 100 µg of selenium, 15 mg of zinc, 1 mg of vitamin A, 2 mg of vitamin B_6, 90 mg of vitamin C, and 15 mg vitamin E for 1 year. The control group (29 patients) received placebo for the same time period. During their hospital stay, none of the participants in the experimental group showed prolongation of the QT interval in comparison to 40% of the control subjects, whose QTC increased 440 milliseconds (about a 10% increase). Although no significant differences in early complications between the two groups were found, six (21%) patients in the control group died of recurrent myocardial infarction, whereas only one patient in the study group (3%) died a noncardiac death. Although selenium is quite safe at levels below 200 µg, excessive selenium can result in alopecia, abnormal nails, emotional lability, lassitude, and a garlic odor to the breath.[72] Skin lesions and polyneuritis have been reported in people taking selenium from health food stores.

A substudy report from the Physician's Health Study showed no relationship between selenium blood levels and the risk of myocardial infarction in well-nourished subjects.[80] However, these findings do not rule out the possibility of an increased risk of myocardial infarction in severe selenium deficiency. Also, questions have been raised about the reliability of plasma selenium levels and other methods to obtain accurate body measurement have been proposed.[81]

Copper is a prooxidant that oxidizes LDL and may contribute to the development of atherosclerosis. Men with high serum copper (>17.6 µmol/L) demonstrate increased thickening in the intima and media of the common carotid arteries.[82] Excessive oral intake of copper may cause nausea, vomiting, diarrhea, and hemolytic anemia. Even higher doses can result in renal and hepatic toxicity as well as central nervous system disturbances similar to those of Wilson's disease. Any multivitamin with higher than the RDA level of copper (2 mg) should be avoided. Excessive levels of copper in drinking water, especially noted in homes with copper pipes, can also contribute to elevated serum copper levels.

OTHER NEUTROCEUTICALS

COENZYME Q10

Coenzyme Q10, present in most foods, especially organ meats and fish, facilitates electron transport in oxidative metabolism. Its reduced form, ubiquinol, protects membrane phospholipids and serum LDLs from lipid peroxidation as well as mitochondrial membrane proteins and DNA from free radical–induced oxidative damage. Ubiquinol's antioxidant effects on membrane phospholipids and LDL directly antagonizes the atherogenesis process. Vitamin E regeneration is significantly improved by the addition of coenzyme Q10 because of the latter's ability to recycle the oxidized form of vitamin E back to its reduced form. Coenzyme Q10 also prevents the prooxidant effect of α-tocopherols. Supplemental coenzyme Q may also improve use of oxygen at the cellular level, hence benefiting patients with coronary insufficiency.[79]

Perhaps coenzyme Q10's most remarkable effects involve tissue protection in the setting of myocardial ischemia and reperfusion.[83] The results of a controlled study of patients with acute MI demonstrated reduction in free-radical indices, infarct size, arrhythmia, and cardiac death in patients who received coenzyme Q10.[84] In addition, coenzyme Q10 supplementation may have a beneficial role in patients with CHF, stable angina pectoris, toxin-induced cardiotoxicity, cerebral ischemia, and peripheral vascular disease. It has also been used as a myocardial preserving agent for cardiac surgery.[84a]

Additional work must be done in determining reliable Q10 levels for clinical purposes. In addition to cholesterol and triglycerides, several other factors— including gender, alcohol consumption, age, and intensity of exercise—can affect coenzyme Q levels. Additional studies with coenzyme Q need to be done regarding dose (300 mg/d is the dose used in most studies) and establishing clinical efficacy before a recommendation can be made regarding its use in treating various cardiovascular disorders as a primary or adjunctive treatment.

Although side effects of coenzyme Q10, such as nausea and abdominal discomfort, are rare, it is not suggested for healthy pregnant or lactating women because the unborn and the newborn both produce sufficient quantities of the compound. However, statin drugs cause profound deficiencies in coenzyme Q10 because HMG-CoA reductase inhibitors (statins) block the endogenous production of coenzyme Q10.[85] Our group has used coenzyme Q10 treatment successfully to counteract the side effect of myalgia associated with statin therapy.

L-CARNITINE

Carnitine is a naturally occurring substance with several physiologic roles. The FDA approved it in 1986 in both its intravenous and oral forms as an orphan drug for the treatment of primary carnitine deficiency. It is also used for patients with conditions known to produce secondary carnitine deficiency, such as renal failure and various cardiovascular diseases. One to two grams daily given orally in divided doses is adequate for most therapeutic purposes. Intravenous doses range from 40 to 100 mg/kg. For children, oral L-carnitine is given at 100 mg/ kg/d.

L-carnitine has a synergistic relationship with coenzyme Q10 because it also penetrates the inner mitochondrial membrane. As a trimethylated amino acid, L-carnitine's primary function is in the oxidation of long-chain fatty acids.

Animal studies and clinical trials indicate that carnitine is effective in treating patients with various cardiovascular diseases, such as ischemic heart disease, CHF, peripheral vascular disease, arrhythmia, and hyperlipidemia. Carnitine appears to boost fatty acid and carbohydrate oxidation in the cell while helping to remove harmful substances, such as excess acyl groups and free radicals, from the cells. However, the exact mechanisms responsible for carnitine's therapeutic actions are not completely agreed upon. Further clinical studies with this substance are warranted.

OMEGA-3 FATTY ACIDS

Omega-3 fatty acids—such as eicosapentaenoic acid (EPA) and docosahexaenoic acid (DHA)—are found in fish oils. They stimulate the production of nitric oxide, which relaxes vascular smooth muscle. Their actions can counteract the impairment of nitric oxide production that is caused by atherosclerotic plaques. In addition, consumption of eicosapentaenoic acid stimulates the production of prostaglandin I_3, an antithrombotic and anti–platelet-aggregating agent similar to prostacyclin. As an anticoagulant, omega-3 fatty acids can increase bleeding time, inhibit platelet adhesiveness, decrease platelet count, and reduce serum thromboxane levels. Omega-3 fatty acids can also blunt the vasopressor effects of angiotensin II and norepinephrine and may reduce blood pressure and the risk of arrhythmia.[8]

In one recent placebo-controlled trial, an average systolic reduction of 5 mm Hg and a mean diastolic decrease of 3 mm Hg was realized in those participants taking DHA.[86] The triglyceride-lowering effect of these fish oil components may be one of many factors that inhibit the progression of atherosclerosis.[87,88] Data from studies are conflicting regarding the role of omega-3 fatty acids in the reduction of arterial restenosis after coronary angioplasty.[89,90]

In a recent landmark decision, the FDA reported that it would allow products containing omega-3 fatty acids to claim heart health benefits. The FDA based its decision on the wealth of scientific evidence that suggests a correlation between omega-3 fatty acids such as EPA and DHA and a reduced risk of CAD. In the GISSI-Prevenzione trial, Italian investigators reported overwhelming health benefits for participants who were placed on 1 gram of omega-3 essential fatty acids a day.[8] After the initial study had been reevaluated, participants on the omega-3 program experienced a 20% reduction in all-cause mortality and a 45% decrease in sudden cardiac death.[91] One case-controlled study showed that participants who ate the equivalent of one fish meal a week had a 50% less chance of sudden cardiac death in comparison to counterparts whose daily menus did not contain these vital fish oils.[92] Recently fish consumption was shown to be associated with a decreased heart rate in men, which may explain, at least in part, the lower risk of death among fish consumers.[93,94]

L-ARGININE

L-arginine is an essential amino acid that serves as the substrate for the enzyme nitric oxide synthetase (NOS), which converts L-arginine to l-citrolline and produces nitric oxide. L-arginine is also known to be the substrate for other processes, including arginine decarboxylase, which catalyzes the synthesis of agmantine. The latter is an endogenous noncatecholamine α_2 agonist that decreases peripheral sympathetic outflow by an effect in the nucleus tractus solitarius and therefore might be involved in the antihypertensive effect of L-arginine.[95]

Intracoronary infusion of L-arginine has been shown to normalize the defective acetylcholine-induced vasodilation of coronary microvessels in patients with hypercholesterolemia[96] and in those with microvascular angina pectoris.[97] In patients with CAD and hypertension, no such effect was observed.[98] Unlike the coronary dilation seen with nitrates, no significant beneficial effect of L-arginine on the large epicardial arteries has been observed.[99]

Thirteen weeks of oral administration of L-arginine was shown to result in an increased generation of vascular nitric oxide, a reduced endothelial release of superoxide anions, and regression of intimal atherosclerotic lesions in rats on a high-cholesterol diet.[100] Another group, however, supplemented rabbits on a high-cholesterol diet for 7 to 14 weeks with oral L-arginine and found a significant effect on the extent of atherosclerotic lesions limited to the descending aorta of males but no effect in the ascending aorta or in females.[101] In this study, plasma L-arginine levels remained only transiently elevated in the supplemented group of animals; also, effects on acetylcholine-induced hindlimb conductance were transient, thus raising questions on the long-term benefit of dietary L-arginine in the prevention of atherosclerosis.

Previous studies have demonstrated that an intracoronary infusion of L-arginine normalizes the defective acetylcholine-induced vasodilation of coronary microvessels in patients with hypercholesterolemia[96] and in patients with microvascular angina pectoris[97] as well in those with atherosclerosis.[102] A 1997 study by Lerman et al examined the effects of 6 months of oral L-arginine supplementation (3 grams tid).[103] They demonstrated that the chronic oral L-arginine supplementation improved coronary small vessel endothelial function in association with a significant improvement in symptoms and a decrease in plasma endothelin concentrations. However, in a study by Blum et al, 30 patients with coronary artery disease on appropriate medical therapy were orally supplemented with 9 g/day for 1 month of L-arginine.[104] This study concluded that chronic oral L-arginine supplementation does not improve nitric oxide bioavailability in this population of patients. Possible explanations for the discrepant study results in the Blum Study include the limited cellular uptake of arginine, a competitive inhibition of eNos, or a limited co-factor availability for eNos.[105]

Quyyumi recently examined the topic of stereospecificity and concluded that parenteral arginine produces nonstereospecific peripheral vasodilation and improves endothelium-dependent vasodilation in patients with stable coronary artery disease.[106]

The doses of L-arginine employed in clinical trials were 8 to 21 grams daily. Adverse reactions associated with L-arginine include nausea, abdominal cramps, and diarrhea.

TAURINE

Taurine is an essential sulfonic amino acid that is present in large quantities in the myocardium. A deficiency of taurine in the diet (animal food and seaweed) can cause cardiomyopathy, and replacement will lead to recovery of myocardial function. Taurine in supplementary doses of 500 mg to 3 mg/d has been used in the treatment of CHF in pilot studies, with apparent hemodynamic benefit. Additional clinical study is needed. Taurine has also been shown to have possible antiatherosclerotic effects.[106a] No adverse reactions have been reported with supplemental taurine treatment.[107]

AMINO ACID MIXTURES

Rather than specific amino acids, the use of various amino acid mixtures has been proposed as a treatment for patients with chronic heart failure, systolic dysfunction, and diabetes mellitus. It is thought by the proponents of this nutritional supplement that amino acids would shift the energy preference away from fatty acids, which would enhance adenosine diphosphate production, with favorable effects on cellular metabolism.[107a,107b] A double-blind clinical study (Effects of Diatrofen on Myocardial Function in Patients with Chronic Heart Failure [D-CHF trial]) is now in progress evaluating the effects of an oral amino acid mixture in patients with chronic heart failure.[107a]

Amino acid supplementation may also have benefits in enhancing myocyte survival and preserving mitochondrial function during ischemia-perfusion injury.[107c,107d]

β-SITOSTEROL (PLANT STEROLS)

β-Sitosterol is a plant sterol with a structure similar to that of cholesterol except for the substitution of an ethyl group at C-24 of its side chain. Despite this structural relation to cholesterol, it is poorly absorbed from the intestine. β-Sitosterol is known to compete with cholesterol for incorporation into mixed micelles, thereby reducing intestinal cholesterol absorption. β-Sitosterol is also thought to inhibit absorption of endogenous biliary cholesterol.[108-110] The importance of dietary intake of plant sterols on cholesterol absorption and serum cholesterol has been demonstrated in human beings; dietary intake of plant sterols is negatively related to fractional cholesterol absorption and overall cholesterol synthesis.[111,112] Sitosterol may also inhibit 7α-hydroxylase.

β-Sitosterol is used for treatment of hypercholesterolemia in Europe. It is quite effective in reducing cholesterol by 5% to 15%.[112] It is a very safe substance, although a high dose is required (6 grams) and is taken before meals and at bedtime. Another plant sterol, β-sitostanol, reduces serum cholesterol more effectively than sitosterol at a lower dose.

Miettinen and colleagues reported on the use of sitostanol ester, a derivative of the plant sterol sitosterol, which reduces the intestinal absorption of cholesterol and serum cholesterol more than sitosterol.[110] In this study, sitostanol ester was dissolved in margarine in a double-blind, randomized trial of men with moderate hypercholesterolemia. The formulation achieved a reduction in serum LDL-cholesterol of 14% with 2.6 g of sitostanol. A more recent study showed significant reduction of serum total cholesterol and LDL-cholesterol even at a dose of 1.6 g of stanol.[113] Although the dose of 2.4 grams resulted in a slightly greater reduction of serum cholesterol than the dose of 1.6 grams, the actual difference was not statistically significant.

Because the inhibition of dietary cholesterol could increase endogenous cholesterol synthesis, several studies investigated the combination of sitostanol with HMG-CoA reductase inhibitors.[114] Combined administration of a sitostanol ester margarine with a statin increased the net reduction in LDL-cholesterol from 38% to 44% in non–insulin-dependent diabetics[115] and from 35% to 46% in postmenopausal women with coronary heart disease.[108] A larger, more recent study confirmed the effective reduction of total cholesterol and LDL from the administration of a stanol with a stable dose of statin. The study showed a 10% reduction in LDL-cholesterol from the combined therapy of a plant stanol ester spread with either atorvastatin, pravastatin, simvastatin, or lovastatin.[116]

In children with hypercholesterolemia, sitostanol is effective and could be considered a treatment of choice. Replacement of regular daily fat intake by a margarine with a soluble ester form of stanol reduced total cholesterol and LDL cholesterol levels by 11% and 15%, respectively, and increased HDL cholesterol by 4% in children with heterozygous familial hypercholesterolemia.[117] The study suggests that familial hypercholesterolemic children with high baseline lathosterol proportions in serum can be expected to be good responders to LDL cholesterol lowering by dietary sitostanol ester.

Another group of plant compounds, the saponins, also interfere with cholesterol absorption by causing cholesterol precipitation, interference with micelle formation, or bile acid absorption. A synthetic saponin, β-tiogenin cellobioside, was found to reduce plasma cholesterol and LDL cholesterol in men with hypercholesterolemia.[118] β-Ketotiogenin cellobioside, a derivative, selectively inhibits cholesterol absorption and is being evaluated as a potential replacement for bile acid resins.[118]

DIETARY FIBER

Dietary fiber is a collective term for a variety of plant substances that are resistant to digestion by human GI enzymes.[119] Fiber may be obtained either from dietary sources or from extradietary supplements. The chemical components of naturally occurring dietary fiber include cellulose, lignins, hemicelluloses, pectins, gums, and mucilages. Dietary fibers can be classified into two major groups based on their water solubility.[119] The structural or matrix fibers (lignins, cellulose, and some hemicelluloses) are insoluble. The natural gel-forming fibers (pectins, gums, mucilages, and the rest of the hemicelluloses) are soluble in humans.

Psyllium hydrophilic mucilloid, a well-known bulk laxative, is a potential cholesterol-lowering agent. Its effectiveness relates to its ability in delivering five times more soluble fiber than oat bran and its ease of administration as a dietary supplement to patients with hypercholesterolemia.

Psyllium is a soluble gel-forming fiber derived from the husks of blond psyllium seeds of the genus *Plantago*, plants grown in the Mediterranean region and in India. The processing of psyllium involves the initial separation of the seeds from the plant husks and then grinding the husks to make the final psyllium substance. The seed husk is then enriched with mucilloid, a hydrophilic substance that forms a gelatinous mass when mixed with water. The unused seed extracts are marketed as health foods or as animal feed.[120] The chemical composition of psyllium is based on its being broken into an 85% mucilage polysaccharide and a 15% nonpolysaccharide component. The polysaccharide fraction is the active one and is made of 63% D-xylose, 20% L-arabinose, 6% rhamrose, and 9% D-galacturonic acid, as derived by acid hydrolysis and methylation analysis. Structural features of this component are those of a highly branched acidic arabinoxylan; xylan backbone with sugar 1:4 and 1:3 linkages.[121] The nonpolysaccharide component has nitrogen and other nonactive components.[121]

Several investigators have studied the activity of psyllium as a cholesterol-reducing agent. It is the universal impression from clinical trials that psyllium is a hypocholesterolemic agent with and without a modified diet.[122] However, debate as to the degree of cholesterol reduction with psyllium remains.

The mechanism by which psyllium and other soluble fiber lower serum cholesterol is currently uncertain. Available information suggests that one or more of the following mechanisms may be operative. First, psyllium has been shown prevent the normal reabsorption of bile acids in the gut.[123] A similar mechanism of action is also seen with cholestyramine and other bile acid sequestran drugs. Secondly, soluble fibers such as psyllium may interfere with micelle formation in the proximal small intestine, thus resulting in decreased absorption of cholesterol and fatty acids.[123] Finally, short-chain fatty acids are produced by bacterial fermentation of soluble fiber in the colon. These fatty acids (predominantly propionate and acetate) are rapidly absorbed into the bloodstream and may inhibit hepatic cholesterol synthesis.[124] Short-chain fatty acids may also decrease hepatic cholesterol concentrations and secretions by interfering with compensatory mechanisms.[124]

Patients tolerate psyllium and other soluble fibers well. In many of the clinical trials, treatment compliance was high. A possible reason for the acceptability of psyllium therapy is that patients will have well-formed stools and a low incidence of side effects. Some patients placed on psyllium report abdominal distention, excessive gas, and flatulence, but these symptoms usually subside after a few weeks. Rarely, allergic reactions to psyllium have been described.[125]

Although reports indicate possible effects of psyllium and soluble fibers on reducing calcium, magnesium, zinc, copper, and iron absorption, other studies have contradicted these findings.[126] Animal studies have revealed the absence of teratogenic effects of psyllium. Some studies have revealed an effect of psyllium on the binding of sodium warfarin. Any potential problem can be avoided by separating the intake of psyllium and drug by 1 to 2 hours. Finally, patients with congestive heart failure may be at risk from an excessive salt load with psyllium ingestion.

The efficacy of psyllium in lowering cholesterol is consistent with that of many other soluble fibers. Studies have found that, in contrast to oat bran, 15 grams of pectin added to the diet lowered cholesterol by an additional 11%. The addition of 100 grams of oat bran to the diet has been shown to lower cholesterol by 19% and LDL cholesterol by 11%.[127] However, the effectiveness of oat bran alone as a long-term hypercholesterolemic intervention has come into question.[127]

The efficiency of psyllium is revealed in its ability to achieve reductions in cholesterol in studies that have used only 10.2 g of the substance daily. It is concluded that psyllium is useful as an adjunct to dietary therapy in the treatment of patients with mild to moderate hyper-cholesterolemia. Clearly, cholestyramine and the HMG-CoA reductase inhibitors have greater efficacy than psyllium alone in reducing cholesterol. However, combining psyllium with the other drug treatments for lowering cholesterol appears to be quite useful.[128,129]

A recent pooled analysis of cohort studies showed that the consumption of dietary fibers from cereals and fruits is inversely associated with risk of CAD.[130]

CONCLUSION

Associations between the use of vitamin and mineral supplements and a lower risk of the development of cardiovascular disease have been reported. Although a sound theoretical basis for using both vitamin and mineral supplementation and other nutriceutical agents to prevent and treat cardiovascular disease often exists, randomized trials are either lacking or have failed to demonstrate any significant benefit of any single vitamin (except for niacin) or vitamin combinations and any other nutriceuticals on the incidence of death from cardiovascular disease.

REFERENCES

1. Drazen JM: Inappropriate advertising of dietary supplements, N Engl J Med 348:777-78, 2003.
2. Morris CD, Carson S: Routine vitamin supplementation to prevent cardiovascular disease: a summary of the evidence for the US Preventive Services Task Force, Ann Intern Med 139:56-70, 2003.
3. Problems with dietary supplements, The Medical Letter 44:84-86, 2002.
3a. Frishman WH, Kruger NA, Nayak DU, Vakili BA: Antioxidant vitamins and enzymatic and synthetic oxygen-derived free-radical scavengers in the prevention and treatment of cardiovascular disease. In Frishman WH, Sonnenblick EH, Sica DA, editors: Cardiovascular pharmacotherapeutics, ed 2, New York, 2003, McGraw Hill, 407-27.
4. Pryor WA: Vitamin E and heart tissue: basic science to clinical intervention trials, Free Radic Biol Med 28:141-64, 2000.
5. Rapola JM, Virtamo J, Haukka JK et al: Effect of vitamin E and beta carotene on the incidence of angina pectoris: a randomized, double-blind, controlled trial, JAMA 275:693-98, 1996.
6. Stephens NG, Parsons A, Schofield PM et al: Randomized controlled trial of vitamin E in patients with coronary disease: Cambridge Heart Antioxidant Study, Lancet 347:781-86, 1996.
7. Yusuf S, Sleight P, Pogue J et al: Effects of an angiotensin-converting-enzyme inhibitor, ramipril, on cardiovascular events in high-risk patients, N Engl J Med 342:145-53, 2000.

8. *Gruppo Italiano per lo Studio della Sopravvivenza nell'Infarto miocardioco:* Dietary supplementation with n-3 polyunsaturated fatty acids and vitamin E after myocardial infarction: results of the GISSI Prevenzione trial, Lancet 354:447-55, 1999.
9. Jialal I, Traber M, Deveraj S: Is there a vitamin E paradox? Curr Opin Lipidol 12:49-53, 2001.
10. Rapola JM, Virtamo J, Ripatti S et al: Randomized trial of alpha-tocopherol and beta carotene supplements on incidence of major coronary events in men with previous myocardial infarction, Lancet 349:1715-20, 1997.
11. Vivekananthan DP, Penn MS, Sapp SK et al: Use of antioxidant vitamins for the prevention of cardiovascular disease: meta-analysis of randomized trials, Lancet 361:2017-23, 2003.
12. Heart Protection Study Collaborative Group: MRC/BHF Heart Protection Study of antioxidant vitamin supplement in 20,536 high-risk individuals: a randomized placebo-controlled trial, Lancet 360:23-33, 2002.
13. Stampfer MJ, Hennekens CH, Manson JE et al: Vitamin E consumption and the risk of coronary disease in women, N Engl J Med 328:1444-49, 1993.
14. Rimm EB, Stampfer MJ, Ascherio A et al: Vitamin E consumption and the risk of coronary disease in men, N Engl J Med 328:1450, 1993.
15. Hodis HN, Mack WJ, LaBree L et al: Serial coronary angiographic evidence that antioxidant vitamin intake reduces progression of coronary atherosclerosis, JAMA 273:1849-54, 1995.
15a. Shekelle P, Morton SC, Jungvig LK et al: Effect of supplemental vitamin E for the prevention and treatment of cardiovascular disease. J Gen Intern Med 19:380-389, 2004.
16. Meagher EA, Barry OP, Lawson JA et al: Effects of vitamin E on lipid peroxidation in healthy persons, JAMA 285:1178-82, 2001.
17. Wolf G: Gamma-tocopherol: An efficient protector of lipids against nitric oxide-initiated peroxidative damage, Nutr Rev 55:376-78, 1997.
18. Freedman JE, Cheney K, Eaney JR: Vitamin E inhibition of platelet aggregation is independent of antioxidant activity, J Nutr 131:374S-77S, 2000.
19. Church TS, Earnest CP, Woods KA, Kampert JB: Reduction of C-reactive protein levels through use of a multivitamin, Am J Med 115:702-07, 2003.
20. Kostner K, Hornykewycz S, Yang P et al: Is oxidative stress casually linked to unstable angina pectoris? a study in 100 CAD patients and matched controls, Cardiovas Res 36:330-36, 1997.
21. Watanabe H, Kakihana M, Ohtsuka S et al: Randomized, double-blind, placebo-controlled study of the preventive effect of supplemental oral vitamin C on attenuation of development of nitrate tolerance, J Am Coll Cardiol 31:1323-29, 1998.

22. Watanabe H, Kakihana M, Ohtsuka S et al: Randomized, double-blind, placebo-controlled study of supplemental vitamin E on an attenuation of the development of nitrate tolerance, Circulation 96:2545-50, 1997.

23. Munzel T, Sayegh H, Freeman B et al: Evidence for enhanced vascular superoxide anion-production in nitrate tolerance, J Clin Invest 95:187-94, 1995.

24. Kritchevsky SB, Shimakawa T, Tell GS et al: Dietary antioxidants and carotid artery wall thickness: the ARIC study, Circulation 92:2142-50, 1995.

25. Osganian SK, Stampfer MJ, Rimm E et al: Vitamin C and risk of coronary heart disease in women, J Am Coll Cardiol 42:246-52, 2003.

26. Kaw KT, Bingham S, Welch A et al: Relation between plasma ascorbic acid and mortality in men and women in EPIC-Norfolk Prospective Study: a prospective population study, Lancet 357:657-63, 2001.

27. Ting HH, Creager MA, Ganz P et al: Vitamin C improves endothelium-dependent vasodilation in forearm resistance vessels of humans with hypercholesterolemia, Circulation 95:2617-22, 1997.

28. Kinlay S, Behrendt D, Fang JC et al: Long-term effect of combined vitamins E and C on coronary and peripheral endothelial function, J Am Coll Cardiol 43:629034, 2004.

29. Kruger NA, Frishman WH, Hussain J: Fish oils, the B vitamins and folic acid as cardiovascular protective agents. In Frishman WH, Sonnenblick EH, Sica DA, editors: Cardiovascular Pharmacotherapeutics, ed 2, New York, 2003, McGraw Hill, 381-405.

30. Chan P, Huang TY, Chen YJ et al: Randomized, double-blind, placebo-controlled study of the safety and efficacy of vitamin B complex in the treatment of nocturnal leg cramps in elderly patients with hypertension, J Clin Pharmacol 38:1151-54, 1998.

31. McCully KS: Vascular pathology of homocysteinemia: implications for the pathogenesis of arteriosclerosis, Am J Pathol 56:111-28, 1969.

32. Gauthier GM, Keevil JG, McBride PE: The association of homocysteine and coronary artery disease, Clin Cardiol 26:563-68, 2003.

33. Matetzky S, Freimark D, Ben-Ami S et al: Association of elevated homocysteine levels with a higher risk of recurrent coronary events and mortality in patients with acute myocardial infarction, Arch Intern Med 163:1933-37, 2003.

34. Soinio M, Marniemi J, Laakso M et al: Elevated plasma homocysteine level is an independent predictor of coronary heart disease events in patients with type 2 diabetes mellitus, Ann Intern Med 140:94-100, 2004.

35. Vasan RS, Beiser A, D'Agostino RB et al: Plasma homocysteine and risk for congestive heart failure in adults without prior myocardial infarction, JAMA 289:1251-57, 2003.

36. Anderson JL, Jensen KR, Carlquist JF et al: Effect of folic acid fortification of food on homocysteine-related mortality, Am J Med 116:158-64, 2004.

37. Malinow RM, Nieto J, Szklo M et al: Carotid artery intimal-medial wall thickening and plasma homocyst(e)ine in asymptomatic adults: the Atherosclerosis Risk in Communities Study, Circulation 87:1107-13, 1993.

38. Selhub J, Jacques PF, Bostom AG et al: Association between plasma homocysteine concentrations and extracranial carotid artery disease, N Engl J Med 332:286-91, 1995.

39. Ridker PM, Manson JE, Buring JE et al: Homocysteine and risk of cardiovascular disease among post-menopausal women, JAMA 281:1817-21, 1999.

40. Rodrigo R, Passalacqua W, Araya J et al: Homocysteine and essential hypertension, J Clin Pharmacol 43:1299-1306, 2003.

41. Al-Obaidi MK, Stubbs PJ, Collinson P et al: Elevated homocysteine levels are associated with ischemic myocardial injury in acute coronary syndrome, J Am Coll Cardiol 36:1217-22, 2000.

42. Lowering plasma homocysteine, The Medical Letter 45:85-86, 2003.

43. Toole JF, Malinow MR, Chambless LE et al: Lowering homocysteine in patients with ischemic stroke to prevent recurrent stroke, myocardial infarction, and death: the Vitamin Intervention for Stroke Prevention (VISP) randomized controlled trial, JAMA 291:565-75, 2004.

44. Hankey GJ, Eikeboom JW: Homocysteine and vascular disease, Lancet 354:407-13, 1999.

45. Homocysteine Lowering Trialists' Collaboration: Lowering blood homocysteine with folic acid based supplements: meta-analysis of randomized trials, BMJ 316:894-98, 1998.

46. Meyers CD, Carr MC, Park S, Brunzell JD: Varying cost and free nicotinic acid content in over-the-counter niacin preparations for dyslipidemia, Ann Intern Med 139:996-1002, 2003.

47. Morgan JM, Capuzzi DM, Guyton JR: A new extended-release niacin (Niaspan): efficacy, tolerability, and safety in hypercholesterolemic patients, Am J Cardiol 82:29U-34U, 1998.

48. Goldberg A, Alagona P Jr, Capuzzi DM et al: Multiple-dose efficacy and safety of an extended-release form of niacin in the management of hyperlipidemia, Am J Cardiol 85:1100-05, 2000.

49. Goldberg AC: Clinical trial experience with extended-release niacin (Niaspan) dose escalation study, Am J Cardiol 82:35U-38U, 1998.

50. Seed M, O'Connor B, Perombelon N et al: The effect of nicotinic acid and acipimox on lipoprotein(a) concentration and turnover, Atherosclerosis 101:61-68, 1993.

51. Greenberg ER, Baron JA, Karagas MR et al: Mortality associated with low plasma concentration of beta carotene and the effect of oral supplementation, JAMA 275:699-703, 1996.

52. Jialal I, Norkus EP, Cristol L et al: B-carotene inhibits the oxidative modification of low-density lipoprotein, Biochem Biophys Acta 1086:134-138, 1991.

53. Reaven PD, Khouw A, Belz WF et al: Effects of dietary antioxidant combinations in humans. Protection of LDL by vitamin E but not by beta carotene, Arterioscler Thromb 13(4):590-600, 1993.
54. Gaziano JM, Hatta A, Flynn M et al: Supplementation with beta carotene in vivo and in vitro does not inhibit low density lipoprotein oxidation, Artherosclerosis 112:187-95, 1995.
55. Gey FK, Puska P: Plasma vitamin E and A inversely correlated to mortality from ischemic heart disease in cross-cultural epidemiology, Ann NY Acad Sci 570:268-82, 1989.
56. Kardinaal AF, Kok FJ, Ringstad J et al: Antioxidants in adipose tissue and risk of myocardial infarction: the EURAMIC study, Lancet 342:1379-84, 1993.
57. The Alpha-Tocopherol, Beta-Carotene Therapy Cancer Prevention Study Group: The effect of vitamin E and beta carotene on the incidence of lung cancer and other cancers in male smokers, N Engl J Med 330:1029-35, 1994.
58. Omenn GS, Goodman GE, Thornquist MD et al: Effects of a combination of beta carotene and vitamin A on lung cancer and cardiovascular disease, N Engl J Med 334:1150-55, 1996.
59. Hennekens CH, Buring JE, Manson JE et al: Lack of effect of long-term supplementation with beta carotene on the incidence of malignant neoplasms and cardiovascular disease, N Engl J Med 334:1145-49, 1996.
60. Howard AN, Williams NR, Palmer CR et al: Do hydroxy-carotenoids prevent coronary heart disease? a comparison between Belfast and Toulouse, Int J Vit Nutr Res 66:113-18, 1996.
61. Maxwell S, Cruickshank A, Thorpe D: Red wine and antioxidant activity in serum, Lancet 344:193-94, 1994.
62. Hertog MC, Feskens EJ, Hollman PC et al: Dietary antioxidant flavonoids and risk of coronary heart disease: the Zutphen Elderly Study, Lancet 342:1007-11, 1993.
63. Freedman JE, Parker C III, Li L et al: Select flavonoids and whole juice from purple grapes inhibit platelet function and enhance nitric oxide release, Circulation 103:2792-98, 2001.
64. Duffy SJ, Keaney JF, Holbrook M et al: Short- and long-term black tea consumption reverses endothelial dysfunction in patients with coronary artery disease, Circulation 104:151-56, 2001.
65. Plotnick GD, Corretti MC, Vogel RA, Hesslink R Jr., Wise JA: Effect of supplemental phytonutrients on impairment of flow-mediated brachial artery vasoactivity after a single high-fat meal, J Am Coll Cardiol 41:1744-49, 2003.
66. Rimm EB, Katan MB, Ascherio A et al: Relation between intake of flavonoids and risk for coronary heart disease in male health professionals, Ann Intern Med 125:384-89, 1996.
67. Sica DA, Frishman WH, Cavusoglu E: Magnesium, potassium, and calcium as potential cardiovascular disease therapies. In Frishman

WH, Sonnenblick EH, Sica DA, editors: Cardiovascular Pharmacotherapeutics, ed 2, New York, 2003, McGraw Hill, 177-89.

68. McLean RM: Magnesium and its therapeutic uses: a review, Am J Med 96:63-76, 1994.

69. Shechter M: Oral magnesium in coronary artery disease: Fresh insight on thrombus inhibition, Magn Rep 1-4, 1999.

70. Shechter M, Merz CN, Paul-Labrador M et al: Oral magnesium supplementation inhibits platelet-dependent thrombosis in patients with coronary artery disease, Am J Cardiol 84:152-56, 1999.

71. Lichodziejewska B, Klos J, Rezler J et al: Clinical symptoms of mitral valve prolapse are related to hypomagnesemia and attenuated by magnesium supplementation, Am J Cardiol 79:768-72, 1997.

72. Kendler BS: Recent nutritional approaches to the prevention and therapy of cardiovascular disease, Prog Cardiovasc Nurs 12:3-23, 1997.

73. Intravenous Magnesium Efficacy in Stroke (IMAGES) Study Investigators: Magnesium for acute stroke (Intravenous Magnesium Efficacy in Stroke trial): randomized controlled trial, Lancet 363:439-45, 2004.

74. Abraham AS, Sonnenblick M, Eini M et al: The effect of chromium on established atherosclerotic plaques in rabbits, Am J Clin Nutr 33:2294-98, 1980.

75. Lefavi RG, Wilson D, Keith RE et al: Lipid lowering effects of a dietary chromium (III)-nicotinic acid complex in male athletes, Nutr Res 13:239-49, 1993.

76. Preuss HG, Wallerstedr' D, Talpur N et al: Effects of niacin-bound chromium and grape seed proanthocyanidins extract on the lipid profile of hypercholesterolemic subjects: a pilot study, J Med 31(5&6):227-46, 2000.

77. Grundy SM: Cholesterol management in the era of managed care, Am J Cardiol 85:3A-9A, 2000.

78. McLaren DS: Vitamin deficiency, toxicity and dependency. In Berkow R, Fletcher AJ, Bondy PK et al, editors: The Merck Manual, ed 16, Rahway NJ, 1992, Merck Research Labs.

79. Kuklinski B, Weissenbacher E, Fahnrich A et al: Coenzyme Q10 and antioxidants in acute myocardial infarction, Mol Aspects Med 15:S143-47, 1994.

80. Salvini S, Hennekens CH, Morris JS et al: Plasma levels of the antioxidant selenium and risk of myocardial infarction among US physicians, Am J Cardiol 76:1218-21, 1995.

81. Kok FJ, Hofman A, Witteman JCM et al: Decreased selenium levels in acute myocardial infarction, JAMA 261:1161-64, 1989.

82. Salonen JT, Salonen R, Seppanen K et al: Interactions of serum copper, selenium, and low density lipoprotein cholesterol in atherogenesis, BMJ 302:756-60, 1991.

83. Langsjoen PH, Langsjoen AM: Overview of the use of CoQ10 in cardiovascular disease, Biofactors 9:273-84, 1999.

84. Singh RB, Wander GS, Rastogi A et al: Randomized, double-blind placebo-controlled trial of coenzyme Q10 in patients with acute myocardial infarction, Cardiov Drugs Ther 12:347-53, 1998.

84a. Berman M, Erman A, Ben-Gal T, et al: Coenzyme Q10 in patients with end-stage heart failure awaiting cardiac transplantation: a randomized, placebo-controlled study. Clin Cardiol 27:295-99, 2004.

85. Bliznakov EG, Wilkins DJ: Biochemical and clinical consequences of inhibiting coenzyme Q biosynthesis by lipid-lowering HMG-CoA reductase inhibitors (statins): a critical overview, Adv Ther 15:218-26, 1998.

85a. Albert C: Fish oil: an appetising alternative to anti-arrythmia drugs? The Lancet 363:1412-13, 2004.

86. Mori TA, Bao DQ, Burke V et al: Docosahexaenoic acid but not eicosapentaenoic acid lowers ambulatory blood pressure and heart rate in humans, Hypertension 34:253-60, 1999.

87. Kenny D, Warltier DC, Pleuss JA et al: Effect of omega-3 fatty acids on the vascular response to angiotensin in normotensive men, Am J Cardiol 70:1347-52, 1992.

88. Kestin M, Clifton P, Belling GB et al: N-3 fatty acids of marine origin lower systolic blood pressure and triglycerides but raise LDL cholesterol compared with n-3 and n-6 fatty acids from plants, Am J Clin Nutr 51:1028-34, 1990.

89. Leaf A, Jorgensen MB, Jacobs AK et al: Do fish oils prevent restenosis after coronary angioplasty? Circulation 90:2248-57, 1994.

90. Dehmer GJ, Popma JJ, van den Berg EK et al: Reduction in the rate of early restenosis after coronary angioplasty by a diet supplemented with n-3 fatty acids, N Engl J Med 319:733-40, 1988.

91. O'Keefe J, Harris W: Omega-3 fatty acids: time for clinical implementation? Am J Cardiol 85:1239-41, 2000.

92. Albert CM, Hennekens CH, O'Donnell CJ et al: Fish consumption and risk of sudden cardiac death, JAMA 279:23-28, 1998.

93. Dallongeville J, Yarnell J, Ducimetiere P et al: Fish consumption is associated with lower heart rates, Circulation 108:820-25, 2003.

94. Simopoulos AP, Leaf A, Salem N Jr et al: Workshop on the essentiality of and recommended dietary intakes for omega-6 and omega-3 fatty acids, J Am Coll Nutr 18:487-89, 1999.

95. Siani A, Pagano E, Iacone R et al: Blood pressure and metabolic changes during dietary L-arginine supplementation in humans, Am J Hypertens 13:547-51, 2000.

96. Drexler H, Zeiher AM, Meinzer K, Just H: Correction of endothelial dysfunction in coronary microcirculation of hypercholesterolemic patients by L-arginine, Lancet 338:1546-50, 1991.

97. Egashira K, Hirooka Y, Kuga T et al: Effects of L-arginine supplementation on endothelium-dependent coronary vasodilation in patients with angina pectoris and normal coronary angiograms, Circulation 94:130-34, 1996.

98. Hirooka Y, Egashira K, Imaizumi T et al: Effect of L-arginine on acetylcholine-induced endothelium-dependent vasodilation differs between the coronary and forearm vasculatures in humans, J Am Coll Cardiol 24:948-55, 1994.

99. Stewart DJ, Holtz J, Bassenge E: Long-term nitroglycerin treatment: effect on direct and endothelium-mediated large coronary artery dilation in conscious dogs, Circulation 75:847-56, 1987.

100. Candipan RC, Wang B, Buitrago R et al: Regression or progression: dependency on vascular nitric oxide, Arteriothromb Vasc Biol 16: 44-50, 1996.

101. Jeremy RW, McCarron J, Sullivan D: Effects of dietary L-arginine on atherosclerosis and endothelium-dependent vasodilation in the hypercholesterolemic rabbit: response according to treatment duration, anatomic site, and sex, Circulation 94:498-506, 1996.

102. Quyyumi A, Dakak N, Diodati J et al: Effect of L-arginine on human coronary endothelium-dependent and physiologic vasodilation, J Am Coll Cardiol 30:1220-27, 1997.

103. Lerman A, Burnett JC Jr, Higano ST et al: Long-term L-arginine supplementation improves small-vessel coronary endothelial function in humans, Circulation 97:2123-28, 1998.

104. Blum A, Hathaway L, Mincemoyer R et al: Oral L-arginine in patients with coronary artery disease on medical management, Circulation 101:2160-64, 2000.

105. Loscalzo J, Welch G: Nitric oxide and its role in the cardiovascular system, Prog Cardiovasc Dis 38:87-104, 1995.

106. Quyyumi A: Does acute improvement of endothelial dysfunction in coronary artery disease improve myocardial ischemia? a double-blind comparison of parenteral D- and L-arginine, J Am Coll Cardiol 32:904-11, 1998.

106a. Oudit GY, Trivieri MG, Khaper N, et al: Taurine supplementation reduces oxidative stress and improves cardiovascular function in an iron-overload marine model, Circulation 109: 1877-85, 2004.

107. Safi AM, Stein RA: Role of nutriceutical agents in cardiovascular diseases: an update—part I, Cardiovasc Rev Rep 24:382-85, 2003.

107a. Pasini E, Opasich C, Pastoris O, Aquilani R: Inadequate nutritional intake for daily life activity of clinically stable patients with chronic heart failure. Am J Cardiol 93 (8A):41A-43A, 2004.

107b. Scognamiglio R, Avogaro A, Negut C, et al: Early myocardial dysfunction in the diabetic heart: current research and clinical applications. Am J Cardiol 93 (8A):17A-20A, 2004.

107c. Pasini E, Scarabelli TM, D'Antona G, Dioguardi FS: Effect of amino acid mixture on the isolated ischemic heart. Am J Cardiol 93 (8A):30A-34A, 2004.

107d. Scarabelli TM, Pasini E, Stephanou A, et al: Nutritional supplementation with mixed essential amino acids enhances myocyte survival, preserving mitochondrial functional capacity during ischemia-reperfusion injury. Am J Cardiol 93 (8A):35A-40A, 2004.

108.   Gylling H, Radhakrishnan R, Miettinen TA: Reduction of serum cholesterol in post-menopausal women with previous myocardial infarction and cholesterol malabsorption induced by dietary sitostanol ester margarine, Circulation 16:4226-31, 1997.

109.   Hallikainen MA, Uusitupa MIJ: Effects of 2 low-fat stanol ester-containing margarines on serum cholesterol concentrations as part of a low-fat diet in hypercholesterolemia, Am J Clin Nutr 69:403-10, 1999.

110.   Miettinen TA, Puska P, Gylling H et al: Reduction of serum cholesterol with sitostanol-ester margarine in a mildly hypercholesterolemic population, N Engl J Med 333:1308-12, 1995.

111.   Miettinen TA, Kesaniemi YA: Cholesterol absorption: regulation of cholesterol synthesis and elimination and within-population variations of serum cholesterol levels, Am J Clin Nutr 49:629-35, 1989.

112.   von Bergmann K: Lipid-lowering drugs working in the intestine, Curr Opin Lipid 1:48, 1990.

113.   Hallikainen MA, Sarkkinen ES, Uusitupa MIJ: Plant stanol esters affect serum cholesterol concentrations of hypercholesterolemic men and women in a dose-dependent manner, J Nutr 130:767-76, 2000.

114.   Nguyen TT, Dale LC, von Bergmann K, Croghan IT: Cholesterol-lowering effect of stanol ester in a U.S. population of mildly hypercholesterolemic men and women: randomized, controlled trial, Mayo Clin Proc 74:1198-1206, 1999.

115.   Gylling H, Miettinen TA: Effects of inhibiting cholesterol absorption and synthesis on cholesterol and lipoprotein metabolism in hypercholesterolemic non–insulin-dependent diabetic men. J Lipid Res 37:1776-85, 1996.

116.   Blair SN, Capuzzi DM, Gottlieb SO et al: Incremental reduction of serum total cholesterol and low-density lipoprotein cholesterol with the addition of plant stanol ester-containing spread to statin therapy, Am J Cardiol 86:46-52, 2000.

117.   Gylling H, Siimes MA, Miettinen TA: Sitostanol ester margarine in dietary treatment of children with familial hypercholesterolemia, J Lipid Res 36:1807-12, 1995.

118.   Davignon J: Prospects for drug therapy for hyperlipoproteinemia, Diabetes Metab 21:139-46, 1995.

119.   Eastwood MA, Passmore R: Dietary fibre, Lancet 2:202-06, 1983.

120.   Chan JKC, Wypyszyk V: A forgotten natural dietary fiber: psyllium mucilloid, Cereal Foods World 33:919, 1988.

121.   Kennedy JF, Sandhu JS, Southgate DAT: Structural data for the carbohydrate of ispaghula husk (ex Plantago ovata Forsk), Carbohydr Res 75:269, 1979.

122.   Levin EG, Miller VT, Muesing RA et al: Comparison of psyllium hydrophilic mucilloid and cellulose as adjuncts to a prudent diet in the

treatment of mild to moderate hypercholesterolemia, Arch Intern Med 150:1822-27, 1990.

123. Pietinen P, Rimm EB, Korhonen P et al: Intake of dietary fiber and risk of coronary artery disease in a cohort of Finnish men: the Alpha Tocopherol, Beta-Carotene Cancer Prevention Study, Circulation 94:2720-27, 1996.

124. Chen WL, Anderson JW, Jennings D: Propionate may mediate the hypocholesterolemic effects of certain soluble plant fiber in cholesterol fed rats, Proc Soc Exp Biol Med 175:215-18, 1984.

125. Lantner RR, Espiritu BR, Zumerchik P, Tobin MC: Anaphylaxis following ingestion of a psyllium-containing cereal, JAMA 264:2534-36, 1990.

126. Behall KM, Scholfield DJ, Lee K et al: Mineral balance in adult men: effect of four refined fibers, Am J Clin Nutr 46:307-14, 1987.

127. Davidson MH, Dugan LD, Burns JH et al: The hypocholesterolemic effects of beta-glucan in oatmeal and oat bran: a dose-controlled study, JAMA 265:1833-39, 1991.

128. Lipsky H, Gloger M, Frishman WH: Dietary fiber for reducing blood cholesterol, J Clin Pharmacol 30:699-703, 1990.

129. Spence JD, Huff MW, Heidenheim P et al: Combination therapy with colestipol and psyllium mucilloid in patients with hyperlipidemia, Ann Intern Med 123:493-99, 1995.

130. Pereira MA, O'Reilly E, Augustsson K et al: Dietary fiber and risk of coronary heart disease, Arch Intern Med 164:370-76, 2004.

CHAPTER 4

Herbal Approach to Cardiac Disease*

William H. Frishman, MD

Stephen T. Sinatra, MD

Mohammed Moizuddin, MD

S ince the beginning of human civilization, herbs have been an integral part of society and have been valued for their culinary and medicinal properties. However, with the development of patent medicines in the early part of the twentieth century, herbal medicine lost ground to new synthetic medicines touted by scientists and physicians to be more effective and reliable. Nevertheless, about 3% of English-speaking adults in the United States still report having used herbal remedies in the previous year. This figure is probably higher among Americans whose first language is not English. The term *herbal medicine* refers to the use of plant structures, known as phytomedicinals or phytopharmaceuticals. Herbal medicine has become an increasing presence and area of interest to pharmacists and other healthcare professionals with the advent of the German commissioned E-monographs, which reported extensive information about the safety and efficacy of herbal preparations.

Herbal medicine has made many contributions to commercial drug preparations manufactured today, including ephedrine from *Ephedra sinica* (ma-huang), digitoxin from *Digitalis purpurea* (foxglove), salicin (the source of aspirin) from *Salix alba* (willow bark), and reserpine from Rauwolfia serpentina (snakeroot)—to name just a few.[1,2] The discovery of the antineoplastic agent paclitaxel (Taxol) from *Taxus brevifolia* (the Pacific yew tree) stresses the role of plants as a continuing resource for modern medicine.

---

*Modified from Sinatra ST, Frishman WH, Peterson SJ, Lin G: Use of alternative/complementary medicine in treating cardiovascular disease. In Frishman WH, Sonnenblick EH, Sica DA, editors: Cardiovascular Pharmacotherapeutics, ed 2, New York, 2003, McGraw Hill, 857-74.

REGULATIONS IN THE UNITED STATES

A number of laws affecting the sale and marketing of drugs exist in the United States. These include the Food and Drug Act (1906) with its Sherley amendment (1912) and the Federal Food, Drug, and Cosmetic Act (1938) with its many amendments. The amendments passed in 1962, also known as the Kefauver-Harris amendments, require that all drugs marketed in the United States be proven both safe and effective. To evaluate the safety and efficacy of drugs, the FDA turned to the Division of Medical Sciences of the National Academy of Sciences—National Research Council, which then organized a drug efficacy study based on reviews of in vitro tests and clinical trials on patients, which were usually supplied by the companies interested in marketing the drugs. At the time, very few herbs had their active ingredients isolated, and even fewer had undergone clinical trials. Hence only a small number of herbs were evaluated—and those that were tested were evaluated only for specific indications.

In 1990, the results of the FDA's study on over-the-counter (OTC) medications, which included many herbs and herbal products, were released to the public. A few plant products, such as *Plantago psyllium* (plantago seed), *Cascara sagrada* (cascara bark, *Rhamnus purshiana*), and *Cassia acutifolia* (senna leaf, *Senna alexandrina*), were judged to be "both safe and effective" (category I) for their laxative actions. However, 142 herbs and herbal products were deemed "unsafe or ineffective" (category II), and "insufficient evidence to evaluate" (category III) existed for another 116 herbs. Many herbs and herbal products in categories II and III had been grandfathered by the 1938 act and 1962 amendments because they were already covered in the 1906 act. Thus they were not subject to the requirements of proving both safety and efficacy to be out on the market. However, to deal with these grandfathered OTC products, the FDA declared that any grandfathered drug with claims of efficacy on the package or in the package insert that did not concur with the FDA's OTC study would be considered misbranded and subject to confiscation.[3]

Unfortunately for the herbal industry, complying with the new FDA regulations meant having to remove all but the names of the herbal products from their labels and marketing them as nutritional supplements or food additives. Therefore consumers who wish to obtain factual information regarding the therapeutic use or potential harm of herbal remedies would have to obtain them from books and pamphlets, most of which based their information on traditional reputation rather than existing scientific research. Another major problem is that the marketing of herbal products under their common names, which is usually the case in healthfood stores and on the internet, does not allow for proper identification because many species of herbs may share the same common name.[4] Another problem is the lack of dose standardization with herbal medicinals having active pharmacologic ingredients.[5,6] These problems will remain until herbal medicinals are recognized as the drugs that they are.[7-9a]

One may wonder why the herbal industry never chose simply to prove their products safe and effective with more in vitro tests or clinical trials. The answer is primarily economic. With the cost and time of developing a new drug estimated at $231 million over 12 years (based on a 1990 report from the Center for the Study of Drug Development at Tufts University), most members of the herbal and pharmaceutical industries shy away from such endeavors, especially with the slim chance of obtaining patent protection for the many herbs that have been in use for centuries.[3] Without financial sponsorship from pharmaceutical companies, very little financial incentive for doing research to evaluate the merits of herbal remedies exists—thus the paucity of scientific data from the United States. One step in the right direction was the decision by the NIH to allocate $2 million each for 1992 and 1993 and 2.4 million in 2000 for research to validate alternative medical practices; however, in comparison to the estimated cost of developing a single new drug, this grant allocation clearly is inadequate.

THE EFFECTS OF HERBAL REMEDIES ON THE CARDIOVASCULAR SYSTEM

The use of herbal medicine has skyrocketed over the last 5 years. Out-of-pocket therapy is estimated at more than $5 billion in the United States alone. The following review of herbal medicinals affecting the cardiovascular system is based on information gleaned from the scientific literature. These herbs are roughly categorized under the primary diseases they are used treat (Table 4-1). Note that most herbal medicinals have multiple cardiovascular effects and that the purpose of this organization is to simplify—not pigeonhole—herbs under specific diseases. In general, the dilution of active components in herbal medicinals results in fewer side effects and toxicities in comparison with the concentration

Table 4-1   SOME CONDITIONS IN WHICH HERBAL MEDICINES ARE USED AS CARDIOVASCULAR TREATMENTS

Conditions	Examples of Herbs Used
Congestive heart failure	*Digitalis purpurea*
	Digitalis lanata
	Crataegus species
	Berberine
Systolic hypertension	*Rauwolfia serpentina*
	Stephania tetrandra
	Veratrum alkaloids
Angina pectoris	*Crataegus* species
	Panax notoginseng
	Salvia miltiorrhiza
Atherosclerosis	Garlic
Cerebral insufficiency	*Ginkgo biloba*
	Rosmarinus officinalis
Venous insufficiency	*Aesculus hippocastanum*
	Ruscus aculeatus

of active components in the allopathic medicines. However, cardiovascular disease is a serious health hazard, and no one should attempt to self-medicate with herbal remedies without first consulting a physician.

CONGESTIVE HEART FAILURE

Cardiac Glycosides

A number of herbs contain potent cardioactive glycosides that have positive inotropic effects on the heart. The drugs digitoxin, derived from either *Digitalis purpurea* (foxglove) or *Digitalis lanata*, and digoxin, derived from *D. lanata* alone, have been used in the treatment of congestive heart failure (CHF) for many decades. Cardiac glycosides have a low therapeutic index, and the dose must be adjusted to the needs of each patient. The only way to control dosage is to use standardized powdered digitalis, digitoxin, or digoxin. Treating CHF with non-standardized herbal agents would be dangerous and foolhardy. Accidental poisonings due to cardiac glycosides in herbal remedies are abundant in the medical literature.[10] Some common plant sources of cardiac glycosides include: *D. purpurea* (foxglove, already mentioned), *Adonis microcarpa* and *Adonis vernalis* (Adonis), *Apocynum cannabinum* (black Indian hemp), *Asclepias curassavica* (red-headed cotton bush), *Asclepias fruticosa* (balloon cotton), *Calotropis precera* (king's crown), *Carissa acokanthera* (bushman's poison), *Carissa spectabilis* (wintersweet), *Cerbera manghas* (sea mango), *Cheiranthus cheiri* (wallflower), *Convallaria majalis* (lily of the valley, convallaria), *Cryptostegia grandiflora* (rubber vine), *Helleborus niger* (black hellebore), *Helleborus viridus*, *Nerium oleander* (oleander), *Plumeria rubra* (frangipani), *Selenicereus grandiflorus* (cactus grandiflorus), *Strophanthus hispidus* and *Strophanthus kombè* (strophanthus), *Thevetia peruviana* (yellow oleander), and *Urginea maritime* (squill). Even the venom glands of the *Bufo marinus* (cane toad) contain cardiac glycosides.[11] Health providers should be aware of the cross-reactivity of cardiac glycosides from herbal sources with the digoxin radioimmunoassay. Treatment of intoxication with these substances is directed at controlling arrhythmias and hyperkalemia, which are the usual causes of fatalities.

Berberine. Berberine is an example of an alkaloid that is distributed widely in nature and used in the Orient for the treatment of CHF. It is reported to also have antihypertensive and antiarrhythmic actions. In a recent placebo-controlled trial, patients with heart failure and significant ventricular ectopy on standard therapy received berberine 1.2 to 2.0 mg/day for up to 24 months.[12] The study found a reduction in mortality and ventricular ectopy, with an improvement in quality of life, in comparison to placebo.

HYPERTENSION

Rauwolfia Serpentina

The root of *Rauwolfia serpentina* (snakeroot), the natural source of the alkaloid reserpine, has been a Hindu Ayurvedic remedy since ancient times. In 1931, Indian literature first described the use of *R. serpentina* root for the treatment of hypertension and psychoses; however, the use of rauwolfia alkaloids in Western medicine did not begin until the mid-1940s. Both standardized whole-root preparations of *R. serpentina* and its reserpine alkaloid are officially monographed in the *United States Pharmacopeia*.[13] A 200- to 300-mg dose of powdered whole root taken orally is equivalent to 0.5 mg of reserpine.

Reserpine was one of the first drugs used on a large scale to treat systemic hypertension. It acts by irreversibly blocking the uptake of biogenic amines (norepinephrine, dopamine, and serotonin) in the storage vesicles of central and peripheral adrenergic neurons, thus leaving the catecholamines to be destroyed by the intraneuronal monoamine oxidase in the cytoplasm. The depletion of catecholamines accounts for reserpine's sympatholytic and antihypertensive actions.

Reserpine's effects are long-lasting because recovery of sympathetic function requires synthesis of new storage vesicles, which takes days to weeks. Reserpine lowers blood pressure by decreasing cardiac output, peripheral vascular resistance, heart rate, and renin secretion. With the introduction of other antihypertensive drugs with fewer central nervous system side effects, the use of reserpine has diminished. The daily oral dose of reserpine should be 0.25 mg or less—and as little as 0.05 mg if given with a diuretic. If the whole root is used, the usual adult dose is 50 to 200 mg per day administered once daily or in two divided doses.

Rauwolfia alkaloids are contraindicated for use in patients with previously demonstrated hypersensitivity to these substances, in patients with a history of mental depression (especially with suicidal tendencies) or an active peptic ulcer or ulcerative colitis, and in those receiving electroconvulsive therapy. The most common side effects are sedation and inability to concentrate and perform complex tasks. Reserpine may cause mental depression, sometimes resulting in suicide, and therefore must be discontinued at the first sign of depression. Reserpine's sympatholytic effect and its enhancement of parasympathetic actions account for its other well-described side effects: nasal congestion, increased secretion of gastric acid, and mild diarrhea.

Stephania Tetrandra

Stephania tetrandra is sometimes used in traditional Chinese medicine (TCM) to treat hypertension. Tetrandrine, an alkaloid extract of *S. tetrandra*, has been shown to be a calcium-channel antagonist that parallels the effects of verapamil. Tetrandrine inhibits T and L calcium channels, interferes with the binding of diltiazem and methoxyverapamil at calcium-associated sites, and suppresses aldosterone production.[14] A parenteral dose (15 mg/kg) of tetrandrine in conscious rats decreased mean, systolic, and diastolic blood pressures for greater than 30 minutes; however, an intravenous dose of 40 mg/kg killed the rats by myocardial depression. In stroke-prone hypertensive rats, an oral dose of 25 or 50 mg/kg produced a gradual and sustained hypotensive effect after 48 h without affecting plasma renin activity.[15] In addition to its cardiovascular actions, tetrandrine has reported antineoplastic, immunosuppressive, and mutagenic effects.[14]

Tetrandrine is 90% protein-bound with an elimination half-life ($t_{1/2}$) of 88 minutes, according to dog studies; however, rat studies have shown a sustained hypotensive effect for more than 48 hours after a 25- or 50-mg oral dose. Tetrandrine causes liver necrosis in dogs that were orally administered 40 mg/kg of tetrandrine thrice weekly for 2 months, reversible swelling of liver cells at a 20-mg/kg dose, and no observable changes at a 10-mg/kg dose. Given the evidence of hepatotoxicity, many more studies are necessary to establish a safe dosage of tetrandrine in humans.

Lingusticum Wallichii

The root of *Lingusticum wallichii* (*chuan-xiong, chuan-hsiung*) is used in TCM as a circulatory stimulant, hypotensive agent, and sedative.[16] Tetramethylpyrazine, the active constituent extracted from *L. wallichii*, inhibits platelet aggregation in vitro and lowers blood pressure by vasodilation in dogs. With its actions independent of the endothelium, tetramethylpyrazine's vasodilatory effect is mediated by calcium antagonism and nonselective antagonism of alpha adrenoceptors. Some evidence suggests that tetramethylpyrazine can selectively act on the pulmonary vasculature.[14] Current information with which to evaluate the safety and efficacy of this herbal medicinal is insufficient.

Uncaria Rhynchophylla

Uncaria rhynchophylla (*gou-teng*) is sometimes used in TCM to treat hypertension.[14] Its indole alkaloids, rhynchophylline and hirsutine, are thought to be the active principles of *U. rhynchophylla*'s vasodilatory effect. The mechanism of *U. rhynchophylla*'s actions is unclear. Some studies point to an alteration in calcium flux in response to activation, whereas others point to hirsutine's inhibition of nicotine-induced dopamine release. One in vitro study has shown that *U. rhynchophylla* extract relaxes norepinephrine-precontracted rat aorta through endothelium-dependent and -independent mechanisms. For the endothelium-dependent component, *U. rhynchophylla* extract appears to stimulate endothelium-derived relaxing factor/nitric oxide release without involving muscarinic receptors.[17] Also, in vitro and in vivo studies have shown that rhynchophylline can inhibit platelet aggregation and reduce platelet thromboses induced by collagen or adenosine diphosphate plus epinephrine.[14] The safety and efficacy of this agent cannot be evaluated at present because of the lack of clinical data.

Veratrum

Veratrum (hellebore) is a perennial herb growing in many parts of the world. Varieties include *V. viride* from Canada and the eastern United States, *V. californicum* from the western United States, *V. album* from Alaska and Europe, and *V. japonicum* from Asia. All *Veratrum* plants contain poisonous veratrum alkaloids, which are known to cause vomiting, bradycardia, and hypotension. Most cases of *Veratrum* poisonings are due to misidentification with other plants. Although once a treatment for hypertension, the use of *Veratrum* alkaloids has lost favor because of a low therapeutic index and unacceptable toxicity as well as the introduction of safer antihypertensive drug alternatives.

Veratrum alkaloids enhance nerve and muscle excitability by increasing sodium conductivity. They act on the posterior wall of the left ventricle and the coronary sinus baroreceptors, thus causing a reflex hypotension and bradycardia via the vagus nerve (Bezold-Jarisch reflex). Nausea and vomiting are secondary to the alkaloids' actions on the nodose ganglion.

The diagnosis of *Veratrum* toxicity is established by history, identification of the plant, and strong clinical suspicion. Treatment is mainly supportive and is directed at controlling bradycardia and hypotension. *Veratrum*-induced bradycardia usually responds to treatment with atropine; however, the blood pressure response to atropine is more variable and may require the addition of pressors. Electrocardiographic changes may be reversible with atropine but are sometimes not. Seizures are a rare complication and may be treated with conventional anticonvulsants. For patients with preexisting cardiac disease, the use of beta agonists or pacing may be necessary. Nausea may be controlled with phenothiazine antiemetics. Recovery is usually within 24 to 48 hours.

ANGINA PECTORIS

Crataegus

Hawthorn, a name encompassing many *Crataegus* species (such as *C. oxyacantha* and *C. monogina* in the West and *C. pinnatifida* in China), has acquired the reputation in the modern herbal literature as an important tonic for the cardiovascular system, particularly useful for angina.[18] *Crataegus* leaves, flowers, and fruits contain a number of biologically active substances such as oligomeric procyanidins, flavonoids, and catechins. From current studies, *Crataegus* extract appears to have antioxidant properties and can inhibit the formation of thromboxane A_2.[19] Also, *Crataegus* extract antagonizes the increases in cholesterol, triglycerides, and phospholipids in low-density lipoprotein (LDL) and very low-density lipoprotein (VLDL) in rats fed a hyperlipidemic diet; thus it may inhibit the progression of atherosclerosis.[20] According to one study, *Crataegus* extract in high concentrations has a cardioprotective effect on ischemic-reperfused heart without an increase in coronary blood flow.[21] On the other hand, oral and parenteral administration of oligomeric procyanins of *Crataegus* leads to an increase in coronary blood flow in cats and dogs.[22,23] Double-blind clinical trials have demonstrated simultaneous cardiotropic and vasodilatory actions of *Crataegus*.[24] In essence, *Crataegus* increases coronary perfusion, has a mild hypotensive effect, antagonizes atherosclerosis, has positive inotropic and negative chronotropic actions, and as an adjunct therapy, improves the symptoms of CHF.[25,26] A study is in progress assessing the effects of hawthorn extract on mortality as well as on quality of life and hospitalization.[27] The Survival and Prognosis Investigation of Crataegus Extract WS 1442 in Congestive Heart Failure (SPICE) trial has enrolled approximately 2300 patients to evaluate the long-term effects (24 months) of a standard preparation of hawthorn extract in comparison to placebo on hospitalization and mortality in patients with modest heart failure receiving an established medical regimen.[27] Crataegus also lowers blood pressure because of its action in lowering peripheral vascular resistance.

Animal studies have also indicated that peripheral and coronary blood flow increases while arterial blood pressure decreases.[28] Hawthorn is relatively devoid of side effects; however, concomitant use of hawthorn and digoxin can markedly enhance the activity of digitalis.[2] Therefore hawthorn and digitalis should not be given together.

Panax Notoginseng

Because of its resemblance to *Panax ginseng* (Asian ginseng), *Panax notoginseng* (*pseudoginseng; san-qui*) has acquired the common name of pseudoginseng, especially because it is often an adulterant of *P. ginseng* preparations. In TCM, the root of *P. notoginseng* is used for analgesia and hemostasis. It is also often used in the treatment of patients with angina and coronary artery disease.[16]

Although clinical trials are lacking, in vitro studies of *P. notoginseng* suggest possible cardiovascular effects. One study that used purified notoginsenoside R1, extracted from *P. notoginseng*, on human umbilical vein endothelial cells showed a dose- and time-dependent synthesis of tissue-type plasminogen activator without affecting the synthesis of plasminogen activating inhibitor, thus enhancing fibrinolytic parameters.[29]

Another study suggests that *P. notoginseng* saponins may inhibit atherogenesis by interfering with the proliferation of smooth muscle cells.[30] In vitro and in vivo studies using rats and rabbits have demonstrated that *P. notoginseng* may be useful as an antianginal agent because it dilates coronary arteries in all concentrations. The role of *P. notoginseng* in the treatment of hypertension is less certain because it causes vasodilation or vasoconstriction, depending on concentration and the target vessel. The results of these in vitro and in vivo studies are encouraging; however, clinical trials will be necessary to enable more informed decisions regarding the use of *P. notoginseng*. The most common side-effects reported with ginseng were insomnia, diarrhea, and skin reactions.

Salvia Miltiorrhiza

Salvia miltiorrhiza (*dan-shen*), a relative of the Western sage *S. officinalis*, is native to China. In TCM, the root of *S. miltiorrhiza* is used as a circulatory stimulant, sedative, and cooling agent.[16] *S. miltiorrhiza* may be useful as an antianginal agent because, like *P. notoginseng*, it has been shown to dilate coronary arteries in all concentrations. Also, *S. miltiorrhiza* has variable action on other vessels, depending on its concentration, so it may not be as helpful in treating hypertension. In vitro, *S. miltiorrhiza*, in a dose-dependent fashion, inhibits platelet aggregation and serotonin release induced by either adenosine diphosphate or epinephrine, which is thought to be mediated by an increase in platelet cyclic adenosine monophosphate caused by *S. miltiorrhiz*'s inhibition of cAMP phosphodiesterase. *S. miltiorrhiza* appears to have a protective effect on ischemic myocardium, enhancing the recovery of contractile force upon reoxygenation. Qualitatively and quantitatively, a decoction of *S. miltiorrhiza* was as efficacious as the more expensive isolated tanshinones.[29] Clinical trials will be necessary to further evaluate the safety and efficacy of *S. miltiorrhiza*.

ATHEROSCLEROSIS

Allium Sativum

In addition to its use in the culinary arts, *Allium sativum* (garlic) has been valued for centuries in many cultures for its medicinal properties. In recent decades, animal and human data have focused on garlic's use in treating atherosclerosis and hypertension.[31] A number of studies have demonstrated its effects, which include lowering blood pressure, reducing serum cholesterol and triglycerides, enhancing fibrinolytic activity, and inhibiting platelet aggregation. However, some investigators have been hesitant to endorse the routine use of garlic for cardiovascular disease outright despite positive evidence because many of the published studies had methodologic shortcomings.[31-33] For example, in one of the largest collective reviews of randomized controlled trials of garlic lasting 4 weeks or longer, the researchers concluded that the effects of garlic treatment are tainted by an inadequate definition of active constituents in the study preparations.[31] The pharmacologic properties of garlic are extremely complex and comprise a variety of sulfur-containing compounds that include allicin, alliin, diallyl disulfide, ajoene, s-allylcysteines, and gamma-glutamylpeptides, to mention a few. Many of the previous controlled trials of garlic used different preparations containing all or some of these active pharmacologic factors. This may be the major reason for the variability and confusion found in the research.[31] The definition and delineation of the major active garlic ingredients and their specific mechanisms of action are absolutely necessary before future trials are planned and conducted.

Intact cells of garlic bulbs contain an odorless, sulfur-containing amino acid derivative known as *alliin*. When garlic is crushed, alliin comes into contact with alliinase, which converts alliin to allicin. Allicin has potent antibacterial properties but is also highly odoriferous and unstable. Ajoenes, self-condensation products of allicin, appear to be responsible for garlic's antithrombotic activity. Most authorities now agree that allicin and its derivatives are the active constituents of garlic's physiologic activity. Fresh garlic releases allicin in the mouth during the chewing process. Dried garlic preparations lack allicin but do contain alliin and alliinase. Because alliinase is inactivated by acids in the stomach, dried garlic preparations should be enteric-coated so that they pass through the stomach into the small intestine, where alliin can be enzymatically converted to allicin. Few commercial garlic preparations are standardized for their allicin yield based on alliin content, thus making their effectiveness less certain.[3] However, one double-blind, placebo-controlled study involving 261 patients over 4 months and using one 800-mg tablet of garlic powder daily, standardized to 1.3 % alliin content, demonstrated significant reductions in total cholesterol (12%) and triglycerides (17%).[34] In studies that use garlic supplements containing either no allicin or poorly bioavailable allicin, no lipid lowering was realized. Consumption of large quantities of fresh garlic (0.25 to 1 g/kg body weight or about 5 to 20 average-size 4-g cloves in a 175 lb person) does appear to produce beneficial effects. However, in a meta-analysis, garlic, in an amount approximating one-half to one clove per day, was demonstrated to decrease total serum cholesterol by about 9% in the patients studied.[35] The allicin yield of each 800-mg garlic tablet is equivalent to 2.8 g of fresh garlic—less than one average-size 4-g clove; in other words, therapeutic effectiveness may be seen in doses much lower than five cloves of garlic.[3] In 11 large databases collected from January 1966 through February 2000, various garlic preparations did suggest small reductions in total cholesterol, LDL, and triglyceride, but no statistically significant changes were noted in high-density lipoproteins (HDL). Significant reductions in platelet aggregation and insignificant effects on blood pressure outcomes were also observed.[31]

Aside from a garlic odor on the breath and body, moderate garlic consumption causes few adverse effects. Consumption in excess of five cloves daily may result in heartburn, flatulence, and other GI disturbances. Case reports have also described bleeding in patients who ingested large doses of garlic (average of four cloves per day). Because of its antithrombotic activity, garlic should also be used with caution in people taking oral anticoagulants.[3] Some individuals have also reported allergic reactions to garlic.

CEREBRAL AND PERIPHERAL ARTERIAL DISEASE

Ginkgo Biloba

Dating back well over 200 million years, *Ginkgo biloba* (maidenhair tree) was apparently saved from extinction by human intervention, surviving in Far Eastern temple gardens while disappearing for centuries in the West. It was reintroduced to Europe in 1730 and became a favorite ornamental tree.[16] Although the root and kernels of *G. biloba* have long been used in TCM, *Ginkgo* gained attention in the West during the twentieth century for its medicinal value after a concentrated extract of *G. biloba* leaves was developed in the 1960s. At least two groups of substances within *G. biloba* extract demonstrated beneficial pharmacologic actions. The flavonoids reduce capillary permeability and fragility and serve as free-radical scavengers. The terpenes (i.e., ginkgolides) inhibit platelet-activating factor, decrease vascular resistance, and improve circulatory flow without appreciably affecting blood pressure. Continuing research appears to support the primary use of *G. biloba* extract for treating cerebral insufficiency and its secondary effects on vertigo, tinnitus, memory, and mood. In a study evaluating 327 demented patients,[36] 120 mg of *G. biloba* extract produced improvements in dementia, similar to other studies with donepezil and tacrine. However, a more recent study showed no benefit of *G. biloba* on cognitive functioning.[37] In addition, *G. biloba* extract appears to be useful for treating peripheral vascular disease, including intermittent claudication and diabetic retinopathy.[3,38] A meta-analysis of eight randomized placebo-controlled trials of *G. biloba* for intermittent claudication showed a mean improvement in pain-free walking distance of 34 meters. Maximal walking distance improved by 35 to 189 meters.[39]

Although approved as a drug in Europe, *Ginkgo* is not approved in the United States and is instead marketed as a food supplement, usually supplied as 40-mg tablets of extract. Because most investigations of the efficacy of *G. biloba* extracts used preparations such as EGb 761 or LI 1370, the bioequivalence of other *G. biloba* extract products has not been established. The recommended dose in Europe is one 40-mg tablet taken three times daily with meals (120 mg daily).[3] Adverse effects of *G. biloba* extract are rare but can include GI disturbances, headache, and skin rash. Several case reports of bleeding, including subarachnoid hemorrhage, intracranial hemorrhage, and subdural hematoma have been associated with *G. biloba*.[40-42] *G. biloba* should not be used in combination with analgesic agents such as aspirin, ticlopidine, and clopidogrel or anticoagulants such as warfarin and heparin because those agents undermine the effect of the platelet-inhibiting factor.[43]

Rosmarinus Officinalis

Known mostly as a culinary spice and flavoring agent, *Rosmarinus officinalis* (rosemary) is listed in many herbal sources as a tonic and all-around stimulant. Traditionally, rosemary leaves are said to enhance circulation, aid digestion, elevate mood, and boost energy. When applied externally, the volatile oils are supposedly useful for arthritic conditions and baldness.[3]

Although research on rosemary is scanty, some studies have focused on antioxidant effects of diterpenoids, especially carnosic acid and carnosol, isolated from rosemary leaves. In addition to having antineoplastic effects (especially skin), antioxidants in rosemary have been credited with stabilizing erythrocyte membranes and inhibiting superoxide generation and lipid peroxidation.[44,45] Essential oils of rosemary have demonstrated antimicrobial, hyperglycemic, and insulin-inhibiting properties.[46,47] Rosemary leaves contain high amounts of salicylates, and its flavonoid pigment diosmin is reported to decrease capillary permeability and fragility.[48]

Despite the conclusions derived from in vitro and animal studies, the therapeutic use of rosemary for cardiovascular disorders remains questionable, as few if any clinical trials have been conducted using rosemary. Because of the lack of studies, no conclusions can be reached regarding the use of the antioxidants of rosemary in inhibiting atherosclerosis. Although external application may cause cutaneous vasodilatation from the counterirritant properties of rosemary's essential oils, no evidence supports any prolonged improvement in peripheral circulation.[3,48] Although rosemary does have some carminative properties, it may also cause GI and kidney disturbances in large doses. Until more studies are done, rosemary should probably be limited to its use as a culinary spice and flavoring agent rather than as a medicine.

Venous Insufficiency

Aesculus Hippocastanum

The seeds of *Aesculus hippocastanum* (horse chestnut) have long been used in Europe to treat venous disorders such as varicose veins. The medicinal qualities of horse chestnut reside mostly in its large seeds, which resemble edible chestnuts. The seeds contain a complex mixture of saponins, glycosides, and several other active ingredients. The grouping of most interest is called aesculic acid or aescin. In addition to a high level of flavonoids, horse chestnuts contain several minerals including magnesium, manganese, cobalt, and iodine.

The saponin glycoside aescin from horse chestnut extract (HCE) inhibits the activity of lysosomal enzymes, which are thought to contribute to varicose veins by weakening vessel walls and increasing permeability, resulting in dilated veins and edema. In animal studies, HCE, in a dose-dependent fashion, increases venous tone, venous flow, and lymphatic flow. HCE also antagonizes capillary hyperpermeability induced by histamine, serotonin, or chloroform. HCE decreases edema formation of lymphatic and inflammatory origin. HCE has antiexudative properties that suppress experimentally induced pleurisy and peritonitis by inhibiting plasma extravasation and leukocyte emigration. HCE's dose-dependent antioxidant properties can inhibit in vitro lipid peroxidation. Randomized double-blind, placebo-controlled trials using HCE show a statistically significant reduction in edema, as measured by plethysmography.[49] Although still controversial, prophylactic use of HCE does not appear to decrease the incidence of thromboembolic complications of gynecologic surgery.

Standardized HCE is prepared as an aqueous-alcohol extract of 16% to 21% of triterpene glycosides, calculated as aescin. The usual initial dose is 90 to 150 mg of aescin daily, which may be reduced to 35 to 70 mg daily after improvement.[3] Standardized HCE preparations are not available in the United States, but nonstandardized products may be available.

Some manufacturers promote the use of topical preparations of HCE for treatment of varicose veins as well as hemorrhoids; however, at least one study has demonstrated very poor aescin distribution at sites other than the skin and muscle tissues underlying the application site.[50] Moreover, the involvement of arterioles and veins in the pathophysiology of hemorrhoids makes the effectiveness of HCE doubtful because HCE has no known effects on the arterial circulation. For now, research studies have yet to confirm any clinical effectiveness of topical HCE preparations.

Although side effects are uncommon, HCE may cause GI irritation and facial rash. Parenteral aescin has produced isolated cases of anaphylactic reactions as well as hepatic and renal toxicity.[3] In the event of toxicity, aescin is completely dialyzable, with elimination dependent on protein binding.

Ruscus Aculeatus

Like *A. hippocastanum*, *Ruscus aculeatus* (butcher's broom) is known for its use in treating venous insufficiency. *R. aculeatus* is a short evergreen shrub found commonly in the Mediterranean region. Two steroidal saponins, ruscogenin and neurogenin, extracted from the rhizomes of *R. aculeatus* are thought to be its active components.[48] In vivo studies on hamster cheek pouch reveal that topical *Ruscus* extract dose-dependently antagonizes a histamine-induced increase in vascular permeability.[51] Moreover, topical *Ruscus* extract causes dose-dependent constriction on venules without appreciably affecting arterioles.[52] Topical *Ruscus* extract's vascular effects are also temperature-dependent and appear to counter the sympathetic nervous system's temperature-sensitive vascular regulation: Venules dilate at a lower temperature (25°C), constrict at near-physiologic temperature (36.5°C) and further constrict at a higher temperature (40°C); arterioles dilate at 25°C, are unaffected at 36.5°C, and remain unaffected or constricted at 40°C, depending on *Ruscus* concentration.[53] Based on the influence of prazosin, diltiazem, and rauwolscine, the peripheral vascular effects of *Ruscus* extract appear to be selectively mediated by effects on calcium channels and alpha-adrenergic receptors.

Several small clinical trials using topical *Ruscus* extract support its role in treating venous insufficiency. One randomized double-blind, placebo-controlled trial of 18 volunteers showed a statistically significant decrease in femoral vein diameter (median decrease of 1.25 mm) using duplex B-scan ultrasonography 2.5 h after applying 4 to 6 g of a cream containing 64 to 96 mg of *Ruscus* extract.[54] Another small trial (n = 18) showed that topical *Ruscus* extract may be helpful in reducing venous dilatation during pregnancy.[55] Oral agents may be as useful as topical agents for venous insufficiency, although the evidence is less convincing.

Although capsule, tablet, ointment, and suppository (for hemorrhoids) preparations of *Ruscus* extract are available in Europe, only capsules are available in the United States. These capsules contain 75 mg of *Ruscus* extract and 2 mg of rosemary oil.[48] Aside from occasional nausea and gastritis, side effects from using *R. aculeatus* have rarely been reported, even at high doses. Nevertheless, one should be wary of any drug that has not been thoroughly tested. Although ample evidence supports the pharmacologic activity of *R. aculeatus*, a relative deficiency of clinical data to establish its actual safety and efficacy remains. Until more studies are completed, no recommendations regarding dosage can be offered.

OTHER HERBS WITH ADVERSE CARDIOVASCULAR EFFECTS

For the following noncardiovascular herbs, only cardiovascular actions are emphasized (Table 4-2).

Table 4-2   ADVERSE CARDIOVASCULAR REACTIONS OBSERVED WITH HERBAL MEDICINES USED FOR OTHER INDICATIONS

Examples	Herbal Medicines
Hypertension	*Tussilago farfara*
	Ephedra sinica
Hypotension	*Aconitum* species
Digitalis toxicity	Over 20 herbal substances with activity to digitalis radioimmunoassay
Bradycardia	*Aconitum* species
	Jin-bu-huan

TUSSILAGO FARFARA

Tussilago farfara (coltsfoot, *kuan-dong-hua*) is a perennial herb that is grown in many parts of northern China, Europe, Africa, Siberia, and North America. Over the years, *T. farfara* has acquired a reputation as a demulcent antitussive agent because of a throat-soothing mucilage within the herb. Recently, the use of *T. farfara* has lost favor because several studies found senkirkine, a pyrrolizidine alkaloid known to cause hepatotoxicity, in all parts of the herb. In addition, rats fed a diet containing *T. farfara* had a high risk of developing hemangioendothelial sarcoma of the liver.[48]

A diterpene isolated from *T. farfara*, named tussilagone, is shown to be a potent respiratory and cardiovascular stimulant. Administered intravenously, tussilagone produces a dose-dependent increase in the peripheral vascular resistance of dogs, cats, and rats without much effect on ventricular inotropy and chronotropy. The LD_{50} in mice with an acute intravenous administration of tussilagone is 28.9 mg/kg.[56]

EPHEDRA SINICA

Ephedra sinica (joint fir, *ma-huang*), the natural source of the alkaloid ephedrine, has been used in TCM for over 5000 years as an antiasthmatic and decongestant. *Ephedra* has gained recent notoriety stemming from several fatalities of youths and professional athletes who took an excess of *Ephedra*, which is promoted by some as a "legal high," weight-loss aid, energy booster, and aphrodisiac.[57-62] In a review of 140 adverse case reports submitted to the FDA between 1997 and 1999, *Ephedra* alkaloids in dietary supplements caused 10 deaths and 13 permanent disabilities. Most of these fatal events were cardiovascular (e.g., cardiac arrest, arrhythmia) or neurologic (e.g., stroke, seizure). Based on this and other experiences, the FDA has banned *ephedra* as of Spring 2004—a use of their powers from the 1994 Dietary Supplement Health & Education Act. Unlike drugs that must be proven safe and effective to be marketed, herbal supplements such as *ephedra* must only be proven unsafe to get them off the market.

Ephedrine acts by releasing stored catecholamines from synaptic neurons and nonselectively stimulates alpha- and beta-adrenergic receptors. Ephedrine increases mean, systolic, and diastolic blood pressures by vasoconstriction and cardiac stimulation. Ephedrine's bronchodilating actions may be helpful for the chronic treatment of asthma. Ephedrine enhances the contractility of skeletal muscle. It penetrates the central nervous system and can produce nervousness, excitability, and insomnia. Patients taking monoamine oxidase inhibitors or guanethidine should not be receiving any product containing ephedrine alkaloids. Patients with preexisting coronary artery disease, hypertension, and severe glaucoma should also avoid ephedrine alkaloids.[48]

Commercially synthesized ephedrine in the United States is identical with the alkaloid derived from *Ephedra*. Oral preparations of ephedrine sulfate are supplied as capsules and syrups. The usual adult dose is 25 to 50 mg every 6 hours; for children, the dose is 3 mg/kg every 24 hours in four divided doses.

ACONITUM

The roots of *Aconitum* species, such as *A. kusnezoffii* (cao-wu) and *A. carmichaeli* (chuan-wa), are sometimes used in TCM to treat rheumatism, arthritis, bruises, and fractures. In Europe, *A. napellus* (monkshood, wolfsbane) grows in the wild and is sometime cultivated as an ornamental.[63]

Plant parts of *Aconitum* species contain diterpenoid ester alkaloids, including aconitine, which have been linked to several deaths in Hong Kong and Australia. Death usually results from cardiovascular collapse and ventricular tachyarrhythmias induced by aconite alkaloids. These alkaloids activate sodium channels and cause widespread membrane excitation in cardiac, neural, and muscular tissues. Characteristic manifestations of aconite intoxication include nausea, vomiting, diarrhea, hypersalivation, and generalized paresthesias (especially circumoral numbness). Muscarinic activation may cause hypotension and bradyarrhythmias. Transmembrane enhancement of sodium flux during the plateau phase prolongs repolarization and induces after depolarizations and triggered automaticity in cardiac myocytes. Aconite-induced cardiac arrhythmias can also lead to cardiac failure in as little as 5 minutes to as long as 4 days.

Management of aconite intoxication consists of symptomatic relief because no specific antidote exists. Amiodarone and flecainide may be used as antiarrhythmic agents. Intragastric charcoal can decrease alkaloid absorption. A fatal dose can be as little as 5 mL of aconite tincture, 2 mg of pure aconite, or 1 g of plant. Considering their low therapeutic index and unacceptable toxicity, *Aconitum* and its products are not recommended even in therapeutic doses because an erroneous dose can be fatal.

JIN-BU-HUAN

Often misidentified as a derivative of *Polygala chinensis*, jin-bu-huan is most likely derived from the *Stephania* genus. This herbal remedy contains an active alkaloid known as levotetrahydropalmatine, which is a potent neuroactive substance that produces sedation, naloxone-resistant analgesia, and dopamine-receptor antagonism in animals. Jin-bu-huan is used as an analgesic, sedative, hypnotic, and antispasmodic agent as well as a dietary supplement. It is associated with significant cardiorespiratory toxicity, including respiratory failure and bradycardia that requires endotracheal intubation. No specific antidote for the treatment of acute jin-bu-huan overdose exists. Several cases of hepatitis have also been associated with long-term ingestion of jin-bu-huan. Although it is now banned in the United States, jin-bu-huan is still being imported illegally as jin-bu-huan anodyne tablets.[64]

DRUG-HERBAL INTERACTIONS

Increases in the use of alternative medicine in the United States have made information about potential drug-herb interactions very important, especially for medications with a narrow therapeutic index, such as warfarin and digoxin.[65] Suspected drug-herbal interactions should be reported by clinicians to the FDA's Med Watch Program. The FDA has established the Special Nutritionals Adverse Event Monitoring System, a computer database that includes information about suspected adverse effects related to dietary supplements as nutritional products.

Commonly, used herbs that can interact with warfarin are listed in Box 4-1. Evidence also suggests that the herb St. John's wort (*Hypericum perforatum*) acts as an inducer of the cytochrome p450 3A4 enzyme.[66,66a] Cardiovascular drugs such as amiodarone, amlodipine, diltiazem, felodipine, lidocaine, losartan, lovastatin, nifedipine, propafenone, simvastatin, and verapamil are substrates of the enzyme. Patients who receive any of these medications along with St. John's wort would be at risk for exacerbation of an arrhythmia, angina pectoris, or hypertension.[67]

Some herbal remedies (e.g., cola, ginger, licorice) have pharmacodynamic interactions with antihypertensive drugs that will counteract their hypotensive effects. Ginseng has been shown to increase digoxin levels. St. John's wort can reduce digoxin levels.[67a]

CONCLUSION

With the widespread use of alternative medicine in the United States, health practitioners should remember to ask about alternative health practices when they take clinical histories and should stay informed regarding the beneficial or harmful effects of these treatments. Continuing research is elucidating the pharmacologic activities of many alternative medicines and may stimulate future pharmaceutical development; however, such research is lacking in the United States and will require grant support from government agencies.[68-71] Legal surveillance of alternative medicine practices with low safety margins should be

---

Box 4-1   Potential and Documented Interactions of Herbs With Warfarin

Potential Increase in Risk of Bleeding
- Chamomile
- Feverfew
- Garlic
- Ginger
- Ginkgo
- Horse chestnut
- Licorice root

Documented Reports of Possible Decrease in Warfarin's Effects
- Ginseng
- Green tea

instituted for the sake of public health.[72] As more information becomes available regarding the safety and efficacy of alternative medicines, research-supported claims may one day appear on the labels of alternative medicinals.

The integration of proven complementary therapies with conventional treatments in heart disease will allow cardiologists to offer many additional options to their patients.[73] An open mind and a willingness to support conventional methodology while investigating alternatives can improve quality of life and reduce human suffering. Choosing from among the best conventional and complementary options is the only logical and ethical thing to do.

REFERENCES

1. Goldman P: Herbal medicines today and the roots of modern pharmacology, Ann Intern Med 135:594-600, 2001.
2. Sinatra ST, Frishman WH, Peterson SJ, Lin G: Use of alternative/complementary medicine in treating cardiovascular disease. In Frishman WH, Sonnenblick EH, Sica DA, editors: Cardiovascular Pharmacotherapeutics, ed 2, New York, 2003, McGraw Hill, 857-74.
3. Tyler VE: Herbs of choice. In Tyler VE (editor): The Therapeutic Use of Phytomedicinals, New York, 1994, Pharmaceutical Product Press.
4. Morris CA, Avorn J: Internet marketing of herbal products, JAMA 290:1505-09, 2003.
5. Garrard J, Harms S, Eberly LE, Matiak A: Variations in product choices of frequently purchased herbs: *caveat emptor*, Arch Intern Med 163: 2290-95, 2003.
6. Straus SE: Herbal medicines: what's in the bottle? N Engl J Med 347:1997-98, 2002.
7. DeSmet PAGM: Herbal remedies, N Engl J Med 347:2046-56, 2002.
8. Marcus DM, Grollman AP: Botanical medicines: the need for new regulations, N Engl J Med 347:2073-75, 2002.
9. Ang-Lee MK, Moss J, Yuan C-S: Herbal medicines and perioperative care, JAMA 286:208-16, 2001.
9a. DeSmet PAGM: Health risks of herbal remedies: an update, Clin Pharmacol Ther 76:1-17, 2004.
10. Slifman NR, Obermeyer WR, Musser SM et al: Contamination of botanical dietary supplements by *Digitalis lanata*, N Engl J Med 339:806-11, 1998.
11. Radford DJ, Gillies AD, Hinds JA et al: Naturally occurring cardiac glycosides, Med J Aust 144:540, 1986.
12. Zeng X-H, Zeng X-J, Li Y-Y: Efficacy and safety of berberine for congestive heart failure secondary to ischemic or idiopathic dilated cardiomyopathy, Am J Cardiol 92:173-76, 2003.
13. Rauwolfia alkaloids. In USP DI, Vol I: Drug Information for the Health Care Professional, ed 16, Rockville, Md, 1996, United States Pharmacopeial Convention.
14. Sutter MC, Wang YX: Recent cardiovascular drugs from Chinese medicinal plants, Cardiovasc Res 27:1891-1901, 1993.

15. Kawashima K, Hayakawa T, Miwa Y et al: Structure and hypotensive activity relationships of tetrandrine derivatives in stroke-prone spontaneously hypertensive rats, Gen Pharmacol 21:343-47, 1990.

16. Physicians' Desk Reference for Nonprescription Drugs and Dietary Supplements, ed 25. Monvale, NJ 2004, Thomson PDR.

17. Kuramochi T, Chu J, Suga T: *Gou-teng* (from Uncaria rhynchophylla Miquel) induced endothelium-dependent and independent relaxations in the isolated rat aorta, Life Sci 54:2061-69, 1994.

18. Chang Q, Zuo Z, Harrison F, Chow MSS: Hawthorn, J Clin Pharmacol 42: 605-12, 2002.

19. Vibes J, Lasserre B, Gleye J et al: Inhibition of thromboxane A2 biosynthesis in vitro by the main components of Crataegus oxyacantha (hawthorn) flower heads, Prostaglandins Leukot Essent Fatty Acids 50:173-75, 1994.

20. Shanthi S, Parasakthy K, Deepalakshmi PD et al: Hypolipidemic activity of tincture of Crataegus in rats, Indian J Biochem Biophys 31:143-46, 1994.

21. Nasa Y, Hashizume H, Hoque AN et al: Protective effect of Crataegus extract on the cardiac mechanical dysfunction in isolated perfused working rat heart [German], *Arzneimittelforschung* 43:945-49, 1993.

22. Roddewig C, Hensel H: Reaction of local myocardial blood flow in nonanesthetized dogs and anesthetized cats to the oral and parenteral administration of a Crataegus fraction (oligomere procyanidines) [German], *Arzneimittelforschung* 27:1407-10, 1977.

23. Taskov M: On the coronary and cardiotonic action of crataemon, Acta Physiol Pharmacol Bulg 3:53-57, 1977.

24. Blesken R: Crataegus in cardiology [German], *Fortschr Med* 110:290-92, 1992.

25. Baughman KL, Bradley DJ: Hawthorn extract: is it time to turn over a new leaf? Am J Med 114:700-01, 2003.

26. Pittler MH, Schmidt K, Ernst E: Hawthorn extract for treating chronic heart failure: meta-analysis of randomized trials, Am J Med 114:665-74, 2003.

27. Holubarsch CJ, Colucci WS, Meinertz T et al: Survival and prognosis: investigation of *Crataegus* extract WS 1442 in congestive heart failure (SPICE)—rationale, study design, and study protocol, Eur J Heart Fail 2:431-37, 2000.

28. Schussler M, Holzl J, Fricke U: Myocardial effects of flavonoids from *Crataegus* species, Arzneim Forsch 45:842-45, 1995.

29. Zhang W, Wojta J, Binder BR: Effect of notoginsenoside R1 on the synthesis of tissue-type plasminogen activator and plasminogen activator inhibitor-1 in cultured human umbilical vein endothelial cells, Arterioscler Thromb 14:1040-46, 1994.

30. Lin SG, Zheng XL, Chen QY et al: Effect of Panax notoginseng saponins on increased proliferation of cultured aortic smooth muscle cells stimulated by hypercholesterolemic serum, *Chung Kuo Yao Li Hsueh Pao* 14:314-16, 1993.

31. Ackermann RT, Mulrow CD, Ramirez G et al: Garlic shows promise for improving some cardiovascular risk factors. Arch Intern Med 161:813-24, 2001.

32. Silagy CA, Neil HA: A meta-analysis of the effect of garlic on blood pressure, J Hypertens 12:463-68, 1994.

33. Silagy C, Neil A: Garlic as a lipid lowering agent: a meta-analysis, JR Coll Physicians Lond 28:39-45, 1994.

34. Mader FH: Treatment of hyperlipidaemia with garlic-powder tablets: evidence from the German Association of General Practitioners multicentric placebo-controlled, double-blind study. Arzneimittelforschung 40:1111-16, 1990.

35. Warshafsky S, Kamer R, Sivak S: Effect of garlic on total serum cholesterol, Ann Intern Med 119:599-605, 1993.

36. Stevermer JJ, Lindbloom EJ: Ginkgo biloba for dementia, J Fam Pract 46:20, 1998.

37. Solomon PR, Adams F, Silver A et al: Ginkgo for memory enhancement: a randomized controlled trial, JAMA 288:835-40, 2002.

38. Ernst E: The risk-benefit profile of commonly used herbal therapies: Ginkgo, St. John's wort, ginseng, echinacea, saw palmetto, and kava, Ann Intern Med 136:42-53, 2002.

39. Pittler MH, Ernst E: Ginkgo biloba extract for the treatment of intermittent claudication: a meta-analysis of randomized trials, Am J Med 108:276-81, 2000.

40. Vale S: Subarachnoid haemorrhage associated with Ginkgo biloba, Lancet 352:36, 1998.

41. Matthews MK: Association of Ginkgo biloba with intracerebral hemorrhage, Neurology 50:1933-34, 1998.

42. Rowin J, Lewis SL: Spontaneous bilateral subdural hematomas associated with chronic Ginkgo biloba ingestion, Neurology 46:1775-76, 1996.

43. Gianni L, Dreitlein WB: Some popular OTC herbals can interact with anticoagulant therapy, US Pharm 23:80, 1998.

44. Offord EA, Mace K, Ruffieux C et al: Rosemary components inhibit benzo(a)pyrene-induced genotoxicity in human bronchial cells, Carcinogenesis 16:2057-2062, 1995.

45. Haraguchi H, Saito T, Okamura N et al: Inhibition of lipid peroxidation and superoxide generation by diterpenoids from *Rosmarinus officinalis*, Planta Med 61:333-36, 1995.

46. Larrondo JV, Agut M, Calvo-Torras MA: Antimicrobial activity of essences from labiates, Microbios 82:171-72, 1995.

47. al-Hader AA, Hasan ZA, Aqel MB: Hyperglycemic and insulin release inhibiting effects of Rosmarinus officinalis, J Ethnopharmacol 43:217-21, 1994.

48. Tyler VE: The honest herbal: a sensible guide to the use of herbs and related remedies, ed 3, New York, 1993, Pharmaceutical Product Press.

49. Diehm C, Vollbrecht D, Amendt K et al: Medical edema protection—clinical benefit in patients with chronic deep vein incompetence: a placebo-controlled double-blind study, Vasa 21:188-92, 1992.
50. Lang W: Studies on the percutaneous absorption of 3H-aescin in pigs, Res Exp Med 169:175-87, 1977.
51. Bouskela E, Cyrino FZ, Marcelon G: Possible mechanisms for the inhibitory effect of *Ruscus* extract on increased microvascular permeability induced by histamine in hamster cheek pouch, J Cardiovasc Pharmacol 24:281-85, 1994.
52. Bouskela E, Cyrino FZ, Marcelon G: Possible mechanisms for the venular constriction elicited by *Ruscus* extract on hamster cheek pouch, J Cardiovasc Pharmacol 24:165-80, 1994.
53. Bouskela E, Cyrino FZ, Marcelon G: Effects of *Ruscus* extract on the internal diameter of arterioles and venules of the hamster cheek pouch microcirculation, J Cardiovasc Pharmacol 22:221-24, 1993.
54. Berg D: Venous constriction by local administration of ruscus extract [German]. Fortschr Med 108:473-76, 1990.
55. Berg D: Venous tonicity in pregnancy varicose veins [German]. Fortschr Med 110:67, 71, 1992.
56. Li YP, Wang YM: Evaluation of tussilagone: a cardiovascular respiratory stimulant isolated from Chinese herbal medicine, Gen Pharmacol 19:261-63, 1988.
57. Shekelle PG, Hardy ML, Morton SC et al: Efficacy and safety of ephedra and ephedrine for weight loss and athletic performance: a meta-analysis, JAMA 289:1537-45, 2003.
58. Fontanarosa PB, Rennie D, DeAngelis CD: The need for regulation of dietary supplements: lessons from ephedra [editorial], JAMA 289:1568-70, 2003.
59. Samenuk D, Link MS, Homoud MK et al: Adverse cardiovascular events temporally associated with *ma huang*, an herbal source of ephedrine, Mayo Clin Proc 77:12-16, 2002.
60. Commentary: American Society for Clinical Pharmacology and Therapeutics position statement on the public health risks of ephedra, Clin Pharmacol Ther 74:403-05, 2003.
61. Gardner SF, Franks AM, Gurley BJ et al: Effect of a multicomponent, ephedra-containing dietary supplement (Metabolife 356) on Holter monitoring and hemostatic parameters in healthy volunteers, Am J Cardiol 91:1510-13, 2003.
62. Bent S, Tiedt TN, Odden MC, Shlipak MG: The relative safety of ephedra compared with other herbal products, Ann Intern Med 138:468-71, 2003.
63. Chan TYK, Chan JCN, Tomlinson B et al: Chinese herbal medicines revisited: the Hong Kong perspective, Lancet 342:1532-34, 1993.
64. Horowitz RS, Feldhaus K, Dart RC et al: The clinical spectrum of *Jin Bu Huan* toxicity, Arch Intern Med 156:899-903, 1996.

65.   Izzo AA, Ernst E: Interactions between herbal medicines and prescribed drugs, Drugs 61:2163-75, 2001.

66.   Wang Z, Gorski C, Hamman MA et al: The effects of St. John's wort (*Hypericum perforatum*) on human cytochrome P450 activity, Clin Pharmacol Ther 70:317-26, 2001.

66a. Tannergran C, Engman H, Knutson L, et al: St John's wort decreases the bioavailability of R- and S-verapamil through induction of first-pass metabolism, Clin Pharmacol Ther 75:298-309, 2004.

67.   Ernst E: The risk-benefit profile of commonly used herbal therapies: ginkgo, St. John's wort, ginseng, Echinacea, saw palmetto and kava, Ann Intern Med 136:42-53, 2002.

67a. Mueller SC, Uehleke B, Woehling H, et al: Effect of St John's wort dose and preparations on the pharmacokinetics of digoxin, Clin Pharmacol Ther 75:546-57, 2004.

68.   Knipschild P: Alternative treatments: do they work? Lancet 356:S4, 2000.

69.   Lin MC, Nahin R, Gershwin E et al: State of complementary and alternative medicine in cardiovascular, lung, and blood research: executive summary of a workshop, Circulation 103:2038-41, 2001.

70.   Vandenbroucke JP, de Craen AJM: Alternative medicine: a "mirror image" for scientific reasoning in conventional medicine, Ann Intern Med 135:507-13, 2001.

71.   Bent S, Ko R: Commonly used herbal medicines in the United States: a review. Am J Med 116:478-85, 2004.

72.   Stein CM: Are herbal products dietary supplements or drugs?: an important question for public safety, Clin Pharmacol Therap 71:411-13, 2002.

73.   Stys T, Stys A, Kelly P, Lawson W: Trends in use of herbal and nutritional supplements in cardiovascular patients. Clin Cardiol 27: 87-90, 2004.

PART III

Mind-Body
Approaches

CHAPTER 5

Mind-Body Approach To Cardiac Illness

James G. Grattan, MD

Cardiovascular disease is the most prevalent disease in Western societies and the major cause of early morbidity and mortality. The process of atherosclerosis with its multitude of risk factors accounts for the majority of cardiovascular disorders and is the most promising target for therapeutic applications. Tremendous strides have been made in the last 2 decades in interventional cardiology, pharmacologic therapy, and preventative strategies, including risk factor modification, all of which have contributed to lowering the rate of new cardiovascular events. The success of some therapies often overshadows the lack of efficacy in the majority of patients. For example, the tremendous success of statin drug therapy with 30% cardiovascular event reduction is celebrated with a seemingly lack of appreciation of the fact that this also represents a 70% failure rate. This has not gone unnoticed by the scores of patients who have been treated for various cardiovascular problems and who have shown a surge of interest in alternative therapies for the management of these diseases. In a random national survey, 18.9% of adults in the United States used mind-body medical therapies; meditation, imagery, and yoga are the most common.[1] Thus astute clinical physicians are taking notice and seeking evidence-based medicine studies to evaluate and potentially validate alternative methodologies, which may enhance and complement conventional therapy. The potential for mind/body medicine approaches to bridge an important gap in our healthcare is tremendous. Even in the era of modern medicine, a quote from Plato seems decidedly appropriate: "This is the great error of our day in the treatment of the human body: that physicians separate the soul from the body."[2]

HISTORICAL PERSPECTIVES

Ancient Greek philosophers first began to explore the relationship between physical and spiritual reality. Heraclitus in the fifth century BC, best known for his description of Cosmos, was also the first metaphysical philosopher. He explored the relationship between opposites and concluded, "It is sickness which makes health pleasant."[3] The relationship between the mind and the body and health has been recognized since the time of the Chinese Emperor Huang Ti (the Yellow Emperor, 2697-2597 BC). He said, "people... should not weary during the day time, and they should not allow their minds to become angry."[4] Without even the simplest understanding of anatomy, he understood the mind-body relationship. The first systematic definition of the mind-body relationship, however, is attributed to René Descartes, the French philosopher, mathematician, and physiologist. He is credited with formulating the reflex theory but also posited that the mind could affect the body via the soul, which he concluded resided in the pineal gland. By the 19th century, much of the philosophy of Descartes and others was rejected by such imminent scholars as Thomas Huxley, who felt that feelings, no matter how intense, were simply molecular changes in the brain incapable of affecting the nervous system or the body. To Huxley and others, what had been accepted and considered intuitive by philosophers for millennia, was discounted in its entirety. This attempt to separate consciousness from physical reality was short-lived, and the concept of the mind-body relationship was rescued, in part, through the works of Jean-Martin Charcot,[4a] who demonstrated the scientific aspects of hypnosis in relieving functional nervous disorders (**see Chapter 6**). Although hypnosis has been much maligned and misunderstood through its misuse, the therapeutic benefits that Charcot demonstrated continue to be used in the 20th century. By the time William James wrote *Principles of Psychology* in 1890, the mind/body connection was beginning to become comprehensible as an integration of science and philosophy. William James, older brother of Henry James, the novelist, was trained as a physician yet established himself as the preeminent psychologist and philosopher of the late 19th century. His godfather, Ralph Waldo Emerson, had initiated his training in intuitive psychology and higher consciousness. James focused his attention upon the relationship of attitude upon health and disease and was a strong proponent of the theory that emotions could create pathology. Much of the credit for the current concepts of mind-body medicine belongs to Herbert Benson of Harvard Medical School, who authored such scientific treatises as the *Relaxation Response* (1975) and *The Mind/Body Effect* (1979).

From the simplistic anatomic standpoint, it is quite clear the cerebral cortex via the pyramidal pathways can induce muscle movement through pure volition. In addition, autonomic and neuroendocrine modulators perform this role in organ tissues. It therefore becomes obvious that thought not only can induce voluntary motions, but also through the autonomic pathways can also influence functional disorders of pathologic interest. Stress-induced headaches and abdominal pain are well known to both physicians and the general public. No example is more obvious than the anxious student suffering a bout of diarrhea before an examination. Physicians commonly see patients with "functional" complaints such as palpitations, fatigue, and dyspnea, all which have a scientific basis in confirming a negative impact physiologically from the mind-body connection. A prime example is the evidence that type-A personality is a harbinger of cardiovascular disease. This concept not only has scientific merit but has been distilled down to the concept of "hostility" as being the prime risk.[5] Many studies have shown an increase in myocardial infarction in relation to hostility. However, Iribarren et al also related the early preclinical phase of coronary artery disease to hostility.[5] In a 10-year follow-up, patients 30 years of age and younger with high hostility scores had a nearly 10-fold increase in the finding of significant calcium in their coronary arteries, even after adjusting for other risk factors. As originally defined, type-A behavior encompassed ambitiousness, aggressiveness, hostility, competitiveness, and a sense of urgency. The absence of these characteristics has been defined as type-B behavior.[6] The Western Collaborative Group Study demonstrated that type-A behavior caused a two-fold increase in the risk of coronary heart disease.[6] Ragland and Brand, however, were able to show some positive attributes of this behavior: type A patients clearly showed an improved survival after myocardial infarction.[7] This is probably due to enhanced coping ability and compliance with medical therapy and lifestyle changes exhibited by these patients. Nevertheless, the component of hostility in type A patients remains a major stressor, increasing cardiovascular risk. In fact, a pessimistic attitude has itself been associated with an increased mortality rate in comparison to being optimistic.[8] Using the Minnesota Multiphasic Personality Inventory in an observation of 19,781 person years, Maruta et al found a 19% increase in mortality for every 10-point T-score increase.[8] They theorized that learned helplessness has a negative psychologic and physiologic impact that may lower immune system responses. Among stable heart patients, feelings of tension, frustration, and sadness have been associated with a greater risk of acute myocardial ischemia during activities of daily living.[9] One first must examine the potential for the mind-body connection to alter physiological function to the point of creating disease and then to realize that the same process can be used to ameliorate disease. Further examination of this hypothesis requires that the available evidence be evaluated in particular regard to the inducement of cardiovascular disorders related to imbalance of the mind-body relationship.

STRESS AND CARDIOVASCULAR DISEASE RISK

Hans Selye first described the stress response as "fight or flight" and further characterized it as "a response to a physical or psychological event perceived as a threat to well being and an inability to cope with perceived outcomes."[9a] Major acute psychological stressors—including divorce, business loss, interpersonal conflict, death of a spouse, and humiliation—are well known to be associated with sudden cardiac death. Nearly half the victims of sudden cardiac death died within minutes to hours of a major psychological stress.[10] Although stress has long been considered the provocative factor in inducing acute myocardial infarction, it is recently recognized as a clear risk factor in the etiology of coronary artery disease from its early stages. Endothelial dysfunction, which is clearly the initial stage of the atherosclerotic process, can be linked to chronic stress.[11]

Social support structures, such as being married and having close contact with friends and relatives, have been shown to decrease cardiovascular mortality by enhancing a sense of well-being. People who live alone or who are not married are demonstrated to have a higher 5-year mortality and risk of recurrent myocardial infarction than those with social support.[12] These findings are completely independent of other cardiovascular risk factors and demonstrate a direct connection between attitude and cardiovascular risk. Job strain has also been linked directly to cardiovascular risk. High job demands or lack of autonomy are among the conditions that negatively impact cardiovascular health.[13] In comparison to those with low job stress, both men and women who demonstrated high job stress in a cross-sectional study had a significantly increased risk of acute myocardial infarction.[14] Prospective studies have also confirmed an increased risk of acute myocardial infarction among both men and women with high job stress.[15] In addition, death from acute myocardial infarction has been noted to be significantly increased in the first month after the death of a spouse or loved one.[16]

In a retrospective review of patients presenting with acute myocardial infarction, a single episode of intense anger was found to double the risk of an acute myocardial infarction in the ensuing 2-hour period.[17] Depression, anxiety, and anger have been established as contributing factors to the risk for coronary disease.[18,19] People who exhibit hostility respond to conflict with a much greater increase in blood pressure than do those who exhibit lower hostility tendencies. Hypertensive patients in general exhibit high levels of anger or suppressed anger than do those who are nonhypertensive.[20] The most startling evidence appears to indicate that hostility is a stronger predictor of coronary heart disease than other traditional risk factors such as hyperlipidemia and smoking.[21] Niaura et al studied 2280 men and measured hostility with the Cook-Medley-Ho Scale, taken from the Minnesota Multiphasic Personality Inventory.[21] They found that the hostility measure was a stronger predictor of coronary heart disease than all the other risk factors with the exception of low level high-density lipoprotein cholesterol.

The highest levels of emotional distress have been correlated with the youngest age of presentation among coronary disease patients.[19] This implies a greater need for treatment of psychosocial stress disorders for both primary and secondary prevention beginning at younger ages. Ketterer et al demonstrated that although depression, anxiety, hostility, somatization, and obsessive compulsive disorders all correlate with the risk of coronary disease, the entry of the hostility scale emerges as the major predictor.[19] In fact, these investigators demonstrated that the genetic basis as a risk factor for cardiovascular disease may in fact be more related to inherited psychosocial characteristics than to inherited physiologic traits. The heritability aspect of anxiety and depression has been described in a study of twins by Bouchard et al.[22] In addition, Carmelli et al described the heritability of hostility.[23] Ketterer et al went on to analyze the potential heritability of coronary artery disease and found a strong correlation with psychosocial/emotional distress.[24] Among men with proven coronary artery disease, the presence or absence of family history was completely independent of other risk factors. The standard risk factors exhibited no significant difference in these two groups. More specifically, they noted that anger reported by a spouse or friend accounted for 68% of the variance. Ketterer et al further indicated that early onset of coronary artery disease should raise greater clinical suspicion of psychosocial/emotional distress, even in the face of denial by the patient.[24] Although familial hyperlipidemia is a well known genetic risk factor, it accounts for only a minority of patients who develop cardiovascular disease. Surprisingly, the major family risk may be the psychosocial milieu that results from familial stress patterns.

PATHOPHYSIOLOGY OF STRESS

The evidence that acute mental stress can precipitate myocardial ischemia is well established.[25] Hostility has been associated with a decrease in parasympathetic activity and an overexpression of sympathetic tone.[26] The etiology of acute cardiovascular events appears to be stress-induced vasoconstriction and enhanced platelet aggregability and plaque rupture.[27,28] A more chronic stress pattern leads to continuous mild vasoconstriction and endothelial dysfunction, which presages the development of the true atherosclerotic process. In fact, chronic stress is associated with an accelerated progression of atherosclerosis.[29,30] The mechanism appears to be through increased oxidative stress, free-radical activity, and lipid peroxide levels. The scientific evidence of stress as an etiologic factor in cardiovascular disease is obviously well established. Given the mind-body relationship, it would seem that reduction of stress empirically would reduce cardiovascular disorders. Nevertheless, an evidence-based medicine approach is required to support this theory—just as with the more traditional therapies, which have demonstrated success. Attempts to modify behavior and reduce stress in cardiac events actually antedated the evidence of causality. The theory of inducing the mind to heal the body, however, has now been validated by a number of scientific studies. Relaxation therapy has been shown to reduce anger as well as cardiovascular mortality and disability.[31] Efforts to target reduction of type-A behavior and hostility have shown moderate success. Teaching patients to manage anger and increase awareness of their negative behavior reduced cardiac events and mortality.[32,33] Focused awareness has been shown to produce beneficial biochemical alterations, including a reduction of catecholamines and cortisol levels.[34-36] The anxiolytic component appears to result from increases in hypothalamic GABAergic tone.[37] This mechanism is similar to the effects of tranquilizing medications such as benzodiazepines. Of major interest are recent studies that have shown that the relaxation response initiates activation of nitric oxide release, which counters the effects of stress hormones and, in particular, the effect of norepinephrine.[38,39] Although many patients undoubtedly have benefited from interventional cardiology, lipid-lowering medications, and antihypertensive treatment, the treatment of mental stress has supporting data that is just as compelling—yet still considered an alternative approach. Stress-management strategies—including meditation, yoga, acupuncture, massage, tai chi, aromatherapy, guided imagery, healing touch, Qi Gong, Reiki, prayer, and behavioral therapy—have demonstrated benefit in the treatment of cardiovascular disorders.

THE POWER OF PLACEBO

Placebo therapy is undoubtedly one of the earliest medicinal therapies incorporated by clinicians invoking the mind-body connection. Although placebo therapy is not well understood, its importance cannot be underemphasized (see Chapter 1). This fact is best demonstrated by the adherence to placebo-controlled clinical trials prevalent in modern medical research. Compliance to placebo alone has been associated with survival. In a 5-year study of 1103 men who were treated with clofibrate, patients who were adherent to drug therapy demonstrated a substantially lower mortality rate than those who were poorly adherent to the drug.[40] Strikingly, however, very similar findings were noted in those patients taking the placebo, in that those who faithfully took the placebo had a lower mortality than those with low levels of adherence. This demonstrates that a simple belief in placebo enhances the power of standard medical therapies to work. This message understates the importance of a positive outlook and encouragement by physicians to promote the healing process. In no way does this support the past practice of subterfuge by which physicians provided prescriptions for "sugar pills." It merely coalesces information that supports the observation that a positive, caring, and nurturing attitude on the part of a physician has a powerful mind-body influence upon the patient. As Coleridge said, "the best inspirer of hope is the best physician."[41]

BEHAVIORAL THERAPY

Studies by Blumenthal et al perhaps best exemplify the potential impact of stress reduction in cardiovascular mortality.[42,43] In a 5-year follow-up study, stress management training significantly lowered the risk of cardiovascular events compared to controls.[42] One-hundred-thirty-six patients with documented coronary artery disease were followed over 5 years. They participated in the Duke Stress Management Program and received a total of 16 90-minute sessions in which they learned skills to reduce stress. This included a graded task assignment, monitoring irrational automatic thoughts, and generating alternative interpretations of situations with unrealistic thought patterns. The patients were instructed in progressive muscle relaxation techniques as well as in biofeedback training. Over a 5-year period, total cardiac events—including cardiac catheterization, coronary angioplasty, bypass surgery, myocardial infarction, and cardiac death—were reduced by 50% in the treatment group in comparison to the usual care group. The physiologic changes of stress reduction have been linked to the autonomic nervous system, musculoskeletal system, psychologic-neurologic-endocrine system, and the limbic system.[44] The acute beneficial changes can be seen in the impact upon respiratory and heart rate as well as upon blood pressure and muscle tension and by the physiologic measurements of corticosteroid release and platelet aggregation.

Dusseldorp et al, in a meta-analysis of psychoeducational programs for coronary disease patients, found an overall 34% reduction in cardiovascular mortality, including a 29% reduction in the recurrence rate of myocardial infarction..[18] In addition, significant positive effects were observed in blood pressure, lipid levels, smoking behavior, exercise, and body weight. Schneider et al showed the significant ability of stress reduction to lower blood pressure over a sustained treatment period.[45]

MEDITATION AND PRAYER

The effects of meditation can be accomplished through the transcendental technique, mindfulness, walking meditation or Tai Chi (see Chapters 9, 10, and 11). Recognition of the benefits of meditation upon health and well-being appears to have originated long before the current mind-body awareness: as far back in the Vedic ages of 3000 BC. It can be followed through the times of Buddha, the early Christians, and Jewish Kabbalism. The resurgence of interest in meditation as a therapy in the United States dates to the arrival of transcendental meditation (TM) with Maharishi Mahesh Yogi in 1967. In the 1970s Jon Kabat-Zin popularized mindfulness, and Benson championed the relaxation response. A supportive study on mindfulness-based stress reduction showed clinically significant relief of physical symptoms, anxiety, and stress over a 1-year period.[46] Mindfulness-based cognitive therapy for depression resulted in a clinically significant reduction in relapse.[47] The mechanism by which TM benefits cardiovascular disease is due in part to stress reduction associated with reduced oxidative stress. Schneider et al reported that patients who used TM had significantly lower levels of lipid peroxide than did a control group.[48] In a comparison between TM and eyes-closed relaxation, the TM group demonstrated a significantly lower blood pressure response and decrease in vasoconstrictive tone.[48] Not surprising, therefore, was the finding that TM was effective in controlling angina in patients with cardiac syndrome X.[49] In a 4-year trial that used a combination of meditation and breathing exercises, fatal myocardial infarction was significantly reduced.[50] In a review of the subject, King et al discussed the benefits of TM in decreasing hypertension and atherosclerosis.[51] At this time, whether TM has unique benefits that may separate it from standard meditation or other stress reduction strategies remains unknown. In a direct comparison between TM and progressive muscle relaxation, both methods were effective in providing sustained lowering of blood pressure; however, TM was found to be twice as effective as the relaxation technique.[47]

Many people use prayer to help cope with everyday stresses of life. Prayer has been reported to result in improvement of perceived stress and control of mild hypertension.[52] In addition, private prayer appears to significantly reduce depression during the year after coronary artery bypass surgery.[53] However, when studied in randomized controlled trials, intercessory prayer still lacked convincing evidence for its benefit (see Chapter 22). In one such study, Harris et al reported improvement in CCU course with no difference in length of hospital stay.[54] In a second large randomized controlled trial, the Mayo Clinic reported no significant effect on medical outcomes in those who used intercessory prayer.[55] Krucoff et al demonstrated in the original MANTRA Pilot Study an improvement in clinical outcomes among patients who underwent percutaneous coronary interventions by use of off-site intercessory prayer, bedside imagery, touch therapy, and relaxation techniques.[56] In a more extensive investigation, The MANTRA II Study randomized 750 patients in nine centers across the United States and compared standard therapy to a combination of off-site prayer, music therapy, guided imagery, and touch therapy. A reduction of mortality from 5.4% to 1.9% was achieved in the treatment group.[57] Although this result narrowly missed statistical significance, it remains a promising strategy for future research.

TOUCH/MASSAGE THERAPY

Massage therapy has been available for centuries; however, the idea of therapeutic or healing touch was strongly promoted in the 1970s by Dolores Krieger at New York University's Division of Nursing.[58] Although the theory of "energy transfer" to patients with cardiovascular disease has been postulated, no scientific substantiation of this concept exists. Some evidence suggests a potential anti-anxiety effect, which bears further scrutiny. A study by Song et al analyzed electroencephalograms and electrocardiograms in 22 subjects who focused attention on their heartbeats with and without kinesthetic (touch) biofeedback.[59] Heart-focused attention and awareness of creative pulsations revealed increased electroencephalographic activities synchronized with the electrocardiogram, possibly reflecting increased baroreceptor and somatosensory feedback. This suggests a homeostatic self-regulation between the brain and the target organ, which may underlie the self-healing mechanisms apparent in mind/body medicine.

Tiller et al demonstrated that patients trained in heart-focused stress-reduction techniques shifted attention away from stress and directly influenced the parasympathetic feedback loop.[60] This information strengthens the hypothesis that self attention to the body has a physiologic basis in the mind-body connection. These and other studies on the physiology of self-attention provide a crossover reference to the effects demonstrated with therapeutic touch.[61] Heidt studied 90 patients who were hospitalized in a cardiovascular unit and compared the effects of therapeutic touch, casual touch, or no touch with all patients receiving a 5-minute intervention.[62] Preintervention and postintervention anxiety scores showed a significantly greater reduction in post-touch anxiety among the patients receiving therapeutic touch. An extensive review of the literature concludes that evidence supports the practice of therapeutic touch for the reduction of both pain and anxiety.[62] Nine of eleven studies analyzed showed statistically significant results from this treatment. Currently, a variety of therapeutic touch techniques are taught in dozens of universities, and future direction should include multidisciplinary studies and standardization.

Massage therapy has a long history of use for musculoskeletal and orthopedic complaints with a variety of positive responses reported (see Chapter 24). Relatively few studies in regard to cardiovascular patients and any long-term benefit have been conducted. McNamara et al studied back massage before diagnostic cardiac catheterization and found some benefit to a 20-minute massage intervention.[63] In the treatment group, systolic blood pressure was reduced a mean 8.6mmHg and perceived psychological distress was reduced as well. For a short-term acute stress intervention, massage seemed to benefit these patients. The mechanism of benefit in massage therapy appears to be both a reduction of anxiety levels and an increase in cardiac parasympathetic activity.[64] In a randomized controlled trial that compared therapeutic massage to the management of stress by using relaxation tapes, both methods were equally effective in lowering stress in preoperative and postoperative settings.[65] Interestingly, however, patients strongly have preferred therapeutic massage over the use of relaxation tapes. At present no controlled trials are evaluating the potential benefit from massage therapy in cardiac event reduction. Such trials seem warranted, as is evidenced by the validity of massage therapy to reduce stress, which is a major provocative factor in coronary artery disease.

ACUPUNCTURE

The ancient Chinese art of acupuncture dates back to the Han dynasty. References to the use of stone or bamboo needles dates back to 2697 BC. Acupuncture is deeply rooted in traditional Chinese medicine although only recently appreciated in Western medicine (see Chapter 15). Although many disciplines of Western medicine have accepted acupuncture, skepticism about many of its proclaimed benefits continues. The World Health Organization has attempted to stratify the myriad of medical conditions treated by some acupuncturists into categories of proven benefit, possible benefit, or unproven benefit. Among those conditions considered to have proven benefit from acupuncture are pain, depression, nausea and vomiting, hypertension, hypotension, and cerebrovascular accidents.[66] The standard acupuncture nomenclature uses a meridian system consisting of 400 acupuncture points and 20 meridians. Researchers, including Pomeranz, have demonstrated a correlation between these acupuncture points and areas of high electrical conductance on the body's surface.[67] The therapeutic effect of acupuncture can be achieved by a variety of stimuli including electricity, temperature variation, needling, mechanical pressure, and laser.[68-70] Although acupuncture has been studied more thoroughly in the alleviation of pain, it has also been studied in regard to the influencing of neuromechanisms in myocardial ischemia.[71] Using a feline model, Longhurst demonstrated that electroacupuncture of the pericardial meridian over the median nerves for 30 minute periods substantially reduced myocardial ischemia, measured as an improvement in regional myocardial wall thickening.[71] This effect lasted up to 90 minutes. Electroacupuncture was also shown to work through the endogenous opioid system—demonstrated by the fact that naloxone injected into the ventral lateral medulla prevented the response. The mechanism of benefit appeared to be a reduction in oxygen demand rather than an improvement in oxygen supplied to the myocardium.

Some studies published in Western journals have demonstrated potential benefits of acupuncture in cardiovascular disease. The beneficial effect on blood pressure control was seen in a study by Williams et al.[72] Some benefit was demonstrated in patients treated with acupuncture over a several-week period for control of angina pectoris.[73,74] Kurono et al measured the effect of acupuncture on coronary artery dilatation during coronary angiography.[75] The mean dilatation with acupuncture was 68.8% of that caused by isosorbide dinitrate, thereby demonstrating a definite physiologic effect. Although they lack double-blind techniques or sham controls, the results of these small studies are promising enough to warrant further investigation.

The sham effect of acupuncture has been a concern of the National Institutes of Health.[76] A statement from the NIH points out that an acupuncture needle placed in almost any position could elicit a biological response and the possibility of a sham effect; nevertheless, they pointed out that adverse reactions were notably lower than with conventional drug therapies. The conclusion of the panel was that future research was warranted on the biological basis of acupuncture. In this regard, NIH-funded acupuncture studies are underway.

In a more Westernized form of acupuncture, nerve stimulation via transcutaneous electrical nerve stimulation (TENS) has been substituted for electroacupuncture.[77] Some reduction in angina was evident with long-term TENS use when it was studied in the pacing-induced setting. An analysis of the physiological basis for TENS therapy in comparison to acupuncture is required for full acceptance and understanding of this modality.

TAI CHI

Tai Chi represents the blend of ancient Chinese medicinal healing with martial arts as taught by Bodhidarma, the founder of Zen Buddhism. Tai Chi represents an 18-movement technique of body control and breathing techniques for a combination of relaxation and defense (see Chapter 11). Through coordination of body movement with breathing, both heart rate and blood pressure are reduced. Although the rigors of tai chi are not in the realm of standard aerobic exercise and do not achieve levels of exercise often recommended for cardiac fitness, definite benefits are produced. In one study of patients after myocardial infarction, Tai Chi achieved better long-term blood pressure control than did aerobic exercise.[78] In a randomized controlled study that compared Tai Chi to sedentary controls, the Tai Chi group exhibited significant improvement in blood pressure and lipid control.[79] A 12-week training course of Tai Chi resulted in a 15.6 mm Hg drop in systolic blood pressure and a 15.2 mg/dl drop in total cholesterol and a concomitant 4.7 mg/dl increase in high density lipoprotein cholesterol. It is apparent that in mildly hypertensive patients, Tai Chi may be an excellent alternative to drug therapy. In addition, anxiety status was greatly improved in the Tai Chi group. In a literature review, Tai Chi was concluded to be both beneficial and cost-effective when used as an adjunct to cardiac rehabilitation exercise training.[80] In patients after coronary bypass surgery, a group using Tai Chi achieved not only better treatment adherence, but a significant improvement in VO2 peak compared to patients involved in a recommended home exercise program.[81] In a study by Yeh, Tai Chi benefited a group of heart failure patients with low ejection fractions.[82] The low-impact activities were easy for heart failure patients to perform and resulted in improvement in 6-minute walking distance and quality of life. B-type natriuretic peptide levels also fell significantly compared to a control group.

YOGA

Yoga—in Sanskrit, literally "to make whole"—is a vitalistic approach to health combining several mind-body exercises (see Chapter 9). Increasingly popular and widely taught in several formats, yoga has a demonstrated history of improving health.[83-85] Yoga calls upon a variety of techniques including meditation, relaxation, stretching, and control of breathing to achieve a state of relaxation and fitness. Yoga is a mainstay of Ayurvedic medicine, which is the ancient (before 2500 BC) Indian holistic healthcare approach that focuses on yoga, diet, and medicinal plants.

Stress reduction by use of yoga has been shown to produce a significant decrease in blood pressure and heart rate.[86,87] The majority of patients studied were able to significantly reduce their doses of antihypertensive medications. Yoga stress management techniques were an essential part of the Lifestyle Heart Trial, in which Ornish et al were able to demonstrate some reversal of heart disease and control of angina.[88] Stress reduction was only one of several treatments that also included diet and exercise, although the effect of stress reduction was not independently analyzed. Nevertheless, the positive results of this remarkable study were significantly more pronounced with yoga than those seen with diet and exercise alone. After 5 years this study group exhibited some regression of atherosclerosis with a total 7.9% relative improvement, whereas the control group experienced a 5.4% relative worsening. In a separate study, yoga was compared to usual care, which included risk factor control and the American Heart Association step-one diet.[89] The yoga group showed improvement in angina control, exercise capacity, body weight, and serum lipids as well as a significant reduction in the need for revascularization procedures, including coronary bypass surgery or angioplasty. In addition, at 1 year, the results of coronary angiography revealed a 20% regression rate in the yoga group versus 2% in the control group. In this randomized prospective study, yoga was shown to both improve symptomatic status and to retard progression of atherosclerosis independent of other interventions.

GUIDED IMAGERY

Guided imagery may be the ultimate expression of mind-body communication (see Chapter 8). The power of imagination is invoked to produce desired physiologic and psychosocial effect. The mind is a powerful tool. By pure concentration the mind can imagine desirable food and produce salivation. No one can dispute the ability to imagine a sexual experience with the attendant physiologic response. This has been known since the dates of Hippocrates, who believed that images released spirits from the brain and aroused the body. Today imagery is used in health care as well as in daily practice by business people and by athletes who use imagery to enhance performance. Imagery has been used in all cultures and in many religions for centuries. The Navajo Indians, for example, use a healing technique with imagery by visualizing themselves as healthy. In imagery, the mind may invoke all five senses, as imagining oneself on a tropical isle, watching the crash of the ocean waves while smelling the fragrance of the orchids, feeling the sand underneath ones feet, and tasting the salt air. Imagery is a therapeutic tool and encompasses some elements of meditation and hypnosis, as well as the placebo effect.

Imagery has been used successfully as a therapeutic intervention in patients with chronic pain, cancer, and surgery.[90-92] Patients are asked to visualize relaxing scenes and describe them to a therapist. Therapists in return interact with the patient, who would describe the scenes that were most pleasant. Therapists then may help a patient embellish the visualized scenes, adding more details. In most instances, therapists individually tailor imagery to the patient rather than use standardized imagery. The MANTRA Study used guided imagery as part of a multipronged mind-body approach to significantly reduce mortality among cardiac patients undergoing coronary interventions.[55]

Hypnosis (see Chapter 6) is also successful in reducing anxiety and also has some evidence of reducing systolic blood pressure. In a study by Benson et al, hypnosis was compared to meditational relaxation with comparable findings of anxiety reduction and blood pressure–reducing effects.[93] In this study, psychiatric assessment revealed an overall improvement of 34%, although self-rating assessment indicated a 63% improvement. Systolic blood pressure was reduced an average of 4 mm Hg, which was statistically significant. The anxiolytic component of hypnosis has been shown to have an effect on heart rate variability, enhancing parasympathetic activity, while reducing sympathetic tone.[94]

ADVERSE EFFECTS

The inappropriate use of various mind-body therapies can result in direct harm, especially in patients with unstable psychiatric conditions where direct supervision is necessary.[1] In addition, patients may suffer persistent guilt if they have less than expected results from the mind-body therapy and therefore may blame themselves for not trying hard enough. Patients should not forego accepted treatments in favor of proven treatments for cardiovascular disease. Mind-body therapy is a complementary approach to standard treatments—not an alternative.

SUMMARY

The mind-body approach to cardiac illness is best exemplified by the analysis and treatment of stress disorders. Stress is an adaptive phenomenon quite necessary for the physiologic response to ensure survival of organisms. However, as previously discussed, stress can have a negative effect in creating an imbalance in the mind-body system thus promoting disease. This can lead to minor functional disturbances as well as accelerated aging and coronary artery disease, the main cause of morbidity and mortality in Western society. Stress can now be seen not as an innocent bystander once largely ignored by medical practitioners but as a major risk factor, not only for the development but also for the accelerated progression of atherosclerosis. Notwithstanding the tremendous successes of conventional medicine, current therapies still fall short because cardiovascular disease remains the predominant scourge in virtually all Western societies. This leaves room for new approaches to treating this disorder by use of techniques, which are not merely alternatives but are quite complementary to conventional medicine. Techniques that invoke the positive change in mind-body connection as described herein, ranging from meditation to yoga, have demonstrated not only a favorable impact on well-being but also significant reductions in morbidity and mortality when added to or compared to conventional therapies. By seeking the power of the mind, we also empower our patients to take control over their lives and the healing process.

In selecting stress reduction modalities, one must remember that this does not represent a one-size-fits-all phenomenon. Whether a patient will respond to any of the stress reduction techniques depends on the character of the individual patient, on personal perceptions, biases, and motivations. Whereas some will rapidly accept self-discipline techniques, others may require professional help in cognitive behavior therapy. We must be mindful of the fact that patients seldom select stress-reduction techniques of their own volition. These powerful tools deserve a more prominent role in every clinician's strategy to reduce cardiac illness. When it comes to selecting the therapeutic armamentarium with which to treat cardiovascular disease, one must remember that truly the mind is a terrible thing to waste.

REFERENCES

1. Wolsko PM, Eisenberg DM, Davis RB, Phillips RS: Use of mind-body medical therapies: results of a national survey, J Gen Intern Med 19:43-50, 2004.

2.   Plato: Charmides, or temperance, 380 BCE. Translated by Benjamin Jowett. Available at *http://classics.mit.edu/Plato/charmides.html*. Accessed February 15, 2004.

3.   Burnet J: Exploring Plato's dialogues: early Greek philosophy, 1920. Available at *http://plato.evansville.edu/public/burnet/*. Accessed February 15, 2004.

4.   Ti H: Nei Ching Su Wen: The yellow emperor's classic of internal medicine, c. 1697-2598 BCE. Translated by Ilza Veith.

4a. Chertok L: On the centenary of Charcot: hysteria, suggestibility and hypnosis. Br J Med Psychol 57 (Pt 2): 111-20, 1984.

5.   Iribarren C, Sidney S, Bild DE et al: Association of hostility with coronary artery calcification in young adults, JAMA 283:2546-2551, 2000.

6.   Peterson C, Seligman ME: Causal explanations as a risk factor for depression: theory and evidence, Psychol Rev 91:347-374, 1984.

7.   Ragland DR, Brand RJ: Type A behavior and mortality from coronary heart disease, N Engl J Med 318:65-69, 1988.

8.   Maruta T, Colligan RC, Malinchoc M, Offord KP: Optimists vs pessimists: survival rate among medical patients over a 30 year period, Mayo Clin Proc 75:140-143, 2000.

9.   Gullette ECD, Blumenthal JA, Babyak M et al: Effects of mental stress on myocardial ischemia during daily life, JAMA 277:1521-1526, 1997.

9a. Selye H: A syndrome produced by diverse nocuous agents. Nature 138: 72, 1936.

10. Rissanen V, Romo M, Siltanen P: Premonitory symptoms and stress factors preceding sudden cardiac death from ischemic heart disease, Acta Med Scand 204:389-396, 1978.

11. Rozanski A, Blumenthal JA, Kaplan J: Impact of psychological factors on the pathogenesis of cardiovascular disease and implications for therapy, Circulation 99:2192-217, 1999.

12. Williams RB, Barefoot JC, Califf RM et al: Prognostic importance of social and economic resources among medically treated patients with angiographically documented coronary artery disease, JAMA 267:520-524, 1992.

13. Bosma H, Peter R, Siegrist J, Marmot M: Two alternative job stress models and the risk of coronary artery disease, Am J Public Health 88:68-74, 1998.

14. Karasek RA, Theorell TG, Schwartz J et al: Job, psychological factors, and coronary heart disease: Swedish prospective findings and US prevalence findings using a new occupational inference method, Adv Cardiol 29:62-87, 1992.

15. Alfredson L, Spetz CL, Theorell T: Type of occupation and near-future hospitalization for myocardial infarction over some other diagnoses, Int J Epidemiol 4:378-388, 1985.

16. Kaprio J, Koskenvuo M, Rita H: Mortality after bereavement: a prospective study of 95,647 widowed persons, Am J Public Health 77:283-287, 1987.

17. Mittelman MA, Maclure M, Sherwood JB et al: Triggering of acute myocardial infarction onset by episodes of anger: determinants of myocardial infarction onset study investigators, Circulation 92:1720-1725, 1995.

18. Dusseldorp E, van Elderen T, Maes S et al: A meta-analysis of psychoeducational programs for coronary heart disease patients. Health Psychology 18:506-519, 1999.

19. Ketterer MW, Fitzgerald F, Thayer B et al: Psychosocial and traditional risk factors in early ischemic heart disease: cross-sectional correlates, J Cardiovasc Risk 7:409-413, 2000.

20. Smith TW, Gallo LG: Hostility and cardiovascular reactivity during marital interaction, Psychosom Med 61:436-445, 1999.

21. Niaura R, Todaro JR, Stroud L et al: Hostility, the metabolic syndrome, and incident of coronary heart disease, Health Psychol 21:588-593, 2002.

22. Bouchard TJ, Lykken DT, McGue M et al: Sources of human psychological differences: the Minnesota Study of Twins Reared Apart, Science 250:223-228, 1990.

23. Carmelli D, Swan GE, Rosenman RH: The heritibility of the cook and medley hostility scale revisited, J Pers Soc Psychol 5:107-116, 1990.

24. Ketterer MW, Denollet J, Chapp J: Familial transmissability of early age at initial diagnosis in coronary heart disease (CHD): males only, and mediated by psychosocial/emotional distress, J Behav Med 27(1); 1-10, 2004.

25. Blumenthal JA, Jiang W, Waugh RA et al: Mental stress-induced ischemia in the laboratory and ambulatory ischemia during daily life: association and hemodynamic features, Circulation 92:2102-2108, 1995.

26. Sloan RP, Shapiro PA, Bigger JT et al: Cardiac autonomic control and hostility in healthy subjects, Am J Cardiol 74:298-300, 1994.

27. Boltwood MD, Taylor CB, Burke MB et al: Anger report predicts coronary artery vasomotor response to mental stress in atherosclerotic segments, Am J Cardiol 72:1361-1365, 1993.

28. Markovitz JH: Hostility is associated with increased platelet activation in coronary heart disease, J Psychosom Med 60:586-591, 1998.

29. Harris CW, Edwards JL, Baruch A et al: Effects of mental stress on brachial artery flow-mediated vasodilation in healthy normal individuals, Am Heart J 139:405-411, 2000.

30. Ghiadoni L, Donald AE, Cropley M et al: Mental stress induces endothelial dysfunction in humans, Circulation 102:2473-2478, 2000.

31. Frasure-Smith N, Prince R: The ischemic heart disease life stress-monitoring program: impact on mortality, Psychosom Med 47:431-445, 1985.

32. Nunes EV, Frank KA, Kornfeld DS: Psychologic treatment for the type A behavior pattern and for coronary heart disease: a metaanalysis of the literature, Psychosom Med 49:159-173, 1987.

33. Friedman M, Thoresen GE, Gill JJ et al: Alteration of type A behavior and its effect on cardiac recurrences in postmyocardial infarction patients: summary results of the recurrent coronary prevention project, Am Heart J 112:653-665, 1986.

34. Michaels RR, Parra J, McCann DS, Vander AJ: Renin, cortisol, and aldosterone during transcendental meditation, Psychosom Med 41:50-54, 1979.

35. Gallois P, Forzy G, Dhont, JL: Hormonal changes during relaxation, Encephale 10:79-82, 1984.

36. Cooper R, Joffe BI, Lamprey JM et al: Hormonal and biochemical responses to transcendental meditation, Postgrad Med J 61:301-314, 1985.

37. Elias AN, Wilson, AF: Serial hormonal concentrations following transcendental meditation: potential role of gamma aminobutyric acid, Med Hypotheses 44:287-291, 1995.

38. Esch T, Fricchione G, Stefano G: Stress-related diseases: a potential role for nitric oxide, Med Sci Monit (8)6, RA103-118, 2002.

39. Esch T, Fricchione G, Stefano G: The therapeutic use of relaxation response in stress-related diseases, Med Sci Monit (9)2 RA23-34, 2003.

40. Coronary Drug Project Research Group: Influence of adherence to treatment and response of cholesterol on mortality in the Coronary Drug Project, N Engl J Med 303:1038-1041, 1980.

41. Coleridge ST: Table Talk, London, 1884, G Bell and Sons.

42. Blumenthal JA, Babyak M, Wei J et al: Usefulness of psychosocial treatment of mental stress-induced myocardial ischemia in men, Am J Cardiol 89:164-168, 2002.

43. Blumenthal JA, Jiang W, Babyak MA, Krantz DS et al: Stress management and exercise training in cardiac patients with myocardial ischemia, Arch Int Med 157:2213-2223, 1997.

44. Burker EJ, Fredrikson M, Rifai N et al: Serum lipids, neuroendocrine, and cardiovascular responses to stress in men and women with mild hypertension, BehavMed 19:155-161, 1994.

45. Schneider RH, Staggers F, Alexander CN et al: A randomized controlled trial of stress reduction for hypertension in older African Americans, Hypertension 26:820-827, 1995.

46. Reibel DK, Greeson JM, Brainard GC et al: Mindfulness-based stress reduction and health-related quality of life in a heterogeneous patient population, Gen Hosp Psychiatry 23:183-192, 2001.

47. Teasdale JD, Segal ZV, Williams JM et al: Prevention of relapse/recurrence in major depression by mindfulness-based cognitive therapy, J Consult Clin Psychol 68:615-623, 2000.

48. Schneider RH, Nidich SI, Salerno JW et al: Lower lipid peroxide levels in practitioners of transcendental meditation program, Psychosom Med 60:38-41, 1998.

49. Cunningham C, Brown S, Kaski JC: Effects of transcendental meditation on symptoms and electrocardiographic changes in patients with cardiac syndrome, Am J Cardiol 85:653-655, 2000.

50. Patel D, Marmot MG, Terry DJ et al: Trial of relaxation in reducing coronary risk: four-year follow-up, Br Med J (Clin Res Ed) 290:1103-1106, 1985.

51. King MS, Carr T, D'Cruz C: Transcendental meditation, hypertension and heart disease, Aust Fam Physician 31:164-168, 2002.

52. Harmon RL, Myers MA: Prayer and meditation as medical therapies, Phys Med Rehabil Clin N Am 10:651-662, 1999.

53. Al A, Dunkle RE, Peterson C, Bolling SF: The role of private prayer in psychological recovery among midlife and aged patients following cardiac surgery, Gerontologist 38:591-601, 1998.

54. Harris WS, Gowda M, Kolb JW et al: A randomized controlled trial of the effects of remote, intercessory prayer on outcomes in patients admitted to the coronary care unit, Arch Intern Med 159:2278, 1999.

55. Aviles JM, Wheelan SE, Hernke DA et al: Intercessory prayer and cardiovascular disease progression in a coronary care unit population: a randomized controlled trial, Mayo Clin Proc 76:1192-1198, 2001.

56. Krucoff MW, Crater SW, Green CL et al: Integrative noetic therapies as adjuncts to percutaneous intervention during unstable coronary syndromes: monitoring and actualization of noetic training (MANTRA) feasibility pilot, Am Heart J 142:760-767, 2001.

57. Krucoff MW: The MANTRA study project: first look at MANTRA II results, Presentation— American College of Cardiology, Big Island, Hawaii, October 2003.

58. Lewis D: A survey of therapeutic touch practitioners, Nurs Stand 13(30):33-37, 1999.

59. Song LZYX, Schwartz, GER, Russek LGS: Heart-focused attention and heart-brain synchronization: energetic and physiological mechanisms, Altern Ther 4(5):44-62, 1998.

60. Tiller WA, McCraty R, Atkinson M: Cardiac coherence: a new noninvasive measure of autonomic nervous system order, Altern Ther Health Med 2(1):52-65, 1996.

61. Spence JE, Olson MA: Quantitative research on therapeutic touch: an integrated review of the literature 1985–1995, Scand J Caring Sci 11:183-90, 1997.

62. Heidt P: Effect of therapeutic touch on anxiety level of hospitalized patients, Nurs Res 30:32-37, 1980.

63. McNamara ME, Burnham DC, Smith C, Carroll DL: The effects of back massage before diagnostic cardiac catheterization, Altern Ther Health Med 9:50-57, 2003.

64. Delaney JP, Leong KS, Watkins A, Brodie D: The short-term effects of myofascial trigger point massage therapy on cardiac autonomic tone in healthy subjects, J Adv Nurs 37:364-371, 2002.

65. Hanley J, Stirling P, Brown C: Randomised controlled trial of therapeutic massage in the management of stress, Br J Gen Pract 53:20-25, 2003.

66. World Health Organization: A proposed standard international acupuncture nomenclature: report of WHO scientific group. Geneva, 1991, World Health Organization.

67. Pomeranz B: Scientific basis of acupuncture. In Stux G, Pomeranz B, editors: Acupuncture textbook and atlas, Berlin, 1987, Springer-Verlag.

68. Altman S: Techniques and instrumentation, Probl Vet Med 4(1):66-87, 1992.

69. Schlager A, Offer T, Baldissera I: Laser stimulation of acupuncture point P6 reduces postoperative vomiting in children undergoing strabismus surgery, Br J Anaesthesia 81:529-532, 1998.

70. Weintraub M, editor: Alternative and complementary treatment in neurologic illness, New York, 2001, Churchill.

71. Longhurst JC: Central and peripheral neural mechanisms of acupuncture in myocardial ischemia, Intl Congress Series 1238:79-87(9), 2002.

72. Williams T, Mueller, K, Cornwall, MW: Effect of acupuncture-point stimulation on diastolic blood pressure in hypertensive patients: a preliminary study, Phys Ther 71:523-529, 1991.

73. Ballegaard S, Pedersen F, Pietersen A et al: Effects of acupuncture in moderate, stable angina pectoris: a controlled study, J Intern Med 227:25-30, 1990.

74. Richter A, Herlitz J, Hjalmarson A: Effect of acupuncture in patients with angina pectoris, Eur Heart J 12:175-178, 1991.

75. Kurono Y, Egawa M, Yano T, Shimoo K: The effect of acupuncture on the coronary arteries as evaluated by coronary angiography: a preliminary report, Am J Chin Med 30:387-96, 2002.

76. NIH Consensus Development Conference Statement Online 1997: Acupuncture. Available at *http://odp.od.nih.gov/consensus/cons/107/107_statement.html*. Accessed February 10, 2004.

77. Longhurst JC: Acupuncture's beneficial effects on the cardiovascular system, Prev Cardiol 1:21-33, 1998.

78. Channer KS, Barrow D, Barrow R et al: Changes in haemodynamic parameters following Tai Chi Chuan and aerobic exercise in patients recovering from acute myocardial infarction, Postgrad Med J 72:349-351, 1996.

79. Tsai JC, Wang WH, Chan P et al: The beneficial effects of *Tai Chi Chuan* on blood pressure and lipid profile and anxiety status in a randomized controlled trial, J Altern Complement Med 9:747-54, 2003.

80. Taylor-Piliae RE: *Tai Chi* as an adjunct to cardiac rehabilitation exercise training, J Cardiopulm Rehabil 23:90-6, 2003.

81. Lan C, Chan SY, Wong MK: The effect of *Tai Chi* on cardiorespiratory function in patients with coronary artery bypass surgery, Med Sci Sports Exerc 31:634-638, 1999.

82. Yeh, GL, Lorell BH, Stevenson LW, et al. Benefit of Tai Chi as an adjunct to standard care for patients with chronic stable heart failure (abstr). J Cardiac Fail, 9(5) Suppl 1: S1, 2003.

83. Upupa KN, Singh RH: The scientific basis of yoga (editorial), JAMA 220:1365, 1972.

84. Hoenig J: Medical research on yoga, Confin Psychiatr 11:69-89, 1968.

85. La Forge R: Mind-body fitness: encouraging prospects for primary and secondary prevention, J Cardiovasc Nurs 11:53-65, 1997.

86. Raju PS, Prasad KV, Venkata RY et al: Influence of intensive yoga training on physiological changes in 6 adult women: a case report, J Altern Complement Med 3:291-295, 1997.

87. Sundar S, Agrawal SK, Singh VP et al: Role of yoga in management of essential hypertension, Acta Cardiol 39:203-208, 1984.

88. Ornish D, Scherwitz LW, Billings JH et al: Intensive lifestyle changes for reversal of coronary heart disease, JAMA 280:2001-2007, 1998.

89. Manchanda SC, Narang R, Reddy KS et al: Retardation of coronary atherosclerosis with yoga lifestyle intervention, J Assoc Physicians India 48:687-94, 2000.

90. Richardson MA, Post-White J, Grimm, EA et al: Coping, life attitudes and immune responses to imagery and group support after breast cancer treatment, Altern Ther Health Med 3:62-70, 1997.

91. Lyles JN, Burish TG, Krozely MG, Oldham RK: Efficacy of relaxation training and guided imagery in reducing the aversiveness of cancer chemotherapy, J Consult Clin Psychol 50:509-524, 1982.

92. Spiegel D, Moore R: Imagery and hypnosis in the treatment of cancer patients, Oncology 11:1179-1189, 1997.

93. Benson H, Frankel FH, Apel R et al: Treatment of anxiety, a comparison of the usefulness of self-hypnosis and a meditational relaxation technique: An overview, Psychother Psychosom 30:229-42, 1978.

94. DeBenedittis G, Cigada M, Bianchi A et al: Autonomic changes during hypnosis: a heart rate variability power spectrum analysis as a marker of sympatho-vagal balance, Int J Clin Exp Hypn 42:140-52, 1994.

CHAPTER 6

Hypnosis for the Relief of Cardiac Symptomatology

Arthur E. Fass, MD

The profound influence of the psyche on the cardiovascular system is obvious even with ordinary daily activities. We all have experienced rapid increases in pulse rate and exaggerated cardiac action when we are faced with sudden stress. The instantaneous tachycardia, palpitations, and muscle tension, orchestrated by the brain via the autonomic nervous system in a perceived emergency is as inherent to the human condition as our reflexive withdrawal from noxious stimuli. This activation of the cardiovascular system in preparation for "fight or flight" has evolved as a hair-trigger defense against outside threats to life and limb. Its perseverance in the essential mammalian blueprint is a testament to its centrality in the survival scheme.

Our evolutionary heritage, however, when juxtaposed with the exigencies of modern civilization, may not always work to our best advantage. The emergencies of past epochs now take the form of a cancelled airline flight, a deadline at work, an argument at home, or a traffic jam on the road. The cardiovascular responses to these "modern" threats can have decidedly detrimental effects on our health both in the short and long terms.

Sudden psychological stress can produce important hemodynamic and physiological consequences. Characterized by surges in catecholamines and cortisol, the stress response includes increases in pulse rate and blood pressure. The hormonal actions also produce a positive inotropic effect on the ventricular myocardium. In addition, the body's clotting mechanisms are activated with blood platelets, thus demonstrating increased aggregability.[1]

In light of the demonstrable cardiovascular hazards of psychological stress on the cardiovascular system, what defenses are available? Clearly, specific pharmacologic interventions are indicated in a variety of clinical situations.

The treatment of depression, for example, usually requires antidepressive medication as well as other treatment modalities.

However, a variety of nonpharmacological methods have been shown to effectively alleviate stress. Exercise is famous for stress alleviation. Meditation, imagery, yoga, biofeedback, acupuncture, and hypnosis have all been employed. Because of the relatively innocuous nature of these techniques, they can be applied in virtually all clinical situations and to the general population.

This chapter will explore the clinical aspects of the hypnosis approach.

DEFINITION AND HISTORY

The nature of hypnosis and hypnotic suggestion has been the subject of lively debate and controversy for centuries. The phenomenon of a "trance" state was originally popularized by the Austrian physician Franz Anton Mesmer in the late eighteenth century.[2] He achieved some success in inducing hypnotic trances, attributing the phenomenon to "animal magnetism." His concept was eventually labeled a fraud.

The term "hypnotism" from the Greek *hypnos* (sleep) was coined by the English physician James Braid in 1843 who realized that hypnosis was not a result of external forces, but rather of the subject's ability to summon his own powers of focus and concentration. It was not a state of sleep at all, but the term had taken hold. Meanwhile, at around the same time, dramatic clinical effects of hypnosis were demonstrated by the Scottish surgeon James Esdaile, who performed hundreds of surgical procedures and used hypnosis alone for anesthesia. The eminent neurologist Jean Martin Charcot became interested in hypnosis in the latter part of the nineteenth century and stimulated an ongoing debate about the phenomenon. He felt that hypnosis was a pathologic state akin to hysteria. During his early medical career, Sigmund Freud visited Charcot at the Paris Hospital of Salpetriere and became intrigued by hypnosis as a potential tool for diagnosing and treating symptoms of neurosis. Eventually, however, Freud felt that hypnosis was not helpful for uncovering unconscious memories and abandoned the technique.

After Freud's defection, interest in hypnosis among medical professionals waned. Many denounced the practice as quackery. Hypnosis seemed destined to become a historical footnote. However, amidst the suffering and trauma of World War I, hypnosis proved effective in the short-term treatment of posttraumatic stress disorder and in pain relief. At this time and later during World War II, the stress-reducing potential of hypnosis was widely acknowledged.

Subsequently, two scientific societies, the American Society of Clinical Hypnosis and the Society for Clinical and Experimental Hypnosis, were founded, further establishing the scientific credentials of the field. In 1956, hypnosis was endorsed by the American Medical Association as an effective adjunct treatment for medical practitioners and dentists. A 1996 report from the National Institutes of Health concluded that hypnosis is an effective treatment for pain from cancer and was of therapeutic value in other chronic conditions, including irritable bowel syndrome and tension headaches.

HYPNOSIS AS TREATMENT FOR STRESS

The crucial role of emotion in physical symptoms and disease states has gained virtually universal acceptance. Mind-body medicine (see Chapter 5), once felt to be outside the boundaries of traditional medical practice, is now featured in mainstream journals and textbooks. Hypnosis as a therapeutic modality has won recognition by the medical community as an important and effective therapeutic approach for a variety of conditions, including chronic pain syndromes, headaches,[3] insomnia, irritable bowel syndrome,[4,5] asthma, and skin conditions.[6] It has also been applied in preoperative and postoperative surgical management as well as in physiatry.

To the extent that hypnosis can favorably affect the mind-body equilibrium and particularly because of its salutary effects on cardiovascular physiology, it has a potentially important place in the cardiology therapeutic armamentarium.

The nature of the trance state, central to hypnosis theory, is not yet thoroughly defined in scientific terms. Most theorists view the trance state as a separate level of consciousness, differing from both wakefulness and sleep. The trance state—although not completely defined physiologically—is characterized by a number of consistent phenomena. An individual in a trance state experiences *increased* focus and concentration, the result of the filtering out of external stimuli. The capacity to relax is enhanced. Because of a reduced influence of conscious inhibition, the hypnotized individual will be more receptive to suggestion. However, it should be emphasized that a hypnotized person cannot be influenced to behave in a fashion that is contrary to his wishes or beliefs.[7]

Generally, hypnotic methods seek to induce a state of deep relaxation. A variety of induction techniques are employed. The methods, which are surprisingly simple, usually call for the subject to fix his or her gaze on a stationary object. The operator will offer repeated relaxing suggestions relying on deep breathing and mental imagery to achieve progressively deeper levels of relaxation. Specific suggestions and reinforcements are directed to the patient's individual needs. Patients are then given suggestions aimed at encouraging changes in behavior or relief of symptoms. The term *posthypnotic suggestion* refers to suggestions designed to alter behavior or perceptions after coming out of the trance state.[8] Hypnosis is characterized by a temporary suspension of critical resistance to beneficial suggestions.

Hypnosis is recognized as one of the most effective nonpharmacological methods available for pain relief and analgesia.[9] PET-scan analyses suggest a possible physiologic basis of hypnosis-induced analgesia. In one study, scans of the brain were obtained in hypnotized volunteers during hot-water hand immersion.[10] The somatosensory cortex, which processes physical stimuli was similarly activated in a group of subjects given the hypnotic suggestion that the stimulus would be painfully hot versus a group that was told the stimulus would be minimally unpleasant. However, the part of the brain involved in the subjective or "suffering" aspect of pain, the anterior cingulate cortex, was much more active in the "painfully hot" group. Hypnotic suggestion therefore may modify the brain's processing and interpretation of external stimuli.

Individuals exhibit considerable variation in hypnotic susceptibility (hypnotizability).[9] Responsiveness to hypnosis appears to be an inherited trait and is not clearly related to personality type.[10] Various tests of hypnotic susceptibility have been devised, most notably the Stanford Hypnotic Susceptibility Scale. The large majority of individuals can be hypnotized at least to some degree. A smaller percentage is highly hypnotizable.

USE IN PREVENTION AND TREATMENT OF CARDIOVASCULAR DISEASE

Individuals under hypnosis appear to possess an ability to influence their bodily systems normally under autonomic control. This effect offers a potential therapeutic window to the autonomic nervous system and its direct effects on the cardiovascular system. Objective measurements of autonomic nervous system activity in subjects under hypnosis reveal characteristic changes.[11,12] Hypnosis shifts the autonomic balance toward increased parasympathetic activity with a simultaneous reduction in sympathetic nervous system output. Highly hypnotizable individuals exhibit the greatest increase in vagal (parasympathetic) activity.[12]

Ornish et al employed guided imagery (a form of self-hypnosis) as a component of a multifaceted approach to the treatment of coronary atherosclerosis.[13] An exercise program and strict low-fat diet were also used. Coronary angiography revealed a greater tendency for reversal of atherosclerosis in the intervention group versus a "usual care" cohort. The relative contribution of the imagery/relaxation component of the program could not be assessed separately.

A meta-analysis of 23 randomized trials[14] underscored the role of such therapeutic interventions as relaxation and stress-management techniques as adjuncts to standard cardiac rehabilitation. Patients receiving the stress intervention experienced a 41% reduction in all-cause mortality and a 46% reduction in nonfatal coronary events at a 2-year follow-up. Other studies support the role of relaxation techniques in improving long-term prognosis after myocardial infarction.[15]

In several clinical studies, hypnotic methods have been used in conjunction with cardiac surgery. Multiple case reports have shown a potentially beneficial effect of hypnosis in alleviating anxiety in patients scheduled for cardiac surgery.[16,17] Pain medication requirements were reduced postoperatively. Hypnosis also had salutary effects in patients who undergo coronary angioplasty procedures.[16,18] Patients given hypnosis before the angioplasty required less pain medication after the procedure and were able to tolerate longer periods of balloon inflation.

The possible use of hypnotherapy for the control of cardiac arrhythmias was explored in a case report from the Walter Reed Army Medical Center.[19] A patient on multiple drug treatments for ventricular arrhythmias experienced an improvement in ventricular ectopy after a hypnosis training program. At this time no prospective controlled trials are evaluating this approach.

Smoking accounts for approximately 30% of clinical cardiovascular disease.[20] Smoking cessation is perhaps the most effective of all interventions in terms of reduction in cardiovascular morbidity and mortality.[21] More than 70% of smokers want to quit smoking, and almost half attempt to quit in a given year.[22] Success rates for individuals trying to quit on their own without outside treatment, however, have a dismally low 7% success rate. Standard treatments, including cognitive-behavioral counseling, pharmacological therapy, and combination therapies increase the success rate to 15% to 30%.

Hypnosis has long been tried for smoking cessation, and abundant anecdotal reports suggest the effectiveness of this treatment modality. Scientific assessment of its efficacy is less certain because of the lack of controlled clinical trials. A cohort study achieved a 23% abstinence rate 2 years after a single-session intervention with self-hypnosis.[23] Studies that used biochemical verification of smoking cessation report a 17% to 33% success rate with hypnosis.[24] A combination of hypnosis, pharmacotherapy to alleviate nicotine withdrawal symptoms, and exercise to avoid weight gain may offer the best option for long-term success.

PERSONAL EXPERIENCE IN PRACTICE

Several years ago I found myself imploring a patient to quit smoking. The patient, a middle-aged woman who had undergone coronary angioplasty several months before, continued to smoke heavily. I had this discussion numerous times with the patient—without results. I had been interested in hypnosis, especially as an aid to smoking cessation, and had done some reading on the subject. I asked the patient if she would be willing to try it, and she readily consented. I discovered that the induction of a hypnotic state was surprisingly easy. I simply had the patient sit comfortably, take deep breaths, and relax. I asked her to imagine being in a calm, peaceful place. Within minutes the patient appeared to be in a hypnotic trance. At this point I offered repeated suggestions about the negative aspects of smoking, especially the unpleasant taste, smells, etc. I also offered positive suggestions: that after quitting smoking she would gain a renewed sense of confidence and satisfaction about taking charge of her health. After "awakening" from the trance, my patient stated that she found the experience to be very relaxing and pleasant. To my surprise, she phoned the office 2 weeks later to boast that she had not smoked a single cigarette since the office session.

With that initial experience, the potential of hypnosis in cardiovascular disease prevention became very clear. Since that time I have tried to incorporate the technique into my clinical cardiology practice. Although I have had no formal training in hypnosis, I find that in most patients I am able to induce a state of hypnosis (of varying degrees, depending on the individual's susceptibility). I have used the technique in a variety of clinical situations. It is extremely effective for stress reduction. Patients immediately feel relaxed and often report lingering effects for several days or more. There is an almost universal immediate drop in systolic and diastolic blood pressure of varying magnitude during and after the hypnosis sessions.

I have also found that stress reduction achieved through hypnosis can be a very effective tool in relief of cardiac symptoms, especially anxiety-related tachycardia and palpitations. Patients often report relief of insomnia, often for prolonged periods. I cannot yet document any success using hypnosis to relieve the symptoms of myocardial ischemia.

With regard to smoking cessation, I have had some spectacular successes (i.e., achieving immediate results in long-term smokers, some with COPD). The success rate, I believe, is strongly related to the individual's motivation. In strongly motivated subjects, a series of closely spaced hypnosis sessions (i.e., every other day) at the start of treatment with gradual tapering to "maintenance" treatments has often yielded gratifying results.

In general, offering this complementary treatment has been very well received by my patients. They appreciate my willingness to take a few extra minutes to address their symptoms and concerns, and I have not encountered any negative effects of the treatment.

Current medical practice, however, imposes a number of important barriers to the integration of a complementary technique to "traditional" care. In the present practice environment, time is a commodity in short supply. Hypnosis can slow things down a bit (even when one can manage to see other patients during a hypnosis session). Moreover, insurance companies do not yet have a "code" for hypnosis treatments, and the billing for this procedure is therefore problematic. I typically simply incorporate the hypnosis into a regular office visit or make a special arrangement for the patient to pay for the service outside the insurance system.

CONCLUSION

Hypnosis holds great promise as a complementary treatment for the prevention and treatment of cardiovascular disease and symptoms. Its potential use for stress management with restoration of a healthy autonomic balance represents perhaps its greatest role. In spite of a lack of controlled clinical trials regarding hypnosis' effectiveness, the available data suggest a beneficial effect in restoring cardiovascular homeostasis. It is reassuring that the technique appears to be especially free of adverse effects. A need to perform controlled clinical trials to objectively document efficacy clearly exists. These studies should hopefully assess long-term physiologic effects as well as cardiovascular outcomes.

Current "traditional" methods in cardiology practice—with their strong emphasis on invasive procedures—have clearly failed to address all our patients' needs. Preventive cardiology, with attention to lifestyle changes and risk factor modification, must assume a central place in our approach. Hypnosis and other complementary therapies can be important elements in this effort.

REFERENCES

1. Braunwald E, Zipes DP, Libby P: Textbook of cardiovascular medicine, ed 6, Philadelphia, 2001, WB Saunders.
2. Wolberg LR: Hypnosis: what is it, how to use it. 2nd ed. Hollywood, Calif, 1982, Melvin Powers Wilshire Book Company.
3. Millea PJ, Brodie JJ: Tension-type headache, Am Fam Physician 66:797-805, 2002.
4. Talley NJ, Spiller R: Irritable bowel syndrome: a little understood organic bowel disease? Lancet 360:555-564, 2002.
5. Palsson OS, Turner MJ, Johnson DA et al: Hypnosis treatment for severe irritable bowel syndrome, Digest Dis Sci 47:2605-2614, 2002.
6. Shenefeld PD: Hypnosis in dermatology, Arch Dermatol 136:393-399, 2000.
7. Preston MD: Hypnosis: medicine of the mind, ed 2, Spokane, Wa., 2001, Pine Orchard Inc.
8. Raz A, Shapiro T: Hypnosis and neuroscience, Arch Gen Psychiatry 59:85-90, 2002.
9. Barrows KA, Jacobs BP: Mind-body medicine, Med Clinics North Am 86:11-31, 2002.
10. Nash MR: The truth and the hype of hypnosis, Scientific Amer 285(1):46-49, 52-55, 2001.
11. Appel PR: Clinical hypnosis in rehabilitation, Sem Integrat Med 1:90-105, 2003.
12. DeBenedictis G, Cigada M, Bianchi A et al: Autonomic changes during hypnosis: A heart rate variability power spectrum analysis as a marker or sympatho-vagal balance. Int J Clin Exp Hypn 42:140-152, 1994.
13. Ornish D, Scherwitz LS, Doody RS et al: Effects of stress management training and dietary changes in treating ischaemic heart disease, JAMA 249:54-60, 1993.
14. Linden W, Stossel C, Maurice J: Psychosocial interventions for patients with coronary artery disease: a meta-analysis, Arch Intern Med 156:745-752, 1996.
15. Patel C, Marmot MG, Terry DJ et al: Trial of relaxation in reducing coronary risk: four-year follow-up. Br Med J (Clin Res Ed) 290:1103-1106, 1985.
16. Luskin FM, Newell KA, Griffith M et al: A review of mind-body therapies in the treatment of cardiovascular disease, part 1: implications for the elderly, Altern Ther Health Med 4:46-61, 1998.
17. Gruen W: A successful application of systematic self-relaxation and self-suggestion about postoperative reactions in a case of cardiac surgery, Int J Clin Exp Hypn 20:143-151, 1971.
18. Weinstein EJ, Au PK: Use of hypnosis before and during angioplasty, Am J Clin Hyperten 34:29-37, 1991.
19. Wain H, Amen DG, Oetgen WJ: Hypnotic intervention in cardiac arrhythmias: advantages, disadvantages, precautions, and theoretical consideration, Am J Clin Hyperten 27:70-75, 1984.

20. Pickering T, Clemow L, Davidson K et al: Behavioral cardiology: has its time finally arrived? Mt Sinai J Med 7:101-112, 2003.

21. Warner KE: Smoking out the incentives for tobacco control in managed care settings, Tob Control 7 Suppl:50-54, 1998.

22. Kinnunen T: Integrating hypnosis into a comprehensive smoking cessation intervention: comments on past and present studies, Int J Clin Exp Hyperten 49:267-271, 2001.

23. Spiegel D, Frischholz E, Fleiss J et al: Predictors of smoking abstinence following a single-session restructuring intervention with self-hypnosis, Am J Psychiatry 150:1090-1097, 1993.

24. Frank RG, Umlauf RL, Wonderlich SA et al: Hypnosis and behavior treatment in a worksite cessation program, Addiction Behaviors 11:59-62, 1986.

CHAPTER 7

Biofeedback in Cardiovascular Disease

Angele McGrady, PhD

B iofeedback is a mind-body therapy often coupled with relaxation train-ing as a clinical intervention for stress-related disorders. Biofeedback involves monitoring and displaying information about a physiological function such as heart rate, skeletal muscle tension, skin temperature, skin conductance, or brain waves. For example, motor unit potentials generated during muscular contraction are recorded from surface sensors by an elec-tromyograph (EMG), and a tone indicates magnitude of tension. The most commonly monitored EMG sites are the forehead, back of neck, shoulders and back. The subject, given information about fluctuating levels of muscle contraction, learns to associate the signal with lower or higher tension levels. Lower tension and relaxed muscles, the desired response, is reinforced through an operant conditioning paradigm.[1]

The most common types of biofeedback used for stress-related cardiovascu-lar disorders are EMG, direct blood pressure feedback, and thermal feedback. Relaxation provides the skills necessary for the person to utilize the feedback information. Types of relaxation include deep breathing, passive focus on relax-ation of skeletal muscle or warming the hands, meditation, and imagery.[2,3] Depending on the individual's disorder, the treatment plan comprises one or more types of biofeedback, one or more varieties of relaxation training, coping skills training, and psychotherapy if appropriate. Regardless of the type of feed-back and preferred relaxation technique, home practice of relaxation is required to generalize the treatment effects from the clinic to everyday life.

A standard biofeedback intervention protocol comprises 8 to 10 sessions of 50 minutes each, following an initial history and the psychophysiological pro-file. The latter consists of measuring muscle tension, heart rate, blood pres-sure, skin temperature, and skin conductance under conditions of rest-eyes open, eyes closed, stressful images, and while the subject attempts to relax.[1] At least three measurements are made under each condition during a period of 2 to 4 minutes. Excessive responses to the stressful imagery are identified and are used later in the training sessions. It is also important to assess the person's ability to relax so that prior experience with relaxation can be incorporated into learning new skills.

If the provider identifies or learns from the patient's history that a psychiatric disorder is present, a referral for medical management and/or psychotherapy is appropriate. Many biofeedback practitioners are licensed in a mental health discipline and thus can provide counseling or psychotherapy as well as biofeedback. Cognitive behavioral psychotherapy (CBT) is the most frequently used method of psychotherapy in the biofeedback setting; however, CBT will lengthen the treatment period and require additional homework.

As with other stress-related disorders, treatment of cardiovascular diseases is usually multidimensional. Behavioral interventions may include weight loss for obese patients, salt reduction for those sensitive to sodium, smoking cessation, moderating alcohol use, and increasing exercise for sedentary patients. Applied psychophysiologic approaches such as biofeedback and relaxation, the topics of this chapter, may be combined with medical management, psychotherapy, and behavioral interventions in a complete treatment plan. No contraindications prevent combining medical management or psychotherapy with feedback and relaxation for persons with cardiovascular disorders.

ESSENTIAL HYPERTENSION

The theoretical framework for prescribing biofeedback and relaxation therapy (BFRT) as treatment of essential hypertension is that blood pressure is stress-sensitive in some people, similar to the sodium sensitivity of other segments of the population with hypertension. The autonomic nervous system, catecholamines and cortisol, which are central to the stress response, have a major influence in the control of blood pressure. Imbalance in sympathetic and parasympathetic functioning—specifically sympathetic dominance and parasympathetic under-activity—is associated with sustained elevated pressure. Sympathetic hyperactivity maintained for months and years, as seen in cases of chronic unremitting stress, predicts elevated insulin levels, dyslipidemia, and hypertension in young adults.[4] Although a detailed discussion of the psychophysiologic etiology of hypertension is beyond the scope of this chapter, determination of the extent of the impact of stress on blood pressure in persons with essential hypertension facilitates the estimation of the potential benefits of BFRT. A predictor profile comprising psychologic and physiologic factors relevant to hypertension was developed to characterize potential responders to BRFT.[5] Hypertensive individuals with high anxiety, elevated cortisol, rapid heart rate, and cool hand temperatures (which indicate vasoconstriction) are the best candidates for BFRT and would be likely to achieve the largest decreases in blood pressure. The contribution of stress to blood pressure should be considered before medical therapy is initiated so that appropriate referrals for BFRT may be made for patients whose blood pressure is stress-sensitive. At this time, there is no basis for successful treatment of secondary hypertension with BFRT.

BFRT are offered to patients in the clinic in workplace settings or, less frequently, in a paradigm based largely on home practice of relaxation. In contrast to the standard treatment, minimal therapist interventions include only two to three clinic sessions. Patients who are strongly motivated, able to apply the relaxation response to stressful situations, and largely untroubled by psychopathology are good candidates for minimal therapist contact protocols.

CLINIC-BASED TREATMENT PROTOCOLS

The most common setting for BFRT in hypertension is the clinic. A behavioral treatment program based on anxiety management was used as an intervention in unmedicated hypertensive individuals. Thermal BFRT and skill training to decrease anxiety resulted in significant decreases in systolic and diastolic blood pressure that were maintained at 6 months after treatment. Participants learned to reduce their anxiety by using adaptive coping techniques. Specifically, structured rehearsal and identification of increased muscle tension were used as cues for applying the relaxation skills that were learned during active treatment.[6] The effects of thermal biofeedback have been tested in numerous other studies and found to be superior to relaxation alone or to no treatment.[7-9] Blood pressure decreases of 10 mm Hg systolic and 5 mm Hg diastolic are observed in patients who successfully apply the techniques to lower blood pressure.

Forehead EMG feedback and direct blood pressure feedback—combined with relaxation—have also been shown to be beneficial in lowering blood pressure in persons with hypertension, regardless of whether they are on antihypertensive medication. In comparison to a credible control condition, EMG biofeedback was associated with small but consistent decreases both in blood pressure and in antihypertensive medication.[10] Sequencing direct blood pressure feedback and relaxation, instead of combining treatments, was proposed based on a trial of these interventions. Clinically significant decreases in blood pressure were observed and were stable at follow up.[11]

The effects of heart rate biofeedback were contrasted with CBT in 77 hypertensive patients randomized to CBT, biofeedback, or control (no treatment).[12] Seventeen sessions of the feedback or the cognitive method (anger control, stress inoculation to anger) were provided. Results showed that both active interventions reduced blood pressure, but the heart rate feedback was associated with larger changes in blood pressure. Because the groups were formed by random assignment, whether the individuals given anger management necessarily had a problem with controlling their anger is unclear.[12]

Feedback of the R wave to pulse interval was tested in 12 persons with elevated and 10 persons with low blood pressures. In both groups, blood pressure tended to normalize, and significant changes were observed. This paradigm, based on the hypothesis of "visceral learning," presumes that, with training, physiological systems will normalize. Although these results are intriguing and could apply to both hypertension and hypotension, no formal baseline or follow-up was established in this study, and only a small number of training sessions (three in approximately 1 week) were offered.[13]

Controlled trials of stress reduction were performed in older African Americans to test the application of these techniques across a wider age span and in ethnic minorities. Transcendental meditation (TM) and progressive muscle relaxation were compared with a lifestyle modification education program. TM reduced systolic blood pressure by an average of 10.7 mm Hg and diastolic blood pressure by 6.4 mm Hg; individuals in the relaxation alone group lowered blood pressure by 4.7 mm Hg and 3.3 mm Hg (systolic/diastolic).[14] Subsequently, subjects were divided into high- and low-risk subgroups. Risk was defined by using the following established risk factors for hypertension: obesity, alcohol consumption, sedentary lifestyle, high dietary sodium, psychosocial stress, and multiplicity of risk factors. Both the high- and low-risk groups decreased systolic and diastolic blood pressure compared with the control subjects. This study suggests that individuals who are at significant risk for more severe hypertension can also benefit from behavioral interventions.[15]

In another study of TM performed on 32 healthy individuals, the TM group decreased systolic blood pressure, heart rate, and total peripheral resistance. Results are important even though participants were healthy adults, because the change in total peripheral resistance is an indicator of improved overall hemodynamic functioning. Individualized stress management matched to subjects' risk factors and personality characteristics was offered to 27 persons with essential hypertension and were compared to 33 persons on a waiting list. Significant reductions in ambulatory blood pressure (6.1 mm Hg systolic and 4.3 mm Hg diastolic) were observed in the stress management group, particularly those with higher initial blood pressure; the decreases were correlated with improvements in distress and better coping with anger in those subjects who were identified as distressed and angry.[16]

If stress management programs can be incorporated into primary care practices, fewer referrals to other practitioners and other sites are necessary. Services are more efficient and costs decrease. Thus a study of biofeedback was designed and carried out in a general practice setting.[17] Patients were trained in deep breathing and relaxation facilitated by galvanic skin response feedback. At 1-year follow-up, blood pressure in the relaxation groups remained significantly lower than at pretreatment. For primary care physicians to successfully use stress management interventions onsite, office space must be adequate and appropriate for quiet practice of relaxation, both practitioners and patients must be motivated and willing to commit the necessary time to the therapy.

Home-Based Treatment Protocols

In comparison to placebo, a 4-week home-based program of biofeedback that used finger blood-pressure monitoring found significant decreases in blood pressure in mild hypertensive subjects on no medications.[18] Blanchard et al[19] compared the effects of 16 clinic sessions of thermal biofeedback during 8 weeks with a home program of similar length. Subjects were patients with hypertension who were maintained on two antihypertensive drugs. The clinic-based regimen was superior to the home-based program in the number of patients who were consistently able to reach the 95° F criterion temperature and apply the technique to decrease blood pressure. However, some blood pressure decreases were also observed in the group working at home in this more severely hypertensive group.

A feedback device called RestErete provides information about breathing rate and depth. In a study of 17 patients whose blood pressure was poorly responsive to medication, they used RestErete for 15 minutes multiple times per week for 8 weeks. Thirteen of the 17 patients reduced blood pressure significantly when they increased depth and lowered rate of breathing.[20] In a randomized, double-blind, controlled study, 32 patients practiced deep breathing for 10 minutes a day for 8 weeks, whereas another group of 29 listened to quiet music. The former had significant decreases in systolic (11.7 mm Hg), diastolic (15.2 mm Hg), and mean arterial blood pressure (10.0 mm Hg).[21]

A similar feedback device that reinforces slow and regular breathing was tested in 33 patients whose blood pressure was difficult to control on antihypertensive medicine alone. Significant decreases in clinic and home blood pressures were found.[22] When patients achieved a breathing rate slower than 10 per minute, the improved blood pressure generalized to home and ambulatory measures.[23]

WORKPLACE INTERVENTIONS

Stress-management programs have been offered at the workplace to decrease the number of required clinic visits and to assist subjects in generalizing the relaxation techniques to stressful situations. McCraty et al provided a 16-hour program (one full day and two half days) that contained some CBT components, heart rate variability biofeedback, and relaxation.[24] Home practice was encouraged through reminders at work. In comparison, controls were on a waiting list. The trained group showed significant decreases in systolic blood pressure (10.6 mm Hg) but not in diastolic blood pressure (6.3 mm Hg). Improvements in self-reported depression and psychologic distress were also noted.

Thermal BFRT was provided at the worksite in a randomized control paradigm.[25] Fifty subjects with essential hypertension participated in eight group sessions, while controls were wait listed. Forty nine percent of the trained subjects decreased their mean arterial pressure by at least 5 mm Hg. Decreases in anxiety scores on a standard questionnaire, lower plasma aldosterone levels and the ability to increase finger temperature were concomitant with decreases in blood pressure. Caucasians, African Americans, and other groups responded similarly.

EFFECTS OF BIOFEEDBACK ON REACTIVITY

The mental-stress test is a useful means of assessing reactivity to situations commonly found in the course of life. Blood pressure reactivity to stress is related to sustained hypertension over time, so a mental stress test may also be a useful indicator of the long-term effects of BFRT. Twenty mildly hypertensive patients had 10 sessions of skin conductance biofeedback supplemented by regular home practice; at the end of treatment there were significant decreases in the blood pressure and heart rate responses to stress. In addition, state anxiety (the anxiety of the moment) assessed by a standard questionnaire was less apparent after training. Persons who had higher initial stress levels and who were able to achieve deeper relaxation during training benefited more than those who were not able to reduce their skin conductance.[26]

In another study of blood pressure reactivity to mental stress, relaxation training was provided for subjects who were not hypertensive (mildly elevated, casual blood pressure). Naltrexone was given to test the antagonism of the learned relaxation response by opioid blockade and to elucidate a potential mechanism for efficacy of BFRT. Diastolic blood pressure reactivity was significantly increased under naltrexone conditions in trained subjects. Therefore learned relaxation may be correlated with the release of endogenous opioids, and these opioids reduce reactivity of the cardiovascular system to stress.[27]

META-ANALYSES AND REVIEWS

An extensive review of biobehavioral approaches, including BFRT, in the treatment of hypertension was conducted. Biofeedback or relaxation therapy alone was found to have only limited blood pressure-reducing effects.[28] A systematic search of the literature from 1966 to 1997 revealed that multicomponent stress management interventions, however, were associated with significant decreases in blood pressure, with minimal side effects. Single therapies (i.e., biofeedback or relaxation) are less effective than multiple component treatment schemas.[29]

A meta-analysis was conducted of 166 studies that evaluated relaxation therapy interventions, and individualized CBT compared to drug and other behavioral therapies. Drug therapy was usually begun at higher initial pressures than were the nondrug treatments. Starting levels of blood pressure have a critical impact on the magnitude of decrease in blood pressure. Once pretreatment levels of blood pressure are equalized, the magnitude of improvement with behavioral therapy was similar to the effects of antihypertensive medication.[30]

Meta-analytic methods were used to examine 22 studies of the effectiveness of biofeedback in the treatment of Stages 1 and 2 hypertension.[31] Biofeedback, relaxation training, and CBT were the most effective in decreasing blood pressure in comparison to an inactive control. Even small decreases are significant because a decrease in diastolic pressure of 5 to 6 mm Hg is associated with a 35% reduction in stroke and 20% to 25% reduction in coronary artery disease.[32]

WHITE COAT HYPERTENSION

Some individuals show evidence of significantly elevated blood pressure in the doctor's office and near normal pressures at home. The influence of stress on the office pressures suggests that these individuals are ideal candidates for a stress-management program. A small study compared white coat hypertension to a group with essential hypertension and showed significant decreases in systolic and diastolic blood pressures in both groups. The intervention was four sessions of direct blood-pressure feedback using the Finapres (finger BP monitoring) for 4 weeks.[33] In addition to the decreases in blood pressure, significant decreases in the responses to mental stress were found.

AUTONOMIC DYSFUNCTION

The classification of autonomic dysfunction is complex and the etiologies diverse. With regard to syncope, assessment of cardiovascular, noncardiac, and psychiatric diseases must be part of the differential diagnosis.[34] Current systems of classification subsume the autonomic dysfunctions into reflex syncope, dysautonomia, and postural orthostatic tachycardia syndrome (POTS).[35] POTS has been further subdivided into partial dysautonomic, hyperadrenergic, and neurally mediated syndromes.[36] Healthcare providers who have the major responsibility for patients with autonomic dysfunction are well advised to implement a multidimensional therapy plan, including medical and behavioral interventions, and to maintain open lines of communication among providers.[34] Behavioral interventions may include exercise, increased intake of fluid and salt, and use of elastic support hose. Psychological interventions include psychotherapy, relaxation therapy, and biofeedback.

Psychological and Physiological Factors in Syncope

In the hyperadrenergic type of POTS, patients often report anxiety and cold and sweaty hands and feet when they are upright or under conditions of psychological stress. They may have migraine-type headaches and other signs of excessive sympathetic activation. Patients who have experienced neurally mediated syncope often have concurrent health problems; gastrointestinal problems were reported by 61%, mood disturbances by 56%, and headaches by 53%. Additional comorbid conditions symptoms—including debilitating fatigue, dizziness, chest pain, and confusion—add to the distress for patients with syncope.[36]

A correlation was postulated to exist between anxiety as assessed with the Burns Anxiety Inventory and syncope during head-up tilt testing. Patients—particularly women—who were highly anxious were more likely to have a positive tilt test result.[37] Individuals who have blood or injury phobia that results in syncope are highly anxious when presented with triggering stimuli. A distinct and different autonomic pattern was observed in controls, in persons with panic disorder, and in those afraid of blood. Persons with panic disorder had the highest heart rates and the lowest heart-rate variability. Bloodphobic people showed more vagally mediated heart-rate variability than people with panic disorder. However, phobics experienced a clear diphasic response, beginning with sympathetic activation, followed quickly by parasympathetic dominance, bradycardia, and hypotension, only when confronted with the phobic stimulus and not under standard stress test conditions.[38]

An in-depth review characterized healthy men and women who have a tendency to faint during head-up tilt, despite lack of evidence of cardiovascular disease. The hypotension resulted from decreased peripheral resistance and increased levels of plasma epinephrine, while norepinephrine and plasma renin activity remained the same. The decrease in plasma volume is not the trigger that initiates syncope in these subjects. Rather, vasodilation may explain the presyncopal decline in peripheral vascular resistance.[39]

The recommended treatment of syncope is a combination of medical and psychosocial interventions. Psychiatric causes of syncope are common particularly in younger people and are associated with anxiety, depression, and somatoform disorders. Although one third of the young patients had an underlying psychiatric disorder, the elderly were more likely to have cardiovascular or medical problems.[40] In a group of 61 patients referred for evaluation of autonomic symptoms, the tilt positive group was younger and had higher scores on the Beck Depression Inventory in comparison to the tilt negative group. More severe symptoms of depression were associated with lower blood pressure. In a second group of 52 patients, skin temperature, skin conductance level, and forehead muscle tension were monitored during tilt, in addition to blood pressure and heart rate. Although systolic and diastolic blood pressure decreased in the tilt positive group, skin conductance decreased only in the tilt-positive group, thus implying decreased sweating and higher skin resistance. This change may be compensatory to hypotension or may indicate psychophysiologic arousal.[41]

BIOFEEDBACK IN SYNCOPE

A clinical series of 10 patients with repeated syncope was studied to test the effects of BFRT on the frequency of syncope, headache, lightheadedness, and dizziness. Six patients showed a major decrease in symptoms at the end of treatment. Patients who tended to be successful in this program were those who had migraine-type headaches and who showed some improvement after only a few training sessions.[42] In the controlled study of BFRT that followed the clinical series, 10 sessions of BFRT were compared to waitlist controls. The treated group evidenced significant decreases in headache and reduction in number of episodes of syncope in comparison to the waitlist controls. No changes were observed in lightheadedness, dizziness, or fatigue.[43]

Tilt training can be used as a type of biofeedback system for recurrent syncope.[44] Forty-two patients with frequent symptoms of syncope were repeatedly tilted to the same angle used for diagnostic testing. It was hypothesized that repeated exposure of the cardiovascular system to orthostatic stress would promote adaptation and lead to a reregulation of the cardiovascular reflex mechanism. Patients continued at home by standing close to the wall without moving for 30 minutes. At the 15-month follow-up, two-thirds of the 42 were free of syncope and reported a major improvement in quality of life.

Postural changes may assist patients to decrease symptoms of vasovagal syncope. Crossing the legs at the ankle and increasing tension in the large muscles of the lower body were found to have a beneficial effect on frequency of symptoms. Patients learned to predict the onset of presyncopal and syncopal episodes and were instructed to cross their legs and tense their muscles for at least 30 seconds. Thirteen of 20 patients reported that the maneuver had been integrated into their daily lives and that there was a significant reduction in frequency of syncopal episodes. Underlying the beneficial effects seem to be the increased sympathetic activity and peripheral resistance that is concomitant with strong muscle tension.[45]

Medically normal, well-conditioned subjects may experience syncope under conditions of significant orthostatic stress. Jet pilots exposed to microgravity often report varying degrees of motion sickness, including lightheadedness, dizziness, and sometimes near syncope. A training paradigm was designed to offset the effects of low gravity; it included four to nine sessions of autogenic feedback training. The pilots learned to increase blood pressure so that extreme lightheadedness did not occur during and after jet flights; repeated practice with several types of feedback also facilitated control of the autonomic nervous system so that nausea and vomiting was dramatically reduced.[46]

CARDIAC DISEASE

ROLE OF STRESS

The application of biofeedback, relaxation, and other stress management therapies to coronary disease is predicated on the relationship between psychological stress, personality type, hypothalamic-sympatho-adrenal activation, and cardiac function. The evidence to support that link consists of research exploring the relationship between psychologic state or the type-A behavior pattern and cardiovascular disease. Feelings of tension, sadness, and frustration were found to double the risk of myocardial ischemia in the hour after patients' experiencing these emotions.[47] Anxiety and depression predict cardiac events and are related to worsening heart disease.[48,49] Early findings that related the type-A behavior pattern with increased risk for myocardial infarction were refined during the last decade. Specifically, hostility was identified as an independent risk factor for cardiovascular disease.[50]

STRESS-MANAGEMENT PROGRAMS

Stress management programs were designed to assist patients who have had a myocardial infarction or who have heart disease to improve quality of life and reduce risk for future worsening of disease. More than 4 years after behavioral intervention that included relaxation, a trained group demonstrated lower morbidity and mortality than an education-alone group.[51] In a study of blood-pressure reactivity to a mental challenge, blood pressure increases were attenuated in the stress management plus exercise group but not in the exercise alone group. Improvement in perceived health status was also observed after behavioral training in 45 patients who had a prior myocardial infarction or coronary bypass surgery.[52] The effects of stress management were compared to propranolol in a small study of post–myocardial infarction patients who were asked to speak in public. The behavioral intervention was as effective in controlling the reactivity to public speaking as 20 mg of drug.[53]

Heart rate variability is an important index of cardiovascular function. In persons with anxiety disorders, variability is small and is associated with increased risk for cardiovascular morbidity.[54] The goal of heart rate variability feedback is to increase the range of variability, a goal achievable by patients with coronary heart disease by a combination of biofeedback and deep breathing training.[55] Biofeedback of heart rate variability can be incorporated into a treatment program for patients with heart disease. A variety of skills are taught and emphasize stress management and relaxation during stressful situations. A sense of personal control is suggested, and over time, patients are encouraged to rely on psychophysiologic self-regulation instead of relying completely on increasing medication to prevent worsening of disease ("use skills, not pills").[56]

Individualized training in relaxation and deep breathing were added to an exercise rehabilitation program in 76 patients who had experienced myocardial infarction. Increased variability, slower breathing and lower heart rate in comparison to controls who were offered exercise alone were recorded in trained patients.[57] One session of thermal biofeedback was tested in patients with advanced heart failure in comparison to no treatment controls. Patients were able to increase finger and toe temperatures; these changes were associated with a concurrent increase in cardiac output and decreases in systemic vascular resistance and breathing rate.[58] Unfortunately, no follow-up was undertaken in either group of patients, but the rapid learning of the response and the physiological effects in these patients with marked vasoconstriction supports further study of thermal biofeedback in heart failure.

TM was taught to nine women with syndrome X over a 3-month period. Outcome analysis showed a lessening of chest pain and an improved quality of life.[59] Exercise-induced ischemia was also reduced in patients with confirmed coronary artery disease who practiced TM.[60] The effects of TM were tested in a group of African Americans with hypertension by using carotid intima media thickness, an indicator of coronary atherosclerosis, as the outcome variable. The practice of TM was recommended twice a day for 20 minutes for three months. Results pointed to TM as a way of reducing carotid atherosclerosis compared to health education alone, with no additional relaxation skills training.[61]

A review of the literature dealing with psychophysiologic interventions in cardiac rehabilitation produced mixed results. It is difficult to show a clear advantage for adding stress management if subjects are neither anxious nor depressed at the onset. However, patients should be screened for psychological distress so programs can be designed to answer individual needs. Long-term follow-up studies are necessary to establish beneficial effects on morbidity and mortality.[62]

RAYNAUD'S DISEASE

Primary Raynaud's disease is characterized by spasm of arterioles that occurs predominately in the fingers and toes. Attacks that last minutes to hours are triggered by exposure to cold and emotional stress. Vasoconstriction of the arterioles produces color changes in the skin, including blanching, blueness, and redness, sometimes associated with pain. Thermal biofeedback training with home practice has been effectively used for patients with Raynaud's disease. A controlled study with 3-year follow-up supported the advantage of thermal biofeedback over relaxation alone; the biofeedback group sustained a 67% decrease in number of vasospastic episodes, which was consistent at follow-up.[63,64] Based on the strongly positive results described above, a multisite randomized controlled study was designed to compare thermal biofeedback with sustained-release nifedipine. Conclusions were that biofeedback was inferior to the drug. However, only a third of the participants learned to increase finger temperature to criterion.[65] Because the relief of symptoms is based on consciously producing warmer fingers, it is not surprising that inability to raise temperature was associated with poor symptom reduction. Although explanations for these results are beyond the scope of this chapter, one can speculate that omission of home practice and of suggestions to use imagery or breathing to facilitate warming may have contributed to these negative findings.[66]

CONCLUSION

Several biofeedback modalities are appropriate interventions for persons with cardiovascular diseases and may be combined with medical and behavioral management. Biofeedback alone is rarely efficacious in essential hypertension, autonomic dysfunction, and heart disease and is best coupled with relaxation therapy, reinforced by consistent home practice. Evidence for learning specific skills must be confirmed and patients must continue to use the skills after formal therapy has ended. Convincing evidence suggests that clinically significant decreases in blood pressure and in reactivity to stress occur in hypertensive individuals treated with BFRT if the following are true: (A) blood pressure is sensitive to stress; (B) patients learn the relaxation skills; and (C) patients are able to apply them to their personal sources of stress. Identification of characteristics of those most likely to succeed requires more research. Raynaud's disease treatment with thermal biofeedback showed promising results early, with elucidation of mechanism of response supporting the therapeutic effects. However, success depends on the acquisition of the hand-warming response and documented increases in hand temperature to criterion. Despite recent conflicting data on the efficacy of biofeedback in Raynaud's disease, the lack of side effects or complications from the biofeedback protocol shifts the balance toward offering biofeedback to patients before undertaking complicated medical interventions.

Combined medical, behavioral, and psychophysiologic therapies are recommended for those with autonomic dysfunction. When mood or anxiety disorders complicate the clinical picture, treatment must be directed toward alleviation of emotional symptoms before or during active biofeedback therapy. Biofeedback, postural movements, and relaxation skills must first be learned and then applied to specific stages of presyncope, syncope itself, and the accompanying comorbid conditions such as headache and nausea. A rationale to support a relationship between psychologic state, personality, and risk for cardiac disease exists. Stress management, including BFRT, contributes to the overall care of the patient with heart disease, clearly improving quality of life. Confirmation of specific effects on morbidity and mortality require further study.

REFERENCES

1. Schwartz M, Andrasik F: Biofeedback: a practitioner's guide, ed 3, New York, 2003, Guilford.
2. Davis M, Eshelman ER, McKay M: The relaxation and stress reduction workbook, ed 4, Oakland, CA, 1995, New Harbinger Publications.
3. Lehrer P, Woolfolk RL, editors: Principles and practice of stress management, ed 2, New York, 1993, Guilford.
4. Brook RD, Julius S: Autonomic imbalance, hypertension, and cardiovascular risk, Am J Hypertens 13:112S-122S, 2000.
5. McGrady AV, Higgins JT Jr: Prediction of response to biofeedback-assisted relaxation in hypertensives: development of a hypertensive predictor profile (HYPP), Psychosom Med 51:277-284, 1989.
6. Canino E, Cardona R, Monsalve P et al: A behavioral treatment program as a therapy in the control of primary hypertension, Behavior 45:23-30, 1994.
7. Blanchard EB, McCoy GC, Musso A et al: A controlled comparison of thermal biofeedback and relaxation training in the treatment of essential hypertension, I: short-term and long-term outcome, Behav Ther 17:563-579, 1986.
8. Blanchard E: Biofeedback treatments of essential hypertension, Biofeedback and Self Regulation 15:209-228, 1990.
9. McGrady AV, Linden W: Biobehavioral treatments of essential hypertension. In Schwartz M. Andrasik F, editors: Biofeedback: a practitioner's guide, ed 3, New York, 2003, Guilford, 382-408.
10. Goebel M, Viol GW, Orebaugh C: An incremental model to isolate specific effects of behavioral treatments in essential hypertension, Biofeedback and Self Regulation 18:255-280, 1993.
11. Glasgow MS, Engel BT, D'Lugoff BC: A controlled study of a standardized behavioral stepped treatment for hypertension, Psychosom Med 61:10-26, 1989.
12. Achmon J, Granek M, Golomb M, Hart J: Behavioral treatment of essential hypertension: a comparison between cognitive therapy and biofeedback of heart rate, Psychosom Med 51:152-164, 1989.
13. Rau H, Buhrer M, Weitkunat R: Biofeedback of R-Wave-to-Pulse interval normalizes blood pressure, App Phychophy & Biof 28:37-46, 2003.
14. Schneider RH, Staggers F, Alexander CN et al: A randomized controlled trial of stress reduction for hypertension in older African Americans, Hyperten 26:820-827, 1995.
15. Alexander CN, Schneider RH, Staggers F et al: Trial of stress reduction for hypertension in older African Americans, II: sex and risk subgroup analysis, Hyperten 28:228-237, 1996.

16. Linden W, Lenz JW, Con AH: Individualized stress management for primary hypertension: a randomized trial, Arch Intern Med 161:1071-1080, 2001.

17. Patel C, Marmot M: Can general practitioners use training in relaxation and management of stress to reduce mild hypertension? Brit Med J 296:12-14, 1988.

18. Henderson RJ, Hart MG, Lal SK, Hunyor SN: The effect of home training with direct blood pressure biofeedback of hypertensives: a placebo-controlled study, J Hypertens 16:771-778, 1998.

19. Blanchard EB, McCoy GC, McCaffrey RJ et al: Evaluation of a minimal-therapist-contact thermal biofeedback treatment program for essential hypertension, Biofeedback and Self Regul 12:93-103, 1987.

20. Rosenthal T, Alter A, Peleg E, Gavish B: Device-guided breathing exercises reduce blood pressure: ambulatory and home measurements, Am J Hyperten 14(1):74-76, 2001.

21. Schein M, Gavish B, Herz M et al: Treating hypertension with a device that slows and regularizes breathing: a randomized double-blind controlled study, J Human Hyperten 15:271-278, 2001.

22. Grossman E, Grossman A, Schein MH et al: Breathing control lowers blood pressure, J Human Hyperten 15:263-269, 2001.

23. Giannattasio C, Failla M, Meles E et al: Efficacy of self-treatment of hypertension at home with device-guided breathing, Am J Hyperten 5:186A, 2002.

24. McCraty R, Atkinson M, Tomasino D: Impact of a workplace stress reduction program on blood pressure and emotional health in hypertensive employees, J Altern Complement Med 9:355-369, 2003.

25. McGrady AV: Effects of group relaxation training and thermal biofeedback on blood pressure and related psychophysiological variables in essential hypertension, Biofeedback and Self-Regul 19:51-66, 1994.

26. Paran E, Amir M, Yaniv N: Evaluating the response of mild hypertensives to biofeedback-assisted relaxation using a mental stress test, J Behav Ther & Exp Psychiat 27(2):157-167, 1996.

27. McCubbin JA, Wilson JF: Relaxation training and opioid inhibition of blood pressure response to stress, J Consult and Clin Psychol 64:593-601, 1996.

28. Blumental JA, Sherwood A, Gullette ECD et al: Biobehavioral approaches to the treatment of essential hypertension, J Consult & Clin Psychol 70:569-589, 2002.

29. Spence JD, et al: Recommendations on stress management, JAMC 160(9 Suppl.):S46-S50, 1999.

30. Linden W, Chambers L: Clinical effectiveness of non-drug treatment for hypertension: a metaanalysis, Ann Behav Med 16:35-45, 1994.

31. Yucha CB, Clark L, Smith M et al: The effect of biofeedback in hypertension, Appl Nurs Res 14:29-35, 2001.

32. Collins R, Peto R, MacMahon S et al: Blood pressure, stroke and coronary heart disease, Lancet 335:827-838, 1990.

33. Nakao M, Nomura S, Shimosawa T et al: Blood pressure biofeedback treatment of whitecoat hypertension, J Psychosom Res 48:161-169, 2000.

34. Grubb BP, Olshansky B: Syncope: overview and approach to management. In Grubb BP, Olshansky B, editors: Syncope: mechanisms and management, Armonk, NY, 1998, Futura Publishing.

35. Grubb BP, Karas B: Clinical disorders of the autonomic nervous system associated with orthostatic intolerance: an overview of classification, clinical evaluation, and management, PACE 22:798-810, 1999.

36. Kanjwal Y, Kosinski D, Grubb BP: The postural orthostatic tachycardia syndrome: definitions, diagnosis and management, PACE 26:1747-57, 2003.

37. Cohen TJ, Thayapran N, Ibrahim B et al: An association between anxiety and neurocardiogenic syncope during head-up tilt table testing, PACE 23:837-841, 2000.

38. Dahllöf O, Lars-Göran O: The diphasic reaction in blood phobic situations: individually or stimulus bound? Scand J Behav Ther 27:97-104, 1998.

39. Evans JM, Leonelli FM, Ziegler MG et al: Epinephrine, vasodilation and hemoconcentration in syncopal, healthy men and women, Auton Neurosci 93:79-90, 2001.

40. Koenig D, Linzer M, Pontinen M, Divine GW: Syncope in young adults: evidence for a combined medical and psychiatric approach, J Intern Med 232:169-176, 1991.

41. McGrady A, Kern-Buell C, Bush E, Khuder S, Grubb BP: Psychological and physiological factors associated with tilt table testing for neurally mediated syncopal syndromes, PACE 24:296-301, 2001.

42. McGrady AV, Bush EG, Grubb BP: Outcome of biofeedback-assisted relaxation for neurocardiogenic syncope and headache: a clinical replication series, Appl Psychophysiol Biofeedback 22:63-72, 1997.

43. McGrady AV, Kern-Buell, C, Bush E et al: Biofeedback-assisted relaxation therapy in neurocardiogenic syncope: a pilot study, Appl Psychophy & Biof 28:183-192, 2003.

44. Girolamo ED, Di Iorio C, Leonzio L et al: Usefulness of a tilt training program for the prevention of refractory neurocardiogenic syncope in adolescents: a controlled study, Circulation 100:1798-1801, 1999.

45. Krediet CT, van Dijk N, Linzer M et al: Management of vasovagal syncope: controlling or aborting faints by leg crossing and muscle tensing, Circulation 106:1684-1689, 2002.

46. Cowlings PS, Toscano MA, Miller NE et al: Autogenic-feedback training: a potential treatment for orthostatic intolerance in aerospace crews, Pharmacol 34:599-608, 1994.

47. Gullette EC, Blumenthal JA, Babyak M et al: Effects of mental stress on myocardial ischemia during daily life, JAMA 277:1521-1526, 1997.

48. Frasure-Smith N, Lesperance F, Talajic M: The impact of negative emotions on prognosis following myocardial infarction: is it more than depression? Health Psychol 14:388-398, 1995.

49. Khawaja IS, Feinstein RE: Cardiovascular effects of selective serotonin reuptake inhibitors and other novel antidepressants, Heart Dis 5:153-160, 2003.

50. Everson SA, Kauhanen J, Kaplan GA et al: Hostility and increased risk of mortality and acute myocardial infarction, Am J Epidemiol 146:142-152, 1997.

51. Buselli EF, Stuart EM: Influence of psychosocial factors and biopsychosocial interventions on outcomes after myocardial infarction, J Cardiovasc Nurs 13:60-72, 1999.

52. Turner L, Linden W, van der Wal R, Schamberger W: Stress management for patients with heart disease: a pilot study, Heart and Lung 24:145-153, 1995.

53. Gatchel RJ, Gaffney FA, Smith JE: Comparative efficacy of behavioral stress management versus propranolol in reducing psychophysiological reactivity in post-myocardial infarction patients, J Behav Med 9:503-513, 1986.

54. Sullivan GM, Kent JM, Coplan JD: The neurobiology of stress and anxiety. In Mostofsky DI, Barlow DH, editors: The management of stress and anxiety in medical disorders, Boston, 2000, Allyn Bacon.

55. Song HS, Lehrer PM: The effects of specific respiratory rates on heart rate and heart rate variability, Applied Psychophy Biof 28:13-23, 2003.

56. Bhat N, Bhat K: Coronary disease and congestive heart disorder. In Moss D, McGrady A, Davies TC, Wickramasekera I, editors: Handbook of mind-body medicine for primary care, Thousand Oaks, Ca, 2003, Sage Publications.

57. Van Dixhoorn J: Cardiorespiratory effects of breathing and relaxation instruction in myocardial infarction patients, Biol Psychology 49:123-135, 1998.

58. Moser DK, Dracup K, Woo MA, Stevenson LW: Voluntary control of vascular tone by using skin-temperature biofeedback-relaxation in patients with advanced heart failure, Alter Ther Health Med 3:51-59, 1997.

59. Cunningham C, Brown S, Kaski JC: Effects of transcendental meditation on symptoms and electrocardiographic changes in patients with cardiac syndrome X, Am J Cardiol 85:653-655, 2000.

60. Zamarra JW, Schneider RH, Besseghini I et al: Usefulness of the transcendental meditation program in the treatment of patients with coronary artery disease, Am J Cardiol 77:867-870, 1996.

61. Castillo-Richmond A, Schneider RH, Alexander CN et al: Effects of stress reduction on carotid atherosclerosis in hypertensive African Americans, Stroke 31:568-573, 2000.

62. Linden W: Psychological treatments in cardiac rehabilitation: review of rationales and outcomes, J Psychosom Res 48:443-454, 2000.

63. Freedman RR, Ianni P, Wenig P: Behavioral Treatment of Raynaud's disease, J Consult Clin Psych 51:539-549, 1983.

64. Freedman RR, Ianni P, Wenig P: Behavioral treatment of Raynaud's disease: long-term follow-up, J Consult Clin Psych 53:136, 1985.

65. Raynaud's Treatment Study (RTS) Investigators: Comparison of sustained release nifedipine and temperature biofeedback for primary Raynaud's phenomenon: results from a randomized clinical trial with one year follow-up, Arch Intern Med 160:1101-1108, 2000.
66. Middaugh S, Haythornthwaite JA, Thompson B, Hill R et al: The Raynaud's treatment study: biofeedback protocols and acquisition of temperature biofeedback skills, Applied Psycho Biofeed 26:251-278, 2001.

CHAPTER 8

Cognitive-Behavioral Therapy in Cardiac Illness

Alan Witkower, EdD

James Rosado, PhD

This chapter is organized to provide the reader with a conceptualization of cognitive-behavioral therapy (CBT) and its application to the prevention and treatment of cardiac illness. The chapter begins with an overview of CBT and a review of the research literature supporting CBT's efficacy in treating a range of psychological and medical conditions and an outline of the treatment components of CBT. The reader is then introduced to two common conditions associated with cardiac illness that are effectively treated with CBT: (1) behavioral risk factors implicated in the development and outcome of cardiac illness; and (2) noncardiac chest pain. These two conditions are discussed in terms of the research literature's support of CBT as an effective intervention for these problems. This discussion is followed by an outline of how CBT has been applied to each of these conditions.

COGNITIVE-BEHAVIORAL THERAPY

CBT is a form of psychotherapy rooted in learning theory. It focuses on the modification of dysfunctional cognitions, emotions, and behaviors. CBT stresses an active, collaborative relationship between therapist and patient.[1] The cognitive part of CBT concentrates on identifying negative thought patterns, challenging those patterns, and replacing them with constructive thought patterns. The behavioral aspect of CBT encourages increasing the quantity of adaptive behavioral responses. The behavioral component also concentrates on a repeated cycle of identifying small problems, generating multiple solutions, evaluating them, testing out the best solution, and reviewing the results.[2]

Assumptions of CBT

CBT approaches share the following assumptions: (1) that cognitive mediational processes are involved in human learning; (2) cognitions may alter behavior by their influences on both emotional and physiologic responses and in turn, cognitions are equally influenced by emotional, physiological and behavioral events; (3) that cognitive activities, such as expectations, self-statements, and attributions, are important in understanding and predicting psychopathology and psychotherapeutic change; (4) that behaviors may be influenced by the environment and, reciprocally, the individual's behaviors may influence environmental events; (5) that a person will need to learn alternative ways of behaving and feeling in addition to modifying cognitions; (6) that patients can be instrumental in learning adaptive strategies for coping with and managing symptoms; and (7) that patients with similar diagnoses have common dysfunctions and symptoms and may therefore be similar in their response to standardized treatment programs.[3-5]

Goals for CBT

The goals for CBT include the following: (1) modifying patients' views of their medical problems from being overwhelming to being manageable; (2) changing patients' perceptions of themselves as being passive to being active collaborators; (3) requiring patients to monitor their thoughts, feelings, and behaviors in order to yield a connection between these and their symptoms; (4) training patients in the skills necessary to manage their symptoms; (5) encouraging patients to attribute their successes to their efforts at employing those sets of skills; and (6) teaching patients how to anticipate and manage future exacerbations of symptoms or changes in their physical status.[5]

Review of CBT Efficacy

In studies that compared cognitive therapy (CT) and CBT to pharmacological treatments, CT and CBT were concluded to be as effective as medication in reducing depressive symptoms.[6-10] CBT has been well established as an efficacious treatment for a range of depressive disorders.[11,12] For depression of mild to moderate severity, CBT has been shown to be as effective as antidepressant medication. However, the improvement is initially slower than with medication, and the duration of effect has not been clearly established.[13,14]

Additionally, some studies also concluded that CBT provided a preventative effect in reducing relapse rates when treatment with medications is discontinued.[15,16] CBT has also been efficacious in the treatment of another set of common psychiatric disturbances, generalized anxiety disorder, and panic disorder.[17-20]

CBT, with its structured, empirical, and problem-focused approach, is a treatment of choice for behavioral medicine practitioners. CBT has proven to be cost-effective and efficacious in a variety of illnesses and at-risk populations, in terms of modifying health behaviors, promoting effective coping skills, and enhancing psychosocial and physical well-being.[21] CBT has been employed extensively in treating patients with chronic medical problems.[22-26] Of particular relevance to the use of CBT and cardiac illness are the numerous studies supporting it's efficacy in treating the functional somatic or psychophysiologic disorders. These are disorders in which psychological factors and stress are considered primary contributors to the initiation, exacerbation, or maintenance of the symptoms of the disorder.[27-30] CBT has been studied and reviewed in the treatment of chronic fatigue syndrome,[31-34] irritable bowel syndrome,[35-37] hypochondriasis,[38] and mixed functional somatic symptoms.[39] Therefore it is not surprising that CBT is particularly well suited to patients with coronary heart disease.[40,41]

TREATMENT COMPONENTS OF CBT

In general, CBT interventions have several components that follow each other in a logical progression of education and training.[42,43] These components or stages of treatment are generally flexible enough that a patient may move back and forth between stages at the same time that he or she is progressing in the overall management of his or her symptoms or illness.[44] The stages of treatment are commonly subsumed under four overlapping categories: (1) reconceptualization; (2) skills acquisition; (3) cognitive and behavioral rehearsal; and (4) generalization and relapse management.[45]

Reconceptualization

In this phase of treatment the objective is to provide the patient with a rationale for CBT and to elicit and clarify the patient's expectation about treatment.[46] The patient and therapist will engage in an exchange of ideas, information, and questioning. Additionally, the patient is encouraged to be receptive to suggestions by the therapist and at the same time to provide feedback to the therapist regarding what is being asked of the patient.[47] Successful engagement of the patient in the process of the treatment at this point will enhance the likelihood of the patient actively participating in subsequent stages of treatment.[5,45-47]

Skill Acquisition

In this phase the objective is to promote the successful acquisition and use of adaptive coping strategies.[5] These strategies can be broadly grouped into behavioral and cognitive coping strategies. The behavioral strategies are directed at reducing excessive autonomic arousal, eliminating maladaptive behavior patterns, and increasing the patient's self-efficacy for using effective coping strategies. The cognitive strategies focus on maladaptive thoughts, beliefs, and appraisal that create heightened emotional and physical arousal or that interfere with the patient using adaptive coping strategies.[45]

Cognitive and Behavioral Rehearsal

In this stage of CBT the task for patients is to integrate the skills acquired in the previous stage and to practice these skills in their everyday lives. Several techniques are employed in this stage, including stress inoculation and role-playing. Effectively managing the stress in everyday life is clearly applicable to patients experiencing cardiac illness. Role-playing permits the patient to rehearse with the therapist or group members the strategies for modifying risk behaviors.

Relapse Management

In this final phase of cognitive-behavioral treatment patients are asked to focus on the circumstances in which they might be prone to relapse.[48,49] This discussion is not intended to suggest to patients that they are expected to fail in modifying their maladaptive behaviors. Rather, it is to recognize that they will likely experience exacerbations of their symptoms or recurrence of their illnesses and that these situations may challenge their coping resources. Once these high-risk situations are identified, patients are encouraged to problem-solve how they will handle that particular situation. During this final stage of treatment patients are asked to review what they have learned and to compare how they were feeling and functioning at the beginning of treatment with how they are currently feeling and functioning at the moment.[45] Ultimately, the goal of this stage of treatment is to reinforce for patients the following: (1) that they have developed a repertoire of coping strategies that have been effective in reducing their headaches or improving their sleep; (2) that the success of these strategies have been a function of their efforts; and (3) that their continued success depends upon their continued adherence to these strategies.[48,50]

BEHAVIORAL RISK FACTORS

Evidence implicating stress' adverse effect on cardiac health began to emerge nearly 3 decades ago with a study by Rosenman et al[51] that showed that men with type-A behavior were twice as likely as men with type-B behavior or men who lacked type-A characteristics to develop cardiac illnesses over an 8.5-year period. Subsequent research makes a strong case that of the three components of the global type-A behavior pattern, hostility is the one most reliably associated with increased coronary heart disease risk.[52-55] More recent studies provide clear and convincing evidence that psychosocial factors contribute significantly to both the development and expression of cardiac illnesses. Two recent literature reviews have identified four broad domains of psychosocial risk factors for cardiac illness.[56,57] The domain of psychological traits includes type-A behaviors and hostility; the domain of psychological states includes anxiety and depression; the domain of work includes issues of control, demands, and supports; and the domain of social network includes isolation and social supports.[56,57] As a group, these psychosocial risk factors for cardiac illness are associated with unhealthy lifestyle behaviors. When psychosocial risk factors cooccur, cardiovascular risk further increases.[56,58,59] Psychosocial risk factors can impact the development and outcome of cardiac illnesses in two ways:[53,56,58,60] (1) by contributing to health-related behaviors like smoking, poor diet, sedentary lifestyle, and increased alcohol consumption;[61,62] and (2) by causing direct acute or chronic psychophysiologic changes, including increased cardiovascular/neuroendocrine reactivity to stress,[63] increased platelet activation,[64,65] increased release of inflammatory cytokines,[66,67] or increased expression of the metabolic syndrome in nondiabetic persons.[68-70] The introduction of CBT and stress-management educational interventions has demonstrated efficacy in reducing the impact of these psychosocial risk factors.[21,53,58,60,71]

Upon a careful review of the literature, the Cardiac Rehabilitation Guideline Panel[72] concluded that strong scientific evidence supported the efficacy of psychosocial and psycho-educational interventions to attenuate stress (i.e., anxiety, depression, distress, and type-A behavior) and enhance quality of life. Positive outcomes included reducing cholesterol levels,[73,75] systolic blood pressure,[73,75,76] obesity,[73] and cardiovascular reactivity.[75,76] The efficacy of CBT approaches for the treatment of hypertension was also demonstrated in the Treatment of Mild Hypertension Study[77] and reductions in dietary sodium,[78] sedentary lifestyles,[79] and hostility.[21,80] Incorporating a CBT intervention, the Recurrent Coronary Prevention Project has further demonstrated that reducing psychosocial risk factors is associated with a 44% reduction of cardiac events after myocardial infarction compared with usual care.[81]

CBT AND BEHAVIORAL RISK FACTORS

The following is a generalized CBT approach to managing several of the common behavioral risk factors—smoking, obesity, and exercise.

Reconceptualization

At this stage of CBT treatment the goal is to engage patients in identifying their motivations for achieving nicotine abstinence, weight loss, or an increase in physical activity. Patients may present various reasons for wanting to lose weight, such as physical appearance, health, work, functional, and/or sports-related concerns. The same is true for smoking cessation. However, these goals are usually presented without an understanding of the process and commitment involved in making the necessary behavioral changes. During this stage of treatment the focus must be on clarifying and differentiating the truths from fiction regarding reasons for wanting to quit smoking, lose weight, or begin an exercise regimen. This is a time for discussion with patients regarding the medical, psychological, and social implications for smoking cessation, weight loss, and exercise. Patients often have incompatible and unrealistic expectations in terms of what they want and are able to do regarding exercise. A common misperception is that exercise requires vigorous physical activity or membership at a fitness center, when in actuality a simple daily walking routine may suffice. Therefore clarification of a person's personal view, understanding, and expectations is critical. The goal is to increase patients' awareness and understanding of both internal and external determinants of smoking, eating, or avoidance of exercise. Thoughts, feelings, and behaviors most closely linked to smoking, eating, or avoiding exercise can be addressed first and can be followed by others that are less associated or obvious to patients. Shaping of behaviors is a gradual process, particularly with behaviors that have powerful reinforcers such as nicotine or food. Although, the process of behavioral change is difficult to engage in for the first time, educating patients in advance regarding the overall treatment process may increase adherence to the program.

Skill Acquisition

At this stage in treatment, patients' resources and coping skills need to be assessed. Prior attempts at changing health-related behaviors (e.g., previous efforts to quit smoking, to lose weight, or to start an exercise program) are discussed in greater detail to assess the patient's level of awareness, ability, and coping in this regard. Assessing an individual's premorbid and postincident exercise habits is important because most patients present with varying levels of exercise tolerance. During this stage, maladaptive behaviors may be identified for either elimination or modification. For example, patients may have tried controlling the size of the food portions consumed without considering the actual caloric content. Another key aspect of this stage of CBT is establishing a treatment plan that identifies realistic goals and objectives. The treatment plans must include goals and objectives that are commensurate with the patients' abilities and skills, and their motivational, psychological, and physical status. For example, establishing a quit date must take into account the likelihood of achieving this goal when considering patients' stressors, functionality, and the need and availability of social support and other healthy nonsmoking activities. Goals for modification of dietary habits could include increasing healthy behaviors such as regular eating times, adequate food portions and preparations, exercise, medical exams, and education related to proper nutrition and meal planning. Breaking down the expected behavioral changes into manageable, discrete components is particularly helpful, especially when patients experience anxiety regarding their involvement in the activity. For patients whose goal is to increase their physical activity, suggesting they start with simple stretches or brief walks at a local park, mall, or around the block may be sufficient to overcome anxiety or the inertia of a sedentary lifestyle. Encouraging patients to select an exercise partner might also increase the likelihood of the patient engaging in exercise since a companion is generally quite motivating, safe, and fun. Patients need to recognize the environmental (e.g., work, financial difficulties), emotional (e.g., depression, anxiety), and physical (e.g., fatigue) stressors that can increase their likelihood of picking up a cigarette or eating inappropriately. Teaching relaxation techniques such as diaphragmatic breathing, autogenics, or cognitive coping strategies such as a thought stopping technique or mindfulness meditation can replace the previous maladaptive responses to stress.

Cognitive and Behavioral Rehearsal

Although homework is an essential component of all the stages of a CBT approach, it can be best illustrated by its role in the rehearsal stage of treatment. At this point in the treatment patients are being asked to engage in progressively more challenging tasks and activities in their everyday lives. The homework assignments are concrete, observable, and measurable and are established in a graded fashion to parallel patients' progression in treatment. These assignments can be useful in providing opportunities for receiving a critique on their application of the behavioral change strategies or an adjustment of the patient's original goals. An example, early in the treatment process is to request patients keep a log of their daily activity levels or track the amount of food consumed or frequency of eating during the day. Another example for increasing exercise tolerance may begin with walking short distances close to home with gradual increases in distances and speed. As patients demonstrate more proficiency in using adaptive strategies such as relaxation or assertiveness to alter their risk behaviors, the homework assignments become more difficult. Examples of tasks assigned later in the course of CBT treatment include the following: (1) having the patient make reservations at a favorite restaurant but with restrictions on the portions or type of food ordered; or (2) suggesting that the patient spend time with friends who smoke and are likely to offer the patient a cigarette. The more that realistic assignments are successfully completed, the greater the likelihood that the patient will attribute his success to his own efforts and abilities rather than to the help of others.

Cognitive rehearsal is a technique that the patient can do with the CBT clinician, or the patient may be encouraged to use this strategy independently before confronting a potentially stressful situation. In the example above, where the patient is asked to spend time with friends who smoke, he or she could first imagine using a learned strategy, such as assertiveness, to convey his or her determination not to accept a cigarette. Focusing the patient's attention on the successes achieved whether in actual practice or during cognitive rehearsal will serve to reinforce the patient's sense of self-efficacy and confidence.

Relapse Management

In the final phase of a CBT approach to modifying risk behaviors, patients are asked to focus on the circumstances in which they might be prone to relapse. The potential for relapse always exists, but the critical aspect of this stage of treatment is assessing the likelihood for relapse. At this point in treatment patients are taught how to identify the warning signs for an early relapse. For patients who have quit smoking, these signs might include increased feelings of cravings, missing the comfort of the cigarettes, noticing a tendency to avoid verbalizing problems, or not engaging in compensatory strategies such as chewing gum. Individuals who have lost weight may notice the first sign of possible relapse is isolating and withdrawing when anxious or overwhelmed. Using excuses to avoid working out or noticing a decrease in the frequency or duration of the work outs are generally reliable cues of an impending relapse for patients who need to be physically more active. Once these red flags are identified the patients are encouraged to problem solve how they will handle that particular situation.

During this final stage of treatment, patients are asked to review what they have learned and to compare how they were feeling and functioning at the beginning of treatment with how they are currently feeling and functioning.

When patients monitor the money saved by not smoking, noticing how clothing fits more comfortably, or observing how many more stairs can be climbed without being out of breath, they are increasing the likelihood of persisting with these lifestyle changes.

NONCARDIAC CHEST PAIN

Chest pain occurs often and is usually benign.[82] Despite this, myocardial ischemia remains important because it is potentially fatal. This leads to an understandable tendency to over investigate, so that as few as 11% to 44% of patients referred to cardiac outpatient clinics have evidence of organic disease,[30,83,84] and up to 31% of patients receiving coronary angiography are shown to have normal coronary anatomy.[85] Although mortality and morbidity from coronary angiography are small, an erroneous diagnosis of coronary disease is difficult to revoke. Most patients with persistent noncardiac pain are happy to accept that they do not have a serious condition, provided that they are given a satisfactory alternative explanation for the pain.[30,85] Negative physical investigation and reassurance are only effective for a small proportion of patients.[86,87] Patients are frequently not reassured by investigation, and there is some evidence that the process of investigation itself may entrench the idea of cardiac disease.[38] One half remain or become unemployed, one half remain on cardiac medication and about three-quarters continue to experience pain.[88,89] Despite a normal expectation of life and physical prognosis, between 50% and 70% continue to experience symptoms, worry about heart disease, restrict their activities, and seek medical help.[84,85,90-92] However, evidence suggests that a CBT intervention is effective in reducing symptoms and disability caused by the symptoms.[88,93] Klimes and colleagues showed that a CBT intervention involving between seven and 11 1-hour sessions with a clinical psychologist was effective in treating patients recruited from general practice with persistent chest pain despite reassurance by cardiologists.[86] A subsequent trial showed that the same procedures were effective in a cardiac outpatient clinic but that there were some practical problems of acceptability.[94] CBT treatment has also been demonstrated effective in several randomized controlled trials,[86,92-94] including one in a group setting.[95] Patients who underwent the group therapy had significantly improved outcomes in terms of reduction in the frequency and severity of chest pain, reduced functional disability as measured by the SF36, less psychological distress, and improved exercise tolerance. Significantly, patients who continued to attribute their pain to heart disease had poorer outcomes. These findings, which were maintained at 6-month follow-up, have important economic implications for the management of patients with noncardiac chest pain.[85,96]

CBT and Noncardiac Chest Pain

The following is an overview of the application of CBT interventions to address the preoccupation and distress of patients with noncardiac chest pain as reviewed above.

Reconceptualization

Although these patients' chest pains are not cardiac, it is imperative that their worries, thoughts, and associated feelings are acknowledged and validated as legitimate and understandable as a form of human suffering. Afterward, further clarification will introduce other possible explanations for the chest pain. This process can aid in fostering a sense of trust, understanding, and eventual acceptance of the help and explanations being offered. An alternative explanation for noncardiac chest pain may best be provided via experiments that test the patient's hypothesis. The hyperventilation provocation test can be used with patients to demonstrate quite dramatically how minor physiological changes caused by overbreathing can cause distressful symptoms. These symptoms mirror the very same sensations, including chest pain, which the patients misinterpret for a serious cardiac condition. Formulating patients' problems in terms of the interaction between cognitions, emotions, and physiology can reassure patients they are not crazy but that a cognitive-behavioral approach can be helpful. Some patients are able to gain insight when given the opportunity to express and explore psychosocial issues in their lives and to understand and accept alternative explanations for their noncardiac chest pain. However, others may persist in believing that there exists a plausible, physical illness that is the cause of the chest pain.

Skill Acquisition

Given that these patients are responding to symptoms generated by their own misperceptions and misinterpretations, the initial phase of skill training is in the area of cognitive reevaluation and restructuring. The patients are first encouraged to identify the specific worries; then patients and their CBT therapist review the actual facts supporting or refuting these perceptions. More accurate and benign interpretations are created and reintroduced to the patients. Patients are taught how to engage in internal dialogues that routinely challenge catastrophic thinking and misinterpretations. As in the reconceptualization phase of treatment, patients might be encouraged to repeatedly provoke the somatic experiences that frighten them. Eventually a deconditoning effect interferes with patients' conditioned responses to these physiological states.

The behavioral component of a CBT approach to noncardiac chest pain asks patients to visualize themselves experiencing symptoms suggestive of a cardiac event. With coaching and practice, patients begin to identify the early physical cues that result in the amplified and more distressful chest tightening and pain. Concomitantly, patients are instructed in various relaxation techniques, particularly the diaphragmatic breathing and muscle-relaxation strategies. Breathing retraining is particularly useful in forestalling hyperventilation. Patients then apply these relaxation strategies to the early physical cues and ultimately interrupt the escalation of the physiologic symptoms.

Cognitive and Behavioral Rehearsal

Patients are asked to practice the behavioral skills between sessions and are encouraged to try out the behavioral experiments in various settings to further confirm the rational explanations for their symptoms. Monitoring their experiences and recording their thoughts and reactions in various circumstances provides more data for review in the sessions. Diary-keeping also promotes patients' responsibility for collaborating in their treatment and implies that patients have more control over the production and management of their symptoms. Listing and then listening to their maladaptive thoughts provides a concrete illustration and opportunity for the patient to review and more effectively understand their possible distortions. Once patients have some control over their symptoms, they may proceed to creating a hierarchy of activities and places they have avoided for fear of eliciting an attack. Patients are then encouraged to gradually approach these situations or participate in these activities while employing the behavioral strategies to manage their physiologic reactivity.

Relapse Management

Ultimately, patients with noncardiac chest pain need assistance to identify and address lifestyle and personality variables that may contribute to their physiological sensitivity and catastrophic thinking. As with the CBT approach to risk factors for cardiac illness, patients with noncardiac chest pain are encouraged to identify the stressful circumstances in which they are most likely to experience the beginning of the cascade of symptoms (i.e., breathing difficulty, chest tightness and chest pain). As patients begin to resume physical pursuits they had once avoided or engage in social outings that had been severely restricted, they regain their confidence and begin to discount the distraction of their symptoms.

CONCLUSION

CBT has been demonstrated empirically to be a therapeutic intervention for a wide variety of psychiatric and medical disorders. This chapter has attempted to provide a conceptual model of CBT and demonstrate its applicability to two conditions commonly associated with cardiac illness: behavioral risk factors and noncardiac chest pain. The hope is that this chapter has informed the clinician of the efficacy of CBT for intervening with the behavioral risk factors associated with the development and outcome of cardiac illness; and has demonstrated the utility and practicality of CBT for noncardiac chest pain. Additionally, it is hoped that these examples of CBT applied to such conditions will permit the clinician to be confident in introducing and preparing patients with cardiac illness for referral for CBT when appropriate.

REFERENCES

1. Otto MW, Reilly-Harrington NA, Harrington JA: Cognitive-behavioral therapy. In Stern TA, Herman JB, Flavin PL, editors: The MGH guide to psychiatry in primary care, New York, 1998, McGraw-Hill, 543-547.
2. Hollon SD: What is cognitive behavioural therapy and does it work? Curr Opin Neurobiol 8:289-292, 1998.

3. Michenbaum DH, Cameron R: Cognitive behavior therapy. In Wilson GT, Franks CM, editors: Contemporary behavior therapy, New York, 1982, Guilford Press.

4. Turk DC, Okifuji A, Scharff L: Chronic pain and depression: role of perceived impact and perceived control in different age cohorts, Pain 61:93-101, 1995.

5. Witkower A: Behavioral medicine assessment and treatment. In Wittink H, Michel T, editors: Chronic pain management for physical therapists, Boston, Butterworth and Heinemann; 2002:161-177.

6. Hollon SD, Shelton RC, Loosen PT: Cognitive therapy and pharmacotherapy for depression, J Consult Clin Psychol 59:88-99, 1991.

7. Hollon SD, DeRubeis RJ, Evans MD, et al: Cognitive therapy and pharmacotherapy for depression: singly and in combination, Arch Gen Psychiatry 49:774-781, 1992.

8. Murphy GE, Simons AD, Wetzel RD, Lustman PJ: Cognitive therapy and pharmacotherapy: singly and together in the treatment of depression, Arch Gen Psychiatry 41:33-41, 1984.

9. Rush AJ, Beck AT, Kovacs M, Weissenburger J, Hollon SD: Comparison of the effects of cognitive therapy and pharmacotherapy on hopelessness and self-concept, Am J Psychiatry 139:862-866, 1982.

10. Rush AJ, Kovacs M, Beck AT, Weissenburger J, Hollon SD: Differential effects of cognitive therapy and pharmacotherapy on depressive symptoms, J Affect Disord 3:221-229, 1981.

11. Dobson KS. A meta-analysis of the efficacy of cognitive therapy for depression, J Consult Clin Psychol 57:414-419, 1989.

12. Robinson LA, Berman JS, Neimeyer RA: Psychotherapy for the treatment of depression: a comprehensive review of controlled outcome research, Psychol Bul 108:30-49, 1990.

13. Schulberg HC, Katon WJ, Simon GE, Rush AJ: Best clinical practice: guidelines for managing major depression in primary medical care, J Clin Psychiatry 60(Suppl 7):19-26, 1999.

14. DeRubeis RJ, Gelfand LA, Tang TZ, Simons AD: Medications versus cognitive behavior therapy for severely depressed outpatients: mega-analysis of four randomized comparisons [see comment], Am J Psychiatry 156:1007-1013, 1999.

15. Kovacs M, Rush AJ, Beck AT, Hollon SD: Depressed outpatients treated with cognitive therapy or pharmacotherapy: a one-year follow-up, Arch Gen Psychiatry 38:33-39, 1981.

16. Simons AD, Murphy GE, Levine JL, Wetzel RD: Cognitive therapy and pharmacotherapy for depression: sustained improvement over one year, Arch Gen Psychiatry 43:43-48, 1986.

17. Beck AT, Emery G: Anxiety disorders and phobias: a cognitive perspective, New York, 1985, Basic Books.

18. Beck AT, Epstein N, Brown G, Steer RA: An inventory for measuring anxiety: psychometric properties, J Consult Clin Psychol 56:893-7, 1988.

19. Beck AT, Steer RA, Ball R, Ranieri W: Comparison of Beck Depression Inventories IA and II in psychiatric outpatients, J Pers Assess 67:588-597, 1996.

20. Chambless DL, Gillis MM: Cognitive therapy of anxiety disorders, J Consult Clin Psychol 61:248-260, 1993.

21. Landel JL, Yount SE: Cognitive-behavioral therapy: applications and advances in behavioral medicine, Curr Opin Psychiatry 9:439-444, 1996.

22. Compton AB, Purviance M: Emotional distress in chronic medical illness: treatment with time-limited group psychotherapy, Mil Med 157:533-535, 1992.

23. Goodwin PJ, Leszcz M, Koopmans J, et al: Randomized trial of group psychosocial support in metastatic breast cancer: the BEST study: Breast-Expressive Supportive Therapy study, Cancer Treat Rev.22(Suppl A):91-96, 1996.

24. Goodwin PJ, Leszcz M, Quirt G, et al: Lessons learned from enrollment in the BEST study: a multicenter, randomized trial of group psychosocial support in metastatic breast cancer, J Clin Epidemiol 53:47-55, 2000.

25. Kelly JA: Group psychotherapy for persons with HIV and AIDS-related illnesses, Int J Group Psychother 48:143-162, 1998.

26. Spiegel D: Health caring. Psychosocial support for patients with cancer, Cancer 74(4 Suppl):1453-1457, 1994.

27. Sharpe M, Peveler R, Mayou R: The psychological treatment of patients with functional somatic symptoms: a practical guide, J Psychosom Res 36:515-529, 1992.

28. Sharpe M: Cognitive behavior therapy for functional somatic complaints: the example of chronic fatigue syndrome, Psychosomatics 38:356-362, 1997.

29. Kroenke K, Arrington ME, Mangelsdorff AD: The prevalence of symptoms in medical outpatients and the adequacy of therapy, Arch Intern Med 150:1685-1689, 1990.

30. Kroenke K, Mangelsdorff AD: Common symptoms in ambulatory care: incidence, evaluation, therapy, and outcome, Am J Med 86:262-266, 1989.

31. Sharpe M, Chalder T, Palmer I, Wessely S: Chronic fatigue syndrome: a practical guide to assessment and management, Gen Hosp Psychiatry 19:185-199, 1997.

32. Sharpe M, Hawton K, Simkin S et al: Cognitive behaviour therapy for the chronic fatigue syndrome: a randomized controlled trial, BMJ 312(7022):22-26, 1996.

33. Sharpe M: Cognitive behavior therapy for chronic fatigue syndrome: efficacy and implications, Am J Med 105(3A):104S-109S, 1998.

34. Deale A, Chalder T, Marks I, Wessely S: Cognitive behavior therapy for chronic fatigue syndrome: a randomized controlled trial, Am J Psychiatry 154:408-414, 1997.

35. Greene B, Blanchard EB: Cognitive therapy for irritable bowel syndrome, J Consult Clin Psychol 62:576-582, 1994.

36. Blanchard EB, Schwarz SP: Adaptation of a multicomponent treatment for irritable bowel syndrome to a small-group format, Biofeedback Self Regul 12:63-69, 1987.

37. Blanchard EB, Schwarz SP, Suls JM, et al: Two controlled evaluations of multicomponent psychological treatment of irritable bowel syndrome, Behav Res Ther 30:175-189, 1992.

38. Barsky AJ, Ahern DK: Cognitive behavior therapy for hypochondriasis. JAMA 291: 1464-70, 2004.

39. Speckens AE, van Hemert AM, Spinhoven P, et al: Cognitive behavioural therapy for medically unexplained physical symptoms: a randomised controlled trial, BMJ 311(7016):1328-1332, 1995.

40. Allan R, Scheidt S. Group psychotherapy for patients with coronary heart disease, Int J Group Psychother 48:187-214, 1998.

41. Thoresen CE, Bracke P. Reducing coronary recurrences and coronary-prone behavior in groups, In Spira J, editor: Group therapy of the medically ill, New York, 1997, Guilford.

42. Bradley LA: Cognitive-behavioral therapy for chronic pain. In Gatchel RJ, Turk DC, editors: Psychological approaches to pain management: a practitioner's handbook, New York, 1996, Guilford Press.

43. Kendell PC, Braswell L: Cognitive-behavioral therapy for impulsive children, New York, 1985, Guilford.

44. Ott BD: Behavioral interventions in the management of chronic pain. In Aronoff GM, editor: Evaluation and treatment of chronic pain, Baltimore, 1992, Williams and Wilkins.

45. Witkower A: Cognitive-behavioral therapy with neurological disorders. In Weintraub MI, Micozzi MS, editors: Alternative and complementary treatment in neurological illness, New York, 2001, Churchill Livingstone, 183-196.

46. Bernstein DA, Borkovec TD: Progressive relaxation training: a manual for the helping professions, Champaign, IL, 1973, Research Press.

47. Kroger WS, Felzer WD: Hypnosis and behavior modification: imagery conditioning, Philidelphia, 1976, JB Lippincott.

48. Holtzman AD, Turk DC, Kerns RD: The cognitive-behavioral approach to the management of chronic pain. In Holtzman AD, Turk DC, editors: Pain management: a handbook of psychological treatment approaches, Elmsford, NY, 1986, Pergamon Press, 31-50.

49. Turk DC, Michenbaum D, Genest M: Pain and behavioral medicine, New York, 1983, Guilford.

50. Meichenbaum D, Turk DC: Facilitating treatment adherence: a practioner's guidebook, New York, 1987, Plenum Press.

51. Rosenman RH, Brand RJ, Jenkins D et al: Coronary heart disease in Western Collaborative Group Study: final follow-up experience of 8 ½ years, JAMA 233:872-877, 1975.

52. Williams RB, Jr., Haney TL, Lee KL et al: Type A behavior, hostility, and coronary atherosclerosis, Psychosom Med 42:539-549, 1980.

53. Williams RB, Barefoot JC, Schneiderman N: Psychosocial risk factors for cardiovascular disease: more than one culprit at work [Editorial], JAMA 290:2190-2192, 2003.

54. Miller TQ, Smith TW, Turner CW, Guijarro ML, Hallet AJ: A metaanalytic review of research on hostility and physical health, Psychol Bull 119(2):322-348, 1996.

55. Williams JE, Paton CC, Siegler IC et al: Anger proneness predicts coronary heart disease risk: prospective analysis from the atherosclerosis risk in communities (ARIC) study, Circulation 101:2034-2039, 2000.

56. Rozanski A, Blumenthal JA, Kaplan J: Impact of psychological factors on the pathogenesis of cardiovascular disease and implications for therapy, Circulation 99:2192-2217, 1999.

57. Hemingway H, Marmot M: Evidence based cardiology: psychosocial factors in the aetiology and prognosis of coronary heart disease: systematic review of prospective cohort studies, BMJ 318(7196):1460-1467, 1999.

58. Schneiderman N, Antoni MH, Saab PG, Ironson G: Health psychology: psychosocial and biobehavioral aspects of chronic disease management, Annu Rev Psychol 52:555-580, 2001.

59. Watkins LLA, Schneiderman N, Blumenthal JA et al: Cognitive and somatic symptoms of depression are associated with medical comorbidity in patients after acute myocardial infarction, Am Heart J 146:48-54, 2003.

60. Berkman LF, Blumenthal J, Burg M et al: Effects of treating depression and low perceived social support on clinical events after myocardial infarction: the Enhancing Recovery in Coronary Heart Disease Patients (ENRICHD) Randomized Trial [comment], JAMA 289:3106-3116, 2003.

61. Scherwitz LW, Perkins LL, Chesney MA et al: Hostility and health behaviors in young adults: the CARDIA Study, Coronary Artery Risk Development in Young Adults Study, Am J Epidemiol 136:136-145, 1992.

62. Siegler IC, Peterson BL, Barefoot JC, Williams RB: Hostility during late adolescence predicts coronary risk factors at mid-life, Am J Epidemiol 136:146-154, 1992.

63. Suarez EC, Kuhn CM, Schanberg SM, Williams RB, Jr, Zimmermann EA: Neuroendocrine, cardiovascular, and emotional responses of hostile men: the role of interpersonal challenge, Psychosom Med 60:78-88, 1998.

64. Markovitz JH: Hostility is associated with increased platelet activation in coronary heart disease, Psychosom Med 60:586-591, 1998.

65. Markovitz JH, Matthews KA, Kiss J, Smitherman TC: Effects of hostility on platelet reactivity to psychological stress in coronary heart disease patients and in healthy controls, Psychosom Med 58:143-149, 1996.

66. Musselman DL, Miller AH, Porter MR, et al. Higher than normal plasma interleukin-6 concentrations in cancer patients with depression: preliminary findings, Am J Psychiatry 158:1252-1257, 2001.

67. Rothermundt M, Arolt V, Peters M et al: Inflammatory markers in major depression and melancholia, J Affect Disorder 63(1-3):93-102, 2001.
68. Surwit RS, Williams RB, Siegler IC et al: Hostility, race, and glucose metabolism in nondiabetic individuals, Diabetes Care 25:835-839, 2002.
69. Niaura R, Todaro JF, Stroud L et al: Hostility, the metabolic syndrome, and incident coronary heart disease, Health Psychol 21:588-593, 2002.
70. Niaura R, Banks SM, Ward KD et al: Hostility and the metabolic syndrome in older males: the normative aging study, Psychosom Med 62:7-16, 2000.
71. Williams RB, Barefoot JC, Blumenthal JA et al: Psychosocial correlates of job strain in a sample of working women, Arch Gen Psychiatry 54:543-548, 1997.
72. Cardiac Rehabilitation Guideline Panel: US Department of Human Services; National Heart, Lung, Blood Institute, Number 17, 1995.
73. Dusseldorp E, van Elderen T, Maes S, Meulman J, Kraaij V: A meta-analysis of psychoeducational programs for coronary heart disease patients, Health Psychol 18:506-519, 1999.
74. Linden W. Psychological treatments in cardiac rehabilitation: review of rationales and outcomes, J Psychosom Res 48(4-5):443-454, 2000.
75. Linden W, Stossel C, Maurice J: Psychosocial interventions for patients with coronary artery disease: a meta-analysis [erratum appears in Arch Intern Med Nov 11;156(20):2302, 1996], Arch Intern Med 156:745-752, 1996.
76. Mullen PD, Mains DA, Velez R: A meta-analysis of controlled trials of cardiac patient education, Patient Educ Couns 19:143-162, 1992.
77. Elmer PJ, Grimm R, Jr, Laing B et al: Lifestyle intervention: results of the Treatment of Mild Hypertension Study (TOMHS), Prev Med 24:378-388, 1995.
78. Dubbert PM, Cushman WC, Meydrech EF, Rowland AK, Maury P: Effects of dietary instruction and sodium excretion feedback in hypertension clinic patients, Behav Ther 19:721-732, 1995.
79. Miller NH: Physical activity: one approach to the primary prevention of hypertension, AAOHN J 43:319-326, 1995.
80. Gidron Y, Davidson K: Development and preliminary testing of a brief intervention for modifying CHD-predictive hostility components, J Behav Med 19:203-220, 1996.
81. Friedman M, Thoresen CE, Gill JJ, et al: Alteration of type A behavior and its effect on cardiac recurrences in post myocardial infarction patients: summary results of the recurrent coronary prevention project, Am Heart J 112:653-665, 1986.
82. Hannay DR: Symptom prevalence in the community, J R Coll Gen Pract 28:492-499, 1978.
83. Mayou RA, Bass CM, Bryant BM: Management of noncardiac chest pain from research to clinical practice, Heart 81:387-392, 1999.
84. Mayou R, Bryant B, Forfar C, Clark D: Non-cardiac chest pain and benign palpitations in the cardiac clinic, Br Heart J 72:548-553, 1994.

85.   Chambers J, Bass C: Chest pain with normal coronary anatomy: a review of natural history and possible etiologic factors, Prog Cardiovasc Dis 33:161-184, 1990.

86.   Klimes I, Mayou RA, Pearce MJ, Coles L, Fagg JR: Psychological treatment for atypical non-cardiac chest pain: a controlled evaluation, Psychol Med 20:605-611, 1990.

87.   Pearce MJ, Mayou RA, Klimes I: The management of atypical non-cardiac chest pain, Q J Med 76:991-996, 1990.

88.   Mayou R, Sprigings D, Birkhead J, Price J: A randomized controlled trial of a brief educational and psychological intervention for patients presenting to a cardiac clinic with palpitation, Psychol Med 32:699-706, 2002.

89.   Ehlers A, Mayou RA, Sprigings DC, Birkhead J: Psychological and perceptual factors associated with arrhythmias and benign palpitations, Psychosom Med 62:693-702, 2000.

90.   Bass C, Wade C: Chest pain with normal coronary arteries: a comparative study of psychiatric and social morbidity, Psychol Med 14:51-61, 1984.

91.   Bass C, Mayou RA: Chest pain and palpitations. In Mayou RA, Bass C, Sharpe M, editors: Treatment of functional somatic symptom. Oxford, 1995, Oxford University Press, 328-352.

92.   Potts SG, Bass CM: Psychological morbidity in patients with chest pain and normal or near-normal coronary arteries: a long-term follow-up study, Psycholog Med 25:339-348, 1995.

93.   Van Peski-Oosterbaan AS, Spinhoven P, Van der Does AJ, Bruschke AV, Rooijmans HG: Cognitive change following cognitive behavioural therapy for non-cardiac chest pain, Psychother Psychosom 68:214-220, 1999.

94.   Mayou RA, Bryant BM, Sanders D et al: A controlled trial of cognitive behavioural therapy for non-cardiac chest pain, Psychol Med 27:1021-1031, 1997.

95.   Potts SG, Lewin R, Fox KA, Johnstone EC: Group psychological treatment for chest pain with normal coronary arteries, QJM 92:81-86, 1999.

96.   Chambers J, Bass C: Atypical chest pain looking beyond the heart, QJM 91:239-244, 1998.

PART **IV**

Alternative Medicine Practices

CHAPTER 9

Ayurveda and Yoga in Cardiovascular Diseases

Ravinder Mamtani, MBBS, MD, M Sc, FACPM
Ronac Mamtani, BS

Ayurveda is an ancient Asian Indian healthcare system, the origins of which go back about 5000 years to the Vedic civilization of India. Ayurveda is derived from two Sanskrit words—namely, *Ayus* and *Veda*, meaning *life* and *knowledge*, respectively.[1] It literally means *life of science*. The literature, principles, and practices of Ayurveda can be found in *Vedas*, the religious and divine Hindu books of knowledge.

Ayurveda, of which yoga is an integral part, is widely practiced in India and is gaining acceptance in many countries around the world. It is a comprehensive and a holistic system, the focus of which is on the body, mind, and consciousness. Ayurveda considers spirituality an essential element to good health and a noble way of life. Ayurvedic treatment is aimed at the person with a health problem rather than on the problem in a person. The treatment consists of herbal preparations, diet, yoga, meditation, and other practices.

This article briefly describes Ayurveda and examines the scientific evidence concerning the usefulness of Ayurvedic herbal treatments and yoga for cardiovascular health problems. It is beyond the scope of this review to examine the details of the traditional theories of Ayurveda and all of its treatments. The discussions on various topics are brief and focused to give the reader an overview of the subject material, with a special focus on herbs and yoga.

AYURVEDA

THEORY AND PRINCIPLES

The basic philosophy of Ayurveda is that everything in the universe, including life, is composed of five elements, called *panchamahabhutas*. These five elements are space (ether), air, fire, water, and earth. These elements are not recognized as physical elements but rather represent principles unique to the particular element. For example, fire represents the natural force associated with light and heat, and water represents the property of cohesiveness that holds things together, and so on. These elements, in turn, give rise to three basic factors (or energies) that regulate the life cycle and control the entire human body. These factors, called *doshas*, are *vata*, *pitta*, and *kapha*. *Vata* arises from space and air, *pitta* from fire and water, and *kapha* from water and earth. *Doshas* contribute in various proportions to make up *prakruti* (the essential constitution) of an individual. *Prakruti* is the genetic in nature. Just as three *doshas* control regulatory aspects of the body, three *gunas—sattva*, *rajas*, and *tamas*—influence and control the mind. Ayurveda also recognizes seven *dhatus* (tissue elements): plasma, blood, muscle, fat, bone, nerve, and reproductive tissue; three *malas* (excretory products): feces, urine and sweat; and agni (energy metabolism). A disturbance in any of these factors can give rise to disease. Because *dosha* imbalance is at the core of every dysfunction, keeping *doshas* in balance will maintain good health.[2]

Like other alternative medicine systems, Ayurveda emphasizes the intrinsic relationship between the body, mind, and consciousness. According to Ayurveda scholars, any imbalance in consciousness (or awareness) leads to undesirable personal lifestyle practices that result in disharmony and disease process. That is why mind-body interventions such as meditation and yoga are essential to disease treatment and prevention Ayurveda.[3]

DISEASE MANAGEMENT IN AYURVEDA

Disease evaluation and management in Ayurveda are individualized. Diagnosis is made by history taking, observation, palpation, and examining various organs and systems with particular attention to the heart, lungs, and intestines. Particular attention is paid to the examination of the pulse, tongue, eyes, and nails. Urine examination is also performed. The nature and the quality of the assessment are quite different from conventional biomedical assessment to which most physicians are accustomed. The findings have different interpretations and are based on principles described previously. For example, in Ayurveda 12 different pulses are recognizable, and they correlate with the functions of various internal organs.

There are four main categories of disease treatments in Ayurveda. They are *shodan* (cleansing), *shaman* (palliation), *rasayana* (rejuvenation), and *satvajaya* (mental health). These treatments include the use of herbal therapies, physical exercise and dietary regimens, meditation, and the use of certain practices. *Panchakarna purification therapy*, a well-known Ayurvedic cleansing treatment, includes vomiting, purgation, use of medicinal enemas, bloodletting, and administration of certain substances such as milk and herbal extracts via nasal passages.[1,2] Examples of commonly used practices and treatments appear in Box 9-1.

PLANT-BASED FOODS AND HERBS AND THEIR RELEVANCE IN THE TREATMENT OF CARDIOVASCULAR DISEASES

The medicinal and nutritional properties of plant-based foods have been known to the practitioners of Ayurveda and alternative systems of medicine for many

---

Box **9-1**   Common Treatment Strategies in Ayurveda

Cleansing Methods (Shodan)

The purpose of these methods is to remove excess toxins from the body. The main method is *Panchakarma,* which has the following five components. Examples are mentioned for each of the components.
- Therapeutic vomiting (*vaman*). Vomiting is induced by the use of emetics such as licorice.
- Purgation (*virechan*)
- Medicated enema (*basti*). Sesame oil and milk are often used for this method.
- Blood letting (*rakta moksha*). Sometimes leeches may be used. Blood-purifying herbs such as sandalwood and turmeric powders are also used.
- Nasal administration or insufflation (*nasya*). Oils, certain herbs, and nasal massages may be used.

Palliation (Shaman)

This is done by use of herbs such as ginger, cinnamon, and black pepper and practices such as the following:
- Fasting (*ksud nigraha*)
- Observing thirst (*trut nigraha*)
- Exercise: Yoga stretching (*vyayama*), and breathing exercises (*pranayama*)
- Lying in the sun (*atap seva*)

Rejuvenation (*Rasayana*)

Rasayanas are ayurvedic preparations used to revitalize the tissues, promote longevity and memory, and help in rejuvenation. MAK 4 and MAK 5 are examples of *rasayans.*

Spiritual healing (*satvajaya*)

Mantras (sacred recitations) and meditation are examples of this type of treatment.

Data from Gerson S: Ayurveda: The Ancient Indian Healing Art, ed 1, Boston, 1993 (Reprinted 1998), Elements Books Limited; Lad V: An introduction to Ayurveda, Alternative Therapies 1:57, 1995; Sharma H, Clark C: Contemporary Ayurveda: medicine and research in Maharishi Ayurveda, Philadelphia, 1998, Churchill Livingston.

---

centuries. However, the scientific proof—based on acceptable methods of research, establishing direct relationship between food and heath and disease—has become apparent only in recent years. For example, not until 1933 was a direct cause-effect relationship observed between consumption of fruits and vegetable and cancer. Subsequent studies have confirmed lower rates of mortality and incidence of heart disease among those whose diets are rich in plant-based foods such as fruits and vegetables.[4] Many reasons for these reported health benefits exist. Vegetarian foods are rich in vitamins, trace minerals, dietary fiber, and other nonnutritive biologically active compounds called phytochemicals. Herbs commonly used in Asian and other cultures as food and for medicinal purposes possess hypolipidemic, antiplatelet, and immune-stimulating properties that can be useful in reducing the risk of cardiovascular disease. The basic science of cardiovascular disease preventive mechanisms of plant-based diets rich in fruits and vegetables appear in Box 9-2.

> *Box* **9-2** Potential Cardiovascular Disease-Preventive Mechanisms of Plant-Based Foods as Identified in Human Studies
>
> - Antioxidant activity
> - Decrease platelet aggregation
> - Alteration of cholesterol metabolism
> - Blood-pressure reduction
> - Stimulation of the immune system
> - Modulation of detoxification enzymes
> - Modulation of steroid hormones concentration and metabolism
> - Antibacterial and antiviral activity

Modified from Lampe JW: Health effects of vegetables and fruit: assessing mechanisms of action in human experimental studies, Am J of Clinical Nutrition, 70(suppl):475 S-90 S, 1999.

Although there is no such thing as an Ayurvedic food or herb, the use of herbs and plant extracts remains an integral and significant part of the Ayurvedic approach to disease management. These extracts or their mixtures, based on Ayurvedic philosophy and principles, have been the subject of many studies in both animals and humans. Examples of herbs and various plant products of interest to researchers and clinicians in the management of hypertension and heart disease are described in the following discussion. Additionally, a listing of the herbs commonly used by Ayurvedic physicians for the treatment of cardio-vascular diseases appears in Table 9-1.

Allium sativum (Garlic)

Garlic has long been used in India as a medicinal food. It was initially used as an antiinfective agent and subsequently became popular for its antihypertensive and lipid-lowering effects. The sales of garlic products have soared in recent years and generated over $61 million in the year 2000. Garlic has been said to have lipid-lowering, antithrombotic, antihypertensive, antioxidant, immunomodulatory, and antimicrobial effects (see Chapter 4).

Several randomized studies performed in the 1980s and 1990s demonstrated the effectiveness of garlic in reducing total and low-density lipoprotein (LDL)-cholesterol. Reductions of 5% to 12% in total cholesterol values have been documented.[5] Some recent studies, however, have failed to demonstrate and confirm these findings.[5,6] A recent meta-analysis has shown an overall marginal benefit of garlic on lipid levels.[7]

Various mechanisms of garlic's lipid-lowering actions are thought to be related to the following:[5,6]

- The presence of allicin, thiosulphates, and organosulfur compounds found in garlic that inhibit cholesterol synthesis at several steps
- Inhibition of hepatic cholesterol biosynthesis at the level of HMG-CoA reductase
- Increased catabolism of fatty acid containing lipids such as triglycerides
- The presence in garlic of saponins, which may retard the absorption of cholesterol from the intestine

Table 9-1   Human Studies Involving the Use of Ayurvedic Plants/Extracts With Beneficial Cardiovascular Results

Genus, Species, Common Sanskrit Name, Common English Name	Conditions and/or Results for Which Human Studies are Reported (Proposed mechanism of action, if any)
Allium cepa Palandu Onion	Hyperlipidemia. Resulted in low levels of lipids (diuretic, antithrombotic).
*Azadirachta indica** Arishta Neem	Congestive heart failure
*Boerhavia diffusa** Punarnaua Spreading hogweed	Congestive heart failure
Curcuma longa *Haridra (Haldi)* Turmeric	Hyperlipidemia. Improved cholesterol levels noted. (Fatty acid metabolism alteration and decrease in serum lipid peroxides levels).
Commiphora (mukul) guggulu Guggulu Guggulu	Hyperlipidemia. Improved lipid levels noted. (Antagonist of farnesoid X receptors).
Emblica officinalis Amla Emblic myrobala	Hyperlipidemia. Improved cholesterol levels.
Gymnema sylvester Meshasringi Gurmar	Diabetes. Resulted in low lipid and glucose levels.
Saussurca lappa Kushtha Costus	Ischemic heart disease. Reduced angina frequency and lowered diastolic blood pressure.
Terminalia arjuna Arjuna English name unavailable	Congestive heart failure and angina pectoris. Improvement noted in both patient groups.
Trigonella foenum graecum Medhika Fenugreek	Diabetes and hyperlipidemia. Improvements noted in both patient groups.

From Blumental M: *The ABC clinical guide to herbs,* New York, 2003, The American Botanical Council, Thieme Publishers; Ernst E: *The desktop guide to complementary and alternative medicine: an evidence-based approach,* ed 1, Toronto, 2001, Mosby; Khan S, Balick MJ: Therapeutic plants of Ayurveda: a review of selected clinical and other studies for 166 species, *J Altern Complement Therapies* 7:405, 2001.
*Used in conjunction with other herbs. Other herbs for which human studies have been reported include *Withania somnifer, Rubia cordiforia, Picrorhiza kurrooa, Nelumbo mucifera,* and *Gymnema sylvestre.*

Studies concerning the effects of garlic on heart disease are few. In a 4-year placebo-controlled study involving 152 subjects, those in the experimental group receiving 900 mg of garlic as powder experienced an average 2.6% reduction of plaque volume, whereas the placebo group's plaque volume increased 15.6%.[6] The antithrombotic effects and heart disease preventive effects of garlic have been attributed to the following:[5,6]

- Inhibition of platelet aggregation and stimulation of fibrinolysis by allicin and thiosulfinates
- Inhibition of lipoxygenase-dependent pathways, thus resulting in the synthesis of prostaglandins and in the interference of metabolism of arachidonate.

Garlic's antihypertensive effect has also been demonstrated in various epidemiological inquiries. In a meta-analysis of eight randomized, controlled studies, three studies demonstrated significant reductions of systolic pressure and four in diastolic pressure. The antihypertensive effect of garlic is thought to be related to gamma-glutamylcysteines and fructans. Gamma-glutamylcysteines inhibit angiotensin-converting enzyme (ACE), thereby lowering blood pressure. Clearly, more research and evidence will be required to recommend garlic therapy for the treatment of hypertension.

In a recent analysis performed by the Agency for Healthcare Research and Quality (AHRQ), the authors concluded that garlic may have short-term positive lipid lowering and encouraging antithrombotic effects.[8] Their carefully worded conclusion states, "it is not clear if statistically significant positive short-term effects.....but negative longer term effects......are due to systemic differences in studies that have longer or shorter follow-up duration, fewer longer term studies, or time dependent effects of garlic."[8]

Garlic can aggravate the effects of oral hypoglycemic and anticoagulant drugs. The risk of its side effects with the usual and recommended dose of 4 grams of fresh garlic or 600 mg of standardized extract a day is small. Its complementary use in certain patients with high cholesterol levels might be appropriate.[9] Because the lipid-lowering effects of garlic are marginal and cannot be sustained over a prolonged period of time, garlic should not be considered a primary therapy for hyperlipidemia. However, its use as an adjunct to lifestyle measures in selected patients with hypercholesterolemia and possibly in those with heart disease might be appropriate. Fresh garlic and dried powder are recommended for patient use because variations in manufacturing practices cannot ensure quality of the garlic tablets at the present time.

Terminalia arjuna

This Ayurvedic herb, which has cardiotonic property, was tested in a crossover randomized controlled trial involving 12 patients with congestive heart failure (CHF-NYHA Class IV). The experimental group received 500 mg of *Terminalia arjuna* bark every 8 hours for 2 weeks in addition to standard therapy. In comparison to the placebo group, the group receiving the herb showed significant improvement with respect to the symptoms and signs of heart failure. Long-term evaluation of results 28 months later showed continuing clinical improvement in all patients receiving the herb.[10]

In an animal study, rabbits on a high-cholesterol diet received *Terminalia arjuna* and showed a slower increase in total cholesterol and triglycerides levels in comparison to those receiving only a high cholesterol diet. Also, rabbits with high levels of cholesterol receiving the herb showed a significant reduction in their cholesterol than the hypercholesterolemic controls.[11] The results of the studies are encouraging but require further confirmation.

Commiphora mukul (guggulu)

This plant belongs to the family *Burseraceae*. When cut, the plant exudes a gum-like resin. In ancient times the resin was used for the treatment of obesity and skin diseases. In the 1960s, assays performed on the resin showed the presence of antihyperlipoproteinemic compounds called guggulsterones. These substances are effective antagonists of the farnesoid X receptor, which is activated by bile acids. The farnesoid X receptor regulates cholesterol by controlling the level of the bile acid. Guggulsterone's blocking action of farnesoid X receptor helps in reducing the level of cholesterol.[12] Guggulsterones also have an inhibitory effect on platelets.

Several studies have confirmed their hypolipidemic activity.[5,13] Although the results are encouraging, many of these studies have methodological problems. Therefore a definitive conclusion regarding the lipid-lowering effect of *guggulu* is premature. In 1987, guggulipid, which contains the active guggulsterones, was registered as a lipid-lowering agent in India. Subsequently, other substances in the plant with hypolipidemic property have been identified and are undergoing clinical trials.[14]

Curcuma longa (Turmeric)

The active ingredient, curcumin, of this spice commonly used in India has anti-inflammatory and lipid-lowering effects. Curcumin's lipid-lowering effects observed in animal experiments are attributed to changes in fatty acid metabolism and facilitating the conversion of cholesterol to bile acids.[5] Although animal study results are promising, no human randomized trials could be found in prominent peer-reviewed literature. Its use as a primary cholesterol-lowering treatment cannot be made at the present time. However, turmeric's use as a spice in the overall healthy diet is prudent.

Rauwolfia serpentina (sarpaganha)

According to ancient Sanskrit texts this plant has been used for centuries in India for the treatment of "madness."[6] In 1952, a group of scientists isolated an active principle, reserpine, an alkaloid, from the plant. In addition to its tranquilizing effect, the principle was found to possess a blood pressure-lowering effect. Subsequently, in 1953, it was marketed as an effective drug for the treatment of hypertension.[5]

Maharishi Amrit Kalash (MAK)

This ayurvedic preparation comes in two forms: MAK 4 and MAK 5. These formulations are mixtures of many fruits and herbs. Several studies suggest that

MAK may reduce atherosclerotic heart and vascular disease by way of controlling free radicals and or reducing platelet aggregation.[15] More research is needed to confirm these findings.

Phytochemicals

Plant-based foods have a wide range of aromas, colors, and tastes. These qualities make them distinctive and attractive for food consumption. These qualities are thought to be due to the presence of compounds called phytochemicals. Allylic sulfides responsible for the pungent odor of garlic, and anthocyanins, the red pigment in fruits such as strawberries, are examples of phytochemicals.

Many foods and herbs recommended by practitioners of Ayurveda contain phytochemicals, which are possibly involved in optimizing health and preventing and/or treating cardiovascular diseases.[16] Phytochemicals are biologically active compounds present in small quantities in plants. They are not nutrients but seem to play a significant role in the prevention of several chronic diseases.

The health benefits of phytochemicals have not been proven conclusively. However, many herbs commonly used in Asian Indian cuisine and by Ayurvedic practitioners may show promise for disease prevention (Table 9-2).[16]

At the present time, potential health benefits of phytochemicals are not attributed to any single compound but rather to wholesome foods that contain thousands of phytochemicals and other nutrients. Also, no single disease entity or deficiency syndrome has been linked to any one or any group of phytochemicals.

Table **9-2**   PUTATIVE MECHANISMS OF PHYTOCHEMICALS IN PROTECTION AGAINST CARDIOVASCULAR AND OTHER DEGENERATIVE DISEASES

Mechanism	Phytochemical (s)	Food/Herb
Lipid-lowering and antithrombotic activities	Diallyl sulfide, disulfides, and flavonoids	Onion, garlic, soy and other beans, chickpeas, tea and fruit, and vegetables
Antioxidant activity	Phenolic compounds (flavonoids, caffeic, ellalic and ferulic acids, sesamol and vanillin)	Green and colored fruits and vegetables, tea, and grape skin
Antiinflammatory activity	Diallyl sulfides, disufides, catechins, gingerol	Onion, garlic, ginger, tea
Estrogenic activity	Coumestans, lignans, and isoflavons	Soy products, other types of beans and chickpeas
Production of detoxifying enzymes*	Sulforaphanes, indoles, and isothiocyanates	Cruciferous vegetables

From Craig WJ: Health-promoting properties of common herbs, Am J Clinical Nutr 70 (suppl):491S, 1999; Dreosti IE: Recommended dietary intake levels for phytochemicals: feasible or fanciful? Asia Pacific J Clin Nutrit 9 (suppl):S119, 2000; Perry EK, Milner L, Houghton PJ: From ancient texts to modern phytotherapy: plants in mind. In Ernst E, editor: Herbal medicine: a concise overview for health professionals. Woburn, MA, 2000, Butter-Heinemann Publishers, 1-18.
*This mechanism has been shown to be useful in cancer, but its role in cardiovascular disease is not known.

For these reasons, recommendations concerning their use as supplements in place of a well-balanced healthy diet is not appropriate.

Based on the limited number of studies, the evidence concerning the effectiveness of Ayurvedic herbs in the treatment of cardiovascular diseases is not compelling. However, lack of compelling evidence of these herbs is not the same as their ineffectiveness. Although more research is needed, inherent difficulties and problems in conducting research in alternative medicine systems such as Ayurveda exist. A brief description of such problems and difficulties appears later in this chapter.

YOGA

The word *yoga* comes from a Sanskrit word *yug*, meaning *to join*. It connotes "the joining of the lower human nature to the higher."[17] Many claim that yoga allows a person to alter his or her mental and bodily responses, normally thought to be beyond one's control. Simply put, yoga is a mind-body technique involving breath control, physical exercises, and meditation, and it promotes physical, mental, social, and spiritual well-being.

Ancient Sanskrit Vedic texts have described several types of yogic practices. These include *bhakti* yoga (emphasizes spirituality and devotion), *jnana* yoga (emphasizes wisdom), *karma* yoga (emphasizes offering services without selfish motive), *raja* yoga (which emphasizes mastering the mind by focused concentration), *dhyana* yoga (emphasizes meditation), *mantra* yoga (emphasizes repetition of sacred recitations) and *hatha* (emphasizes psychophysical energies of the body).[17,18]

Hatha yoga is the most popular form in the United States. It has the following three essential components: a) physical exercises and postures (called *asanas*); b) breathing techniques (called *pranayamas*); and c) concentration and thinking techniques such as meditation.

Yoga Session

A yoga session can vary in content and time. A typical 45- to 60-minute yoga session begins with breathing exercises requiring long and deep breaths through the nose.[3] Mental concentration of each breath as the air enters and exits the nostril is important. This allows people to relax their bodies and calm their minds. This phase could last anywhere between 15 and 20 minutes and can be done sitting or lying down. The next phase (usually of 20 to 25 minutes) involves gentle exercises and postural movements to facilitate relaxation of joints and muscles. This is followed by somewhat more difficult postures and exercises. Practitioners are advised to exercise gently and slowly and not to stretch beyond their comfort levels. Exercises and movements should be performed with ease. The last phase (10 to 15 minutes) involves meditation or a related technique such as visualization or guided imagery and usually concludes with chanting, such as repeating *Om shanti* ("let there be peace").

Transcendental Meditation

Transcendental Meditation (TM) is a variant of yoga that is devoid of the cumbersome physical and mental exercises usually associated with yoga. Invented by an Indian practitioner, Maharishi Mahesh Yogi, this mind-body method of self-regulating attention has become quite popular in the US. Several reports of its benefits in reducing blood pressure and anxiety and improving quality of life exist.[3]

TM comes in different forms. In its simplistic form, learners are asked to repeat and focus on a mantra over a period of 20 to 30 minutes. Mantra is a phrase, a sentence, or words such as "om" and "shanti". Occasionally learners may choose to simply focus on an object of their liking. For beginners, distractions are not uncommon. In case of distractions, the learner is asked to return to his or her focus on mantra. TM is easy to master, and its repeated use produces relaxation and relieves anxiety.

Evidence Base of Yoga

Many research findings have documented the usefulness of yoga in the treatment of various cardiovascular diseases. A brief summary of the evidence base appears in the following discussion.

Heart Disease and its Risk Factors

Studies conducted abroad indicate regular yoga practice can significantly improve heart disease risk factors such as lipid profiles, body weight, and blood pressure.[18-20] Schmidt et al reported a significant improvement in the levels of blood pressure, LDL cholesterol, and body mass index after a 3-month residential training program consisting of a vegetarian diet and yoga.[19] In another randomized controlled study, similar reductions were achieved in the intervention group receiving yoga.[21]

A recent randomized, observer-blinded study was conducted on 42 angiographically proven coronary artery disease patients not receiving lipid-lowering agents.[20] The experimental group practiced yoga for 90 minutes and experienced a significant reduction in coronary stenosis as compared to the control group. Both groups continued to receive medical treatment and the American Heart Association step-one diet as prescribed. Although these results are encouraging, the study has methodological problems.

Studies performed in the US have shown that the complementary use of various mind-body techniques produce significant improvement in patients with coronary heart disease.[18] In the famous randomized Lifestyle Heart Trial,[21] patients who were prescribed intensive lifestyle changes demonstrated significant regression of coronary artery disease (as determined by numbers of angioplasties and frequency of cardiac events) in comparison to the usual-care control group. The intensive lifestyle program consisted of vegetarian diet, yoga and meditation, aerobic exercise and group psychologic support.

Several controlled and uncontrolled studies have demonstrated the long-term usefulness of yoga in the treatment of hypertension.[15,18,22] In earlier studies that involved *Savasna* (a type of yogic activity), significant reductions in blood pressures were noticed.[18] The sample size of patients in these studies was small.

In a randomized trial of 33 hypertensive patients, subjects were assigned to one of three groups: those receiving yoga, those prescribed antihypertensive medication, or those receiving no treatment. Both yoga and antihypertensive medications were noted to reduce blood pressure over an 11-week period.[23] One randomized, controlled study suggests yoga is capable of producing a long-term beneficial effect in the treatment of hypertension.[3] Other studies involving postural techniques of yoga (*asanas*) have produced significant reductions in blood pressure.[3] Many scientists believe *asanas* can restore baroreflex sensitivity, thereby reducing blood pressure.[23-25]

Other physiological effects. Yoga can also alter various pulmonary, cerebral, mental, and metabolic physiologic functions, thereby producing beneficial effects on the cardiovascular status. These beneficial effects include better breath holding ability, improved tidal volume and vital capacity, an improvement in physical fitness,[26] reduction in anxiety,[27] and improved blood-glucose levels among diabetic patients. An association between increased cerebral blood flow and TM has also been observed.[15,28]

A unique and distinct phase of relaxation known as "the fourth state of consciousness" (the other three being waking, dreaming, and sleeping) has been described during TM.[15,28] This state is characterized by not only the usual changes seen in deep relaxation, such as reduced cortisol and plasma lactate levels, decreased muscle and red cell metabolism, and reduced breath rate but also by an increased alpha brain wave activity and a distinctive pattern of enhanced cerebral blood flow.

The regular practice of yoga has also been shown to have positive effects on mood and emotional well-being.[17] Improved muscle strength and relaxation response have also been described.[3,17]

Recommendations and Cautions

Although yoga cannot be recommended as a primary treatment for patients with hypertension and/or heart disease, its use as an adjunct in such patients can be safely recommended. Adjustment of postures may be required for certain patients. Pregnant women should avoid certain postural yogic techniques. Also, those with a history of psychosis should refrain from yoga. Excessive meditation may lead to mental disturbances.

Yoga is flexible, and its techniques can be custom-tailored to individual needs. It can be self-taught, although it is best learnt with supervision in class situations. Yoga is a safe and inexpensive method for promoting general health and a state of emotional well-being.

AYURVEDA RESEARCH: PROBLEMS AND DIFFICULTIES

Lack of funding, lack of research, and lack of academic infrastructure are common problems facing research in Ayurveda and yoga.[29] Methodological problems also exist.

AYURVEDIC APPROACH AND ITS INCOMPATIBILITY WITH RANDOMIZED CONTROLLED TRIAL METHODOLOGY

Ayurveda and its practices are deeply rooted in day-to-day routine activities of Indian households. Diet, personal habits, hobbies, and spirituality are examples of such activities. In disease states, adjustments of these activities, the use of herbal preparations, and other practices are required to treat the whole person in terms of the mind, body, and spirit to create a balance to optimize health and well-being.

Ayurvedic treatment usually has several components and is not only disease-specific but also person-specific. Two persons with similar disease patterns could receive two entirely different treatments. Such a treatment approach cannot lend itself to a randomized controlled trial (RCT). This is so because in a RCT all patients in the treatment group must receive the same treatment while those in the control group receive an indistinguishable placebo. To fit into this research design, many research workers have chosen to test only specific herbal ingredients or plant products on a particular condition.[30] The reality of good ayurvedic practice is that ayurvedic physicians tend to use a wide range of ayurvedic approaches including the use of herbs, diet, meditative and yoga practices, and a variety of other interventions. Similar variations are seen in yoga.

PROBLEM OF DESIGNING PLACEBOS FOR THE AYURVEDIC APPROACH

Given the wholesomeness and the complexity of the Ayurvedic approach, devising an acceptable placebo intervention is unthinkable. Also, designing placebos for specific Ayurvedic practices such as massage, fasting, vomiting, and yoga would be very cumbersome and difficult. How, for example, could a subject receive a sham massage or yoga? Although complicated procedures can be devised to fool subjects into believing that they are receiving a true treatment, such an approach may work for a treatment or two but not when treatments are spread over a few weeks.

The methodological problems discussed above can have the following effects on Ayurveda research data:

1. The treatment techniques used in RCTs are not representative of those used in the day-to-day practice of Ayurveda.
2. In typical RCTs in which herbal or yoga treatments are compared with placebo and in which only short-term outcomes are assessed, the following questions will still remain unanswered:
   a. What are the long-term effects of Ayurvedic or yoga treatments compared to conventional treatments?
   b. Are the RCT results, when put into practice, helping our patients, and if so, to what extent?

CONCLUSION

Based on the review of available studies, the evidence is not convincing that any Ayurvedic herbal treatment is effective in the treatment of heart disease or hypertension. The use of fresh garlic and turmeric as spices in the overall healthy diet is appropriate. Many studies reported in the literature suffer from methodological problems and inadequate sample size. However, lack of evidence should not necessarily be viewed as lack of effectiveness for commonly used herbal treatments. Several Ayurvedic herbs, such as *guggulu*, might be appropriate for larger randomized trials in the future.

Yoga has been shown to be useful to patients with heart disease and hypertension. Yoga reduces anxiety, promotes well-being, and improves quality of life. Its safety profile is excellent. Its complementary use under medical supervision is appropriate, and may be worth considering.

Ayurveda is the oldest medical system in the world, dating back 5000 years to the Vedic civilization of India. Ayurvedic preparations have valuable medicinal properties, and its practices, such as yoga, can promote health. Ayurveda offers many challenges and opportunities and is worthy of research and our attention.

"Is there anyone so wise as to learn from the experience of another?"

VOLTAIRE

REFERENCES

1. Gerson S: Ayurveda: The Ancient Indian Healing Art, ed 1, Boston, 1993 (Reprinted 1998), Elements Books Limited.
2. Lad V: An introduction to Ayurveda, Alternative Therapies 1:57, 1995.
3. Alternative Medicine: Expanding Medical Horizons: A Report to the NIH on Alternative Medical Systems and Practices in the US, 1992.
4. Drewnowski A, Gomez-Carneros C: Bitter taste, phytonutrients and the consumer: a review. Am J Clin Nutri 72:1424, 2000.
5. Low Dog T, Riley D: Management of hyperlipidemia, Alternative Therap 9:28, 2003.
6. Blumental M: The ABC clinical guide to herbs, New York, 2003, The American Botanical Council, Thieme Publishers.
7. Stevinson C, Pittler MH, Earnst E: Garlic for treating hypercholesterolemia: a meta-analysis of randomized trials, Ann Intern Med 133:420, 2000.
8. Mulrow C, Lawrence V. Ackerman R: Evidence report/ technology assessment number 20-garlic: effects on cardiovascular risks and diseases, protective effects against cancer and clinical adverse effects, Rockville, MD, Oct 2000, Agency for Healthcare Research and Quality (AHRQ); Pub No 01-EO23.
9. Ernst E: The desktop guide to complementary and alternative medicine: an evidence-based approach, ed 1, Toronto, 2001, Mosby.
10. Bharani A, Ganguly A, Bhargava KD: Salutary effect of *Terminalia arjuna* in patients with severe congestive heart failure, Int J Cardiology 49:191, 1995.
11. Tewari AK: Effect of *Terminalia arjuna* on lipid profiles of rabbits fed hypercholesterolemic diet, Int J Crude Res 28:43, 1990.

12. Low Dog T: Herbs in cardiovascular diseases, Botanical Medicine in Modern Clinical Practice , 8th Annual Course, Columbia University, June 9-13, 2003.

13. McGuffin M, Hobbs C, Upton R, Goldberg A: American Herbal Products Association botanical safety handbook, Boca Raton, FL, 1997, CRC Press.

14. Dev Sukh: Ancient-modern concordance in Ayurvedic plants: some examples, Environmental Health Perspectives 107:783, 1999.

15. Sharma H, Clark C: Contemporary Ayurveda: medicine and research in Maharishi Ayurveda, Philadelphia, 1998, Churchill Livingston.

16. Craig WJ: Health-promoting properties of common herbs, Am J Clinical Nutr 70 (suppl):491S, 1999.

17. Ananda S: The complete book of yoga: harmony, of body and mind, Delhi, 1981 (Reprinted 2001), Orient Paperbacks.

18. Raub JA: Psychophysiologic effects of hatha yoga on musculoskeletal and cardiopulmonary function: a literature review, J Altern Complement Med 8:797, 2003.

19. Schmidt T: Wijga A, Von Zur Muhlen A, et al: Changes in cardiovascular factors and hormones during comprehensive residential three months kriya yoga training and vegetarian nutrition, Acta Physiol Pharmacol 42:205, 1998.

20. Manchanda SC, Narang R, Reddy KS et al: Retardation of coronary atherosclerosis with yoga lifestyle intervention, J Assoc Physicians India 48:687, 2000.

21. Mahajan AS, Reddy KS, Sachdeva U: Lipid profile of coronary risk subjects following yogic life style intervention, Indian Heart J 51:37, 1999.

22. Patel C. Twelve month follow-up of yoga and bio-feedback in the management of hypertension, Lancet 1:62, 1975.

23. Marugesan R, Govindarajulu N, Bera TK: Effect of selected yogic practices on the management of hypertension, Indian J Physiol Pharmacol 44:207, 2000.

24. Selvamurthy W, Sridharan K, Ray US et al: A new physiological approach to control essential hypertension, Indian J Physiol Pharmacol 42:205, 1998.

25. Bernardi L, Porta C, Spicuzza L et al: Slow breathing increases arterial baroreflex sensitivity in patients with chronic heart failure, Circulation 105:143, 2002.

26. Benson H: The physiology of meditation, Scientific American 226:84, 1972.

27. Fenwick PB, Donaldson L, Gillis L: Metabolic and EEG changes during transcendental meditation: an explanation, Biological Psych 5:101, 1977.

28. Jevning R, Wilson AF: Behavioral increase of blood flow, Physiologist 21:60, 1978.

29. Bodekar G: Evaluating Ayurveda, J Altern Complement Med 7:389, 2001.

CHAPTER 10

Heart Qi and the Heart of Healing: Qigong for the Prevention and Treatment of Cardiac Disease

Linda C. Nadia Hole, MD

"Each person carries his own doctor inside him. They come to us not knowing the truth. We are at our best when we give the doctor who resides within each patient a chance to go to work."

ALBERT SCHWEITZER, MD

WHAT IS QIGONG?

Qigong is a 5000-year-old energy healing system from China, with over 80 million practitioners worldwide. *Qi,* pronounced "chee," is your breath, or vital life force healing energy, known in other cultures as *prana, shakti, ki,* etc. *Gong,* pronounced "gung," is practice or work. Qigong is the practice of cultivating and working with this vital life force, life-giving, healing energy. Via gentle breathing, stretching, and meditative exercises, Qigong cleanses and revitalizes your body, mind, heart, and spirit. On a philosophical level, Qigong is also about integrating your body, mind, heart, and spirit harmoniously with the universe.

Nearly every culture has some mind-body energy healing practice, ranging from modern-day practices such as reiki therapeutic touch, guided imagery, hypnotherapy, mindfulness, and stress reduction to shamanism and faith healing. As a paradigm shift tool for New Millennium medicine, Qigong takes mind-body medicine a step higher. Qigong is an example of what Larry Dossey, MD, heralds as "New Era," "non-local," "eternal," medicine.[1] Unlike traditional Newtonian medicine, Qigong transcends body, mind, time, space, and matter. Qigong healing may be long distance, spontaneous, and at times even instantaneous.

Qigong practitioners routinely report profound healing and transformation on many levels: in overall health, relief of symptoms, personal and professional growth, sense of well-being, sense of purpose, acceptance, self-love, and in relationships—with oneself, loved ones, and community.[2,2a] In a survey of 226 subjects who practice Qigong, Hayashi reports increased "emotional stability, joy of life, more open attitude, interest, willpower, and care about others".[3] Among others, Wang observed that Qigong practice significantly decreases type-A behaviors.[4]

Qigong is furthermore documented in scientific literature to strengthen the immune system, prevent aging and disease, relieve stress and fatigue, increase energy, reverse paralysis, and promote peak performance.[5] Qigong also potentiates the effectiveness of Western medications, both alleviating side effects and allowing reductions in dosages.[6]

Literally hundreds of different styles and schools of Qigong are taught throughout the world. Although I myself am still a beginner, I've taught Qigong since 1995 and studied closely with a number of recognized Qigong Masters. My formal Qigong training has been primarily with Qigong Grandmaster Effie Poy Yew Chow, PhD, RN, LAc, co-author with Charles McGee, MD of *Qigong Miracle Healing from China* in her Chow Integrated Healing System, also known as Chow Medical Qigong. Among others, my training has also included time with Robert Ibriham Jaffe, MD, who in his own divine inspiration in healing of the heart, teaches "Healing in the Way of Love," with results and Qi as powerful as any I've experienced with any traditional Qigong Master from China. My patients have, of course, been my greatest teachers.

Programs across the country, such as the California Pacific Medical Center in San Francisco and Columbia Presbyterian Hospital in New York, have integrated Qigong into their treatment programs for cardiac patients.[7]

By now, every cardiologist has heard about the work of Dean Ornish, MD and his research on the importance of changing lifestyle in the reversal of heart disease.[8,9] In our experience, Qigong is a powerfully effective tool for changing lifestyles and is well worth considering as a complementary integrative modality for the care of cardiac patients.

We hope in this chapter to take the mystique out of Qigong. The "miracles" of Qigong are freely available to all. Within each and every one of us is a Qigong master healer. In Qigong, our job is simply to awaken to the healer within.

MEDICAL QIGONG AND "SUPERHUMAN" PHENOMENA

Qigong may be categorized as "soft Qi" medical Qigong or "hard Qi" martial arts performance Qigong.

Examples of "soft Qi" medical Qigong "miracles" include Qi-induced surgical anesthesia, spontaneous cancer remissions, reversal of paralysis, and Qi-induced changes in blood pressure, electroencephalogram (EEG) results, and blood levels of various neurotransmitters and hormones.[5,10]

In the "hard Qi" superhuman category, various Qigong Masters, with just their bare hands and Qi, are able to light fluorescent bulbs, charge batteries, set newspaper on fire, bend steel, break concrete slabs, pull trucks with a full load of passengers, balance standing on raw eggs, etc.[5,10-12] Dr. Chow, a petite woman, routinely and seemingly without effort with her Qi pushes the largest and strongest volunteers from the audience, several at a time, across the floor.

Soft Qi "superhuman" abilities include medical x-ray vision, uncanny intuition, precognition, fingertip diagnosis, the ability to direct or emit Qi with measurable physical results, and the ability to heal long-distance. Some Qigong Masters can also affect scientific instrument measurements, petri plate growth cultures, and/or kill laboratory cancer cells across a room.[5,10,12,13] Qigong Master Dr. Yan Xin reportedly is able to change the molecular structure of water and influence the decay rate of radioactive isotope Am-241.[14]

A Qigong Master is someone who has cultivated his Qi—both his inner Nei Qi and outer Wai Qi—and demonstrated extraordinary Qigong healing ability. Nei Qi is healing Qi cultivated by circulating one's own internal Qi via simple breath, movement, and meditative Qigong exercises. In Wai Qi the practitioner brings about healing in a subject by sending or emitting Qi. The discipline of Nei Qi is necessary for the practice of Wai Qi.

SOME CLINICAL STUDIES AND OBSERVATIONS

THE CHALLENGES OF RESEARCH IN QIGONG

There is a wealth of clinical research from China on the efficacy of Qigong in the treatment of cardiac disease. In a worldwide survey of Qigong scientific literature published in English, Dr. Ken Sancier, PhD's *Qigong Institute* computerized database cites over 183 references on Qigong for cardiac disease.[15]

How to conduct research in Qigong presents many obvious challenges, and the quality of much of the research is admittedly uneven. What exactly are we measuring when we measure Qi? How does one perform a double-blind study in Qigong? What about the factor of intention? What about the bias of the researchers? Are the studies rigorously randomly assigned, matched, nonbiased, controlled, made double-blind, and so on, according to rigorous Western scientific standards? What are adequate controls in Qigong research?

Michael Mayer, PhD, has authored thoughtful critiques on the problematic methodology of the clinical studies available in English on Qigong and hypertension and raises questions regarding the scientific validity of the available research to date.[16] More scientifically rigorous studies need to done.

HYPERTENSION AND QIGONG

Mayer's review of clinical studies on Qigong and hypertension, with a total of 5545 subjects, observed that nearly all the studies suggest that Qigong, over time, can lower blood pressure in hypertensive patients.[16]

The most extensive single study on Qigong and cardiovascular disease is Kuang's 20-year study.[17] Kuang followed hypertensive patients who were randomly assigned, 100 to a medication alone group, and 103 to a medication plus Qigong group. The Qigong group practiced Qigong 30 minutes twice a day. Kuang reported that the blood pressure of the control group (medications alone) increased (p <0.01) and that 31% required an increase in their antihypertensive medications, whereas the blood pressure of the Qigong group stabilized, with 48% reducing the dosage of their antihypertensive medications and 30% no longer requiring antihypertensive medications at all.

Many studies likewise report significant lowering of blood pressure with the practice of Qigong, with measurable results over varying periods of time, from one session to 1 year.[18-24] A reduction in blood pressure—even in refractory hypertensive patients unresponsive to medication—has also been reported.[18,20] In a survey of 400 students enrolled in his Qigong School of Australia, Lim reported that of the 22 suffering hypertension, all experienced a lowered blood pressure, with 15 of the 22 entirely eliminating their need for antihypertensive medications.[25] In one particular study of 32 hospitalized hypertensive patients with renal failure, the practitioners reported a significantly greater decrease in blood pressure in patients treated with external "emitted Qi" by a genuine Qigong master than did those treated by a sham Qigong master (p <0.01).[26]

Huang reported the results of a study of hypertensive subjects who practiced Qigong for a period of 1 year and showed an improvement in the electrocardiogram (ECG), carotid artery pulse, and in both systolic and diastolic blood pressure levels.[27] In a study of 2114 cases of hypertension by the Shanghai Institute of Hypertension, Wen reported improved blood circulation to the limbs, fingertips, and brain, as well as an improved cardiac index.[28] Sancier reported that data from the Shanghai Institute of Hypertension indicated that subjects who actively practiced Qigong for a period of 1 year increased their cardiac output, ejection fraction, mitral valve diastolic closing velocity, and mean velocity of circumferential fiber shortening while decreasing total peripheral resistance.[29] The Kuang study also noted a decrease in peripheral vascular resistance.[17]

Other researchers reported improved circulation and capillary microcirculation with Qigong practice in comparison to control groups by using a laser microcirculation blood flow meter,[30-32] with a significant decrease in blood flow resistance and vascular tension with Qigong practice,[33] and improved left-ventricular function.[31]

In Kuang's 20-year study on Qigong and hypertension, the Qigong practice group showed an increased HDL, decreased triglycerides and total cholesterol, decreased incidence of cardiovascular lesions, decreased blood viscosity, and reduced platelet aggregation.[17] Others likewise report that Qigong practice significantly raises HDL blood levels, decreases cholesterol and triglycerides levels, improves circulation, and reduces abnormal clotting.[34-38]

Wang and the Shanghai Institute of Hypertension also report changes in blood chemistries in hypertensive patients, including improvements in plasma fibrinolysis, blood viscosity, the erythrocyte deformation index, plasma tissue type plasminogen activator levels, plasminogen activator inhibitor levels, VII factor–related antigen levels, antithrombin, and enhanced superoxide dismutase activity, thus suggesting that Qigong may play a role in altering the coagulation fibrinolytic system in the prevention of coronary heart disease.[29,31,39]

CORONARY HEART DISEASE AND QIGONG

Many studies have reported the effectiveness of Qigong in the prevention and treatment of coronary heart disease (CHD).[17,27,34,39-50]

Wang studied 120 patients diagnosed with CHD and hypertension. He randomly divided subjects into a Qigong practice group and a control group treated with medication only. After 1 year of treatment, relief of clinical symptoms was observed in 62.6% of the Qigong group versus 34.8% of control subjects. Blood pressure was lowered in 86.7% versus 65%, respectively, and improvement in the ECG was observed in 52.6% versus 22.2%, respectively.[39,51]

After Qigong practice for 1 year, Wang et al observed an increase in cardiac output, decrease in total peripheral resistance, increase in ejection fraction, increase in mean velocity of circumferential fiber lengthening, with an overall improvement in left ventricular function in 30 subjects with CHD.[33,39] Xu observed similar results in a 1-year study, with the Qigong group attaining an increase in cardiac output, decrease in total peripheral resistance, increase in ejection fraction, and increase in mean velocity of circumferential fiber lengthening.[48]

Sun reports a 100% success rate in relieving angina pain in 51 patients with diagnosed CHD, with symptoms markedly improved in 29 of 51, significantly improved in 22 of 51, and documented ECG improvements in 94.12% of subjects.[46] Li reported on a study of 40 CHD patients with symptoms of dyspnea, angina, arrhythmias, palpitations, dizziness, insomnia, numbness, and excess perspiration. With Qigong practice, 18 of the 40 subjects returned to normal function, and 19 of the 40 cases showed marked improvement, both in relief of symptoms and by ECG.[43] Zhuo reports that in 32 CHD subjects treated with Qigong, 96.87% demonstrated a positive response, with symptomatic relief.[50] These were all uncontrolled studies.

Wang et al reported the effect of Qigong on cardiac function after 6 months of Qigong practice twice a day for 30 minutes (n = 67). They measured a significant increase in stroke work index, cardiac index, and vascular compliance, and a significant decrease in total peripheral resistance and systolic and diastolic pressures.[52]

OTHER CARDIAC CONDITIONS AND QIGONG

Various researchers also report successful results with Qigong in reducing the incidence of symptomatic congestive heart failure and acute myocardial infarction[47] and in the successful treatment of myocarditis, arrhythmias,[40] rheumatic heart disease with heart failure, and atrial fibrillation.[53]

SURGICAL QI

For cardiac procedures, Johnson reported that using Qigong preoperatively, postoperatively, and intraoperatively reduces bleeding, enhances immune function, minimizes infections, accelerates recovery, and reduces pain.[54] McGee reported reduction in recovery time by as much as 50%.[5] In a series of 34 minor surgery cases, Lin reported 91.8% success rate with Qigong surgical anesthesia.[55] In Qigong anesthesia "the patient loses his consciousness when the

Qigong master emits his Qi to him."[56] Of note, Machi reports the synchronization between the subject and Qi master in stimulated Qi anesthesia, of alpha and beta brain waves, and heart rate.[57]

THE SCIENCE OF QI: SOME STUDIES AND OBSERVATIONS

WHAT EXACTLY IS QI?

Activating Your Qi

Examine your palms and note the lighter colored area at the center of your palm. This point is the acupuncture point Pericardium 8, also known as the Lao Gung point, or "old worker." Rub your palms together, Lao Gung points meeting, as fast as possible, as if you're about to start a fire. Now notice the feeling between your hands. You may feel a tingling, a warmth, a magnetic sensation, or even a palpable "ball" of energy. What you feel between your hands is Qi. The more you practice Qigong, the more open and clearer you are, and the bigger this healing ball of Qi becomes.

Measuring Qi

Respected scientific laboratories in China such as the National Atomic Energy Lab in Shanghai and the Space Science and National Electro-Acoustics Institute in Beijing demonstrate that the Qi energy that Qigong masters emit is measurable as infrared, magnetic, static electric, and acoustical energy. Seto measured the magnetic field between the hands of healers to be in the range of 1 milligaus.[58] Niu and Liu[59] measured the infratonic sound waves emitted by a Qi master in the range of 45 to 76 decibels, or 100 to 1000 times stronger than that emitted by an ordinary person's 45 to 50 decibels. Via Kirlian photography, Lee beautifully documents the effects of Qi.[60]

Emitted Qi

Have you ever had someone tell you that they feel better just being near you? You're very likely "emitting" Qi. Emitted Qi from a Qigong master's hands has been documented in scientific laboratories to change the color of crystals, light fluorescent bulbs, increase the fluorescence of organisms by 68%,[61] kill in vitro laboratory cancer cells, expose light-sensitive plates, and change magnetic fields.[10]

Subjects' Experience of Qi

When receiving Qi emitted by a Qigong master, subjects may experience sensations of heat; electric current; pressure; pulsing energy; involuntary movement; perspiration; tingling; relaxation; pain relief; and simultaneous measurable changes in body temperature, skin temperature, blood pressure, heart rate, body secretions, nail fold circulation, etc.[13,36,61,62] and healthy weight loss over time.[62a] Subjects at times may also possibly experience temporary nausea, hot flashes, coldness, drowsiness, dizziness, palpitations, heaviness, emotional release, spontaneous tears, and/or some other discomfort as a healing aggravation reaction to the Qi, as part of the healing process.[14]

Non-Local Qi and at-a-Distance Qi Healing

Non-local Qi treatment at a distance is possible by "Yi Nian," which refers to the focus and clarity of the healer's intention, somewhat like prayer. Another kind of Qigong long distance treatment is via inert materials, such as Qi-energized audiotapes, paper, metal, glass, stone, clothes, etc., into which a Qi master has emitted Qi.[62-64]

The Biophysiology of Qi

Improved Circulation

Many studies report improved blood circulation (e.g., to nail fold beds, to the brain, and to diseased or stressed tissues).[34,36] Liu reports that in 68 subjects, Qigong exercises decreased blood levels of the vasoconstrictor 5-hydroxy-tryptamine (5HT) and increased levels of norepinephrine and dopamine, with resulting vasodilatation and increased blood flow.[64a] Increased blood flow both increases the delivery of oxygen, nutrients, and endorphins and the removal of metabolic waste products for pain relief.[65] As mentioned earlier, Qigong may also play a role in the coagulation fibrinolytic system.[66,67]

Sympathetic Parasympathetic Modulation

As mentioned earlier, some studies suggest that Qigong modulates parasympathetic tone.[68] Higuchi found that active Qigong meditation also decreases blood levels of plasma cortisol, adrenalin, and dopamine, which suggests that Qigong meditation may decrease sympathetic nervous system activity.[69]

Neurotransmitter and Hormone Activity

Higuchi found that Qi meditation increases levels of endorphins,[69] with other researchers demonstrating the inhibition of Qi analgesia by naloxone, suggesting the involvement of endogenous opiates.[70,71]

Qi applied to an acupuncture point releases neurotransmitters and hormones such as acetylcholine, methionine enkephalin, beta endorphin, ACTH, secretin, cholecystokinin, norepinephrine, serotonin, GABA, dopamine, dynorphin1-13, prostaglandin E1, serotonin, norepinephrine, and cholecystokinin.[72]

As mentioned earlier, Qigong practice has an effect on estradiol and testosterone levels as well.[73-76]

Immune Activity

There is also evidence for increased immune activity in subjects of emitted Qi,[65,77] with observable Qi-induced increased antibody levels against infections.[10,78]

Acupuncture Meridians and Energy Field

Sancier measured the electrical conductivity of acupuncture meridians and found that the active practice of Qigong balances the acupuncture meridians of internal organs.[79] Lee demonstrated with Kirlian photography the changes in the human energy field when the subject is giving Qi, versus receiving Qi, versus actively practicing Qigong.[10]

THE MYSTERY OF QI

Countless studies have demonstrated the effect of Qi on both living subjects and on inanimate objects. To eliminate the placebo effect, some of these studies have been performed on anesthetized animal subjects.

In Qigong healing, Machi measured simultaneous physiologic changes in both the subject and in the Qi master emitting Qi to the subject, such as synchronization of their heart rates, simultaneous changes in the EEG and ECG, galvanic skin resistance, and skin temperature. In both subject and Qi master, EEG alpha waves increased and beta waves decreased.[57]

Omura likewise found that a simultaneous marked increase in EEG alpha waves in both the patient and in the Qigong master emitting Qi to the patient. He furthermore found that bystanders in the same room who were simply observing the Qigong treatment experienced the same effect, and likewise even for people on different floors of the same building![80]

In one fascinating study, one group of Qigong masters emitted Qi. A second group of Qigong masters sat a distance away from their subjects, eyes closed, and were instructed to simply practice internal Qigong (i.e., focusing on their own "inner tranquility"). The Qigong masters who focused on their own inner state of Qi produced the same results as the masters who actively emitted Qi.[81]

In these and other studies, Qigong masters—without any voice, touch, or eye contact—used Qi to induce changes in their subjects for healing. For some inexplicable reason, Qigong masters and subjects, as healer and patient, somehow come together in unison, in oneness, as their heart rates, EEGs, and other indices become synchronous.

How exactly does Qi work? How does one Qigong master emitting Qi to a subject on one floor of the building have an effect on the people on another floor? What exactly produces the Qi bioelectric magnetic field that somehow, without any physical contact, brings about healing? How does prayer "work"? As in so much of medicine, the healing of Qi still remains somewhat a mystery.

THE *HOW* OF QI: SOME BASIC QIGONG PRACTICES

QIGONG POSTURE AND FINDING YOUR CENTER

"When you have a disease, do not try to cure it. Find your center, & you will be healed."

CHINESE PROVERB

The first step in Qigong is to find your center and *relax*. Different schools may call this "grounding," "centering," or finding your "alignment." In Qigong, paying attention to "correct" posture, how you stand, how you sit, how you walk, how you hold yourself as you walk through life, is key for finding and maintaining your center.

As in the Chinese character for emperor, or master, the correct Qi posture is standing centered, open, and tall, between heaven and earth, open to the heavens above, grounded to the earth below, aligned with the "universal" Qi. Many people stand rigid, tense, or hunched over, carrying responsibilities and the weight of the world on their shoulders and in their bodies. Correct Qi posture, centered between heaven and earth, allows the burdens to roll off your shoulders and is vital for the good flow of Qi.

THE BREATH OF QI

"Be still and know that I am."

PSALMS 46:10

The breath, as a catalyst for healing, is central to Qigong. With each breath, you can actively and consciously breathe in the universal vital life force, life-giving, energy of Qi. When I think of the Qigong breath, I think of the Sistine Chapel painting by Michelangelo of God breathing life into Adam and the fact that the words "inspire" and "spirit" come from the same root, *spiritus.* As there are many schools of Qigong, there are many different methods of breathing—at least 118, according to some Qigong texts.[14]

One of the most effective basic Qigong breathing techniques is deep diaphragmatic breathing, or breathing as a baby breathes: from the belly. On a physical level, the deep diaphragmatic breath of Qigong brings in more oxygen and facilitates the release of carbon dioxide and toxins. On another level, shallow breathing is related to non-permission and buried emotions, such as fear. Consciously breathing in Qi as positive life-force energy, with an open heart of compassion, and soft belly of letting go, can catalyze the release of these walled-off emotions. With each breath, remember to breathe out bad Qi and breathe in good Qi. On the in breath, allow each breath of life-giving Qi to wash, restructure, and reorder you—your body, your mind, your spirit, and your heart—down to the cellular DNA level in whatever way necessary to bring you into harmony with the Oneness of the universe.

"GOOD QI," "BAD QI"

"Pain is eliminated when the block is removed."

CHINESE MEDICINE PRINCIPLE

In Qigong, "bad Qi"—stagnant or blocked Qi—is the root cause of pain and *dis*ease. One way of dispelling bad Qi is to simply replace it with good Qi. On the in breath, breathe in good Qi, and imagine sending a golden ball of Qi, or a ball of love and light, from your heart to any area of discomfort in your body or to any ache in your heart. On the out breath, breathe out the bad, stagnant, or blocked Qi. To prevent the bad Qi from reentering, always remember to fill the space where the bad Qi used to be with good Qi.

QI EXERCISES: FREE YOUR BODY; FREE YOUR SPIRIT

"A day without dancing is a day lost."

UNKNOWN

The purpose of the physical Qigong exercises is to open your body and spirit to the healing of Qi. The exercises help open and bring into balance your meridian energy channels—for greater Qi, awareness, healing, and healing ability. Hundreds of different Qigong exercises are available for a wide range of different purposes. For those suffering from some medical illness and seeking alleviation of symptoms, and perhaps even healing, the Chow Medical Qigong set of exercises is superb. For serious students of Qigong, it is best to study under a Qigong master because even a slight adjustment in performing a specific exercise can make a tremendous difference in the flow of Qi.

Those new to Qigong will appreciate an easy-to-learn Qi exercise: shaking Qigong. Find your center, open your base, check your posture, and align yourself. Now simply shake your body from head to toe, vertebra by vertebra. With a gentle "inner smile" of self-love, shake out all your worries, troubles, tension, discomfort, and disease. Allow yourself to shake yourself free, let go, and fill with life-giving Qi.

QI MEDITATION

"To forget a thousand useless thoughts, focus on one pure thought."

A QIGONG TEACHER

Qigong meditation encompasses many of the same teachings of other schools of meditation (e.g., mindfulness stress reduction, visualization, hypnosis, transcendental meditation, vipassana, and centering prayer). Qigong, like centering prayer, calls upon a higher source for healing. In Qigong, this greater source is universal Qi.

The ultimate purpose of Qigong meditation is not to just quiet the mind but also to bring one's heart, body, mind, and spirit into harmony with the oneness of the universe, so that the healer is in such a constant state of inner peace, inner knowing, acceptance, centeredness, harmony, and of course love that regardless of any ongoing darkness and chaos, the healer's very *being* or presence is healing. Besides helping you find your center amidst the chaos and stress of day-to-day living, Qigong meditation helps give you the freedom to be who you truly are and the ability to move from your center with greater clarity and power.

THE MICROCOSMIC ORBIT AND FIVE-ELEMENT MEDITATIONS

"The root of all disease is spiritual... in the mind and the emotions."

TAE WOO YOO OMD, PHD, KORYO HAND ACUPUNCTURE

Have you ever had a patient present with a purely somatic complaint, unaware of feelings, and in denial of any possible underlying wound to the psyche? The physical symptom points to a deeper psychospiritual pain and is a call for help. The Qigong microcosmic orbit and five-element meditations help you and your patient become aware of these deeper wounds and help you, as healer, and your patient become free from the pain pictures and concomitant blocked or stagnant, stuck Qi, around these wounds.

The Microcosmic Cycle Meditation

Visualize your Qi as a ball of light circulating from your Dan Tian, the seat of energy 2 inches below your umbilicus; down to your Hui Yin, or perineum; then up the Governing Vessel energy channel along your spine; then through your pelvic Lower Gate, which is related to fear, sexuality, willpower, and your pelvic organs; next through your abdominal Middle Gate, which is about power, control, resistance, judgment, empowerment, and your abdominal organs; then to your thoracic Upper Gate and issues around heart sadness and joy, speaking your truth, surrendering to Divine will, and your thoracic organs; then up to your crown or Bai Hui, your Divine knowing and connection to the heavens; then back down the front of your body along your Conception Vessel to your Dan Tian. As you actively visualize the Qi circulating through the Microcosmic cycle, visualize the Qi washing away any stuck, blocked, or stagnant Qi having do do with the issues of the Lower, Middle, and Upper Gates, and/or your Conception Vessel, Governing Vessel, Dan Tian (belly), Hui Yin (perineum), and Bai Hui (crown).

The Five-Element Meditation

The body is about the five senses. The spirit is about the five elements: fire, earth, metal, water, and wood. Each of the five elements governs a coupled yin yang organ pair (e.g., heart and pericardium), each with a specific energy channel acupuncture meridian "map" on the body. Each of the five elements is associated with a specific set of emotions and a whole set of other characteristics specific to the particular element as well: color, taste, season, etc. For example, the element of the heart is fire, emotion joy or sadness, and color red. An emotional heartache, if not released and cleared, eventually leads to a physical manifestation. The five-element location of presenting symptoms, the five-element color a patient chooses to wear, and so on all provides clues to a patient's deeper wounds and "stuck" Qi.

The microcosmic orbit and five-element meditations are both core to Qigong. Each meditation will help free the spirit, to free the body in a powerful yet gentle way, for healing.

QI MEDICAL INTUITION: PICTURES, MIRRORS, AND AWARENESS

"Stressed is desserts spelled backwards."

UNKNOWN

With regular disciplined Qigong practice and meditation come increased awareness and intuition. Many Qigong masters are natural medical intuitives, with uncanny "x-ray vision." In a moment, they "read" or somehow know the intimate details of your life, details which no ordinary person could possibly know. With Qigong practice and meditation, as the noise of the useless random thoughts become quiet, you may find yourself also becoming more intuitive and aware.

As you yourself become more intuitive and start seeing pain pictures in others, know that on some level every patient is a mirror for you. For every pain picture you recognize in someone else, you yourself have a matching picture for your own pain. This is especially true for those toward whom you feel a strong emotional reaction. The more aware you become of *your* own pain pictures, the more you clear your own blocked, stagnant, bad Qi; the freer, clearer, and greater a vessel you become for greater Qi, the more effective healer you'll be.

THE WAY OF QI: SOME PRACTICAL QI TOOLS FOR HEALING

"The Way that can be spoken is not the Way."

LAO TZE

Many different Qigong techniques are effective. Qigong master Dr. Zhi Gang Sha, OMD, author of *Power Healing*, teaches a one hand close/one hand far technique.[82] For specific techniques for different ailments, Johnson's textbook *Chinese Medical Qigong Therapy* is the most thorough source available in English.[83] Some Qigong masters teach, however, that rather than memorizing techniques, mastering some basic core tools such as learning to feel into your heart, listen for your own inner guidance, and trust that your heart and hands will know where to go is far more valuable. We share with you here some practical easy ways to apply basic core tools.

SCANNING QI

To scan, or diagnose, a patient's Qi, run your hands about 6 to 12 inches over the patient's body and feel his or her energy field. Areas that seem hot and push your hands out have excess Qi. Areas that seem cold and pull in your hands in have deficient Qi. Excess or deficient Qi are signs of blockage, pain, illness, or injury. As you scan, allow yourself to intuitively "see" and "feel" what "pictures" or emotions may underlie your subject's presenting symptoms and complaints.

DIRECTING QI

For treatment, brush away the excess Qi, which are the areas that feel hot and/or that push your hands out. Pack the deficient areas, which are those areas that feel cold or empty or pull your hands in, with good Qi. Simply brushing away and packing in Qi as indicated often gives significant relief. With this intentional movement of Qi, the patient may feel Qi sensations such as warmth and tingling.

QI ACUPUNCTURE

One can also transmit Qi through an acupuncture needle or via the fingertips to indicated acupuncture points and meridians, or acupuncture "correspondence" points, for "needle-less" Qi acupuncture.[84,85]

QI-ENERGIZED MATERIAL

Some Qigong masters have found good results with Qi magnetic tapes[64] and audio recorded Qi music tapes as well.[44]

EMITTING QI AND TRANSMITTING QI

In "emitting" Qi, the healer "emits," or beams out the Qi he has cultivated, accumulated, and stored in his/her Dan Tian and other energy centers. In "transmitting" Qi the healer serves as a conduit for Qi to flow through the healer from a higher source to the subject. Qi may be emitted and/or transmitted via your Lao Gong points, which are found at the center of your palm, via your fingertips, and also by your very presence or being.

NON-LOCAL HEALING AND YI NIAN CLEAR INTENTION

Non-local long-distance Qigong healing is by Yi Nian: "so be it" clear intention. Dr. Tae Woo Yoo, PhD, OMD, demonstrates this kind of healing by dispelling a subject's pain, without any direct eye, voice, or physical contact with the subject. On one occasion, Dr. Yoo simply, with Yi Nian clear intention, drew the correct acupuncture prescription for the subject on a blackboard, out of view of the subject, and the subject's chronic pain of years disappeared, only to return in moments when he erased the correct prescription and wrote instead an incorrect prescription. The pain then disappeared again with the correct prescription. As a healer, hold a Yi Nian clear intention of the perfection possible, and without attachment, expect "miracles."

Some Qigong masters, as catalysts for healing, come from such a grounded space of centeredness, clarity, power, surrender, and love, that by their very *being* and "Yi Nian" clear intention are able to command and heal.

QI FOR THE HEART AND SOUL

Regardless of your religious beliefs, and for that matter, regardless of whether you even believe in God, there is a kind of Qi that can touch, feed, and heal your heart and soul. One effective way of opening to this level of Qi is repetition of a "sacred" sound, such as "aaah-lah-hu" or "om." Interestingly, a National Institutes of Health (NIH) panel stated that a variety of techniques work in "lowering one's breathing rate, heart rate, and blood pressure" as long as they had two essential elements, "a repetitive focus of a word, sound, prayer, phrase, or muscular activity, and neither fighting nor focusing on intruding thoughts."[86]

THE ART OF QI: HEALER, HEAL THYSELF

SOME QI MIND-BODY PRINCIPLES: LOVE, LAUGHTER, HUGS, AND TOUCH

"One joy shatters a thousand griefs."

CHINESE PROVERB

"A merry heart doeth good medicine make."

PROVERBS 17:22

Qigong is an attitude. One must continually remind and discipline oneself each moment to have, as Qigong Grandmaster Effie Chow, Ph.D., R.N., LAc would say, a PMA: positive mental attitude. Qigong reframes the challenges of life's day-to-day stresses and crises as opportunities to grow. The Chinese word for *crisis* translates as either "danger" or as "opportunity." In Qigong, your symptoms are your friends, and we intentionally choose to "reframe" the challenges of life in a positive light, look for the blessings in disguise, and simply give thanks.

In the schools of the more enlightened Qigong masters, love is a foundation cornerstone for healing. Although it is indeed possible to reach some degree of mastery in Qigong just with disciplined practice, the key of love expands your healing to a whole new level. One of Qigong Grandmaster Dr. Effie Chow's prescriptions for healing is to "give and receive lots of love." Dr. Jaffe tells his own story of how years ago he developed a serious cardiac condition, with months left to live. His teacher prescribed "love" for the physical healing of his heart, and with love, his heart was indeed physically healed.[87]

On another level, psychoneuroimmunology studies have documented the mind-body connection—how thoughts and emotions affect your immune system. Qigong demonstrates how thoughts and emotions affect Qi via kinesiology. Negative thoughts and feelings decrease your Qi and make you physically weaker. Positive thoughts, feelings, and/or love increase your Qi and make you physically stronger.

To increase positive thoughts, positive feelings, and positive Qi, the Chow Medical Qigong System actively incorporates love, laughter, hugs, and touch in treatment sessions. Qigong Grandmaster Dr. Effie Chow's prescriptions for healing include at least eight hugs a day and "at least three belly-aching laughs a day."

Qigong is thus about intentionally *choosing* and giving thanks for the good, and about cultivating positive thoughts and feelings, ones that make your heart sing, and give you something to live for. One way of making a positive "good Qi" choice in any particular situation is to ask yourself the question, "If I were a messenger of love, what words, thoughts, and/or actions would I choose?"

THE INNER SMILE: SELF LOVE, ACCEPTANCE, FORGIVENESS, AND CONTENTMENT

"Peace starts with a smile."

MOTHER THERESA

Physicians are notorious for being great givers and poor receivers. Remembering to give yourself an "inner smile," a smile of self-love, acceptance, and contentment is core to Qigong healing. The more you love, accept, and *forgive* yourself, the easier it is to love, accept, and forgive others. The more harmonious you are with yourself, the easier it is to be in harmony with your outside circumstances, with the people surrounding you, and with the universe. True self-love, self-acceptance, and self-forgiveness frees you to accept life as is, to open your heart to greater Qi, and as a healer to move in a more powerful, clear, and centered way. Thus with each breath in Qigong, practice giving to yourself, to your heart, to your body, to each five-element organ, down to every cell, an inner smile.

UNIVERSAL QI: EGO, ONENESS, AND SURRENDER

"EGO stands for easing God out."

UNKNOWN

All true healing in Qigong comes from a higher power. Knowing and surrendering to the higher power of universal Qi is key for Qigong healing. To be an effective healer in Qigong, one must, *without ego*, surrender and open to the flow of universal Qi from this higher source, both the big ego of arrogance and the small ego of unworthiness. Anyone who attempts to practice Qigong from ego or for self-serving ends limits and may even lose the ability to heal with Qi.

QIGONG AS A WAY OF LIFE: DE, VIRTUE, AND RIGHT LIVING

"Let Go; Let God; Let Love"

UNKNOWN

Qigong Master Dr. Yan Xin teaches that "observing virtue is the fundamental principle for success in Qigong."[14] In Qigong, *De* is the virtue of your moral character. It comprises 10 aspects: moral attitude or politeness; moral conduct; beneficence or true selfless generosity; fairness; equality; charity or benevolence; respect; truthfulness; self-reflection or self-responsibility; and righteousness.

Thus Qigong is far more than just practicing the Qigong exercises. In Qigong, the way you think, the way you relate to your loved ones, the way you relate to your community, the way you relate to the world, the way you handle your emotions, the way you care for your body, the way you earn a living, the way you stand in the universe, the way you commune with nature, the way you commune with God, and the way you love all determine your peace of mind, your state of health, and your quality and level of Qi. The choices you make about the *way* you live determine *how* you live; how you age; how you love; and how healthy, happy, free, and whole you are.

In Qigong, remember that your symptoms are your friends and that illness is a wake-up call that invites you to take an inventory of your life. Do you really need a heart attack before you wake up to what is truly important in life? Are you living a life of "De" or virtue (i.e., having the right livelihood, right relationships, and right self-care)? Are you living a life that truly and fully nourishes your heart? Are you, in Qi, living life to the fullest?

Confucius taught that first you take care of yourself, then you serve your family, then your community, then the world. In Qigong, the more you live a life true to your heart of hearts, the greater Qi is available to you, and the more effective a healer you'll be. Qigong, at its highest, is a way of life.

INTEGRATING QIGONG INTO YOUR PRACTICE: ONE PHYSICIAN'S PERSPECTIVE

"Start the day with Love. Fill the day with Love. End the day with Love."

SAI BABA

There are many ways of integrating Qigong into your life and practice, from the practice of consciously remembering to *fully breathe* each breath *with Qi* to *fully* living a life of Qi. For our patients, we've offered weekly Qigong classes for the past 9 years and have yet to have any regular attendee suffer a cardiac event. And yes, the class participants are self-selected, and there are no controls.

On a day-to-day level, as physicians, we do our best to teach our patients Qigong PMA (positive mental attitude) mind-body principles; Qigong diaphragmatic breathing; how to breathe in good Qi and breathe out bad Qi; how to ground; how to find their center and alignment; and last but not least, the power of Love. For those willing to do the real work, we teach our patients how to identify their own pain pictures, release the bad Qi around these pictures, and open to the healing of simply breathing in positive Qi. We also frequently use Qi Koryo hand acupuncture, which we find especially effective in relieving chest pain.[85,88]

For patients who are responsive to Qigong, we expect to see results within the first session: patients with blood pressures in the 240/115 mm Hg range may drop their blood pressure to the range of 140-160/80-100 mm Hg.

As an example of how we integrate Qigong into our daily office routine, I once saw a 77-year-old widow for her 2-year history of hypertension after her husband's death. She had blood pressures usually around 200/90 mm Hg and complained of lightheadedness and cough on her antihypertensive medication. During her first appointment, with basic Qigong diaphragmatic breathing and some simple Qi Koryo hand acupressure, her blood pressure dropped immediately from 170/80 to 124/70 mmHg. Upon the mention of her late husband, however, her systolic blood pressure rose to 140/60 mm Hg. Her pain picture was about the 50 years she suffered an abusive marriage. When we taught her how to find and release her buried pain pictures and emotions and focus instead on breathing in positive Qi, her blood pressure dropped within minutes to 120/58 mm Hg.

Upon her 2-week follow-up appointment, she reported that her morning blood pressure without medication was now usually 118-125/53-70 mm Hg but would increase with stress and/or stressful thoughts. On follow-up 1 month later, we guided her again on how to find and release her pain pictures, and her blood pressure dropped from 145/73 to 110/70 mm Hg. On this visit and in a thank-you letter over a year later, she reported that she had learned to lower her own blood pressure with Qigong meditation, had markedly reduced her dosage of antihypertensive medication, slept better, and furthermore no longer suffered medication side effects such as dry cough and lightheadedness.

CONCLUSION: QI HAPPENS!

"Gold is precious, but true Qi is priceless."

CHINESE PROVERB

My teachers and I are the first to admit that much of the material we have presented in this chapter isn't anything new. The principles as taught in Qigong are not by any means unique to Qigong. Different schools, cultures, and teachers throughout the ages have taught from this same universal body of wisdom.

As with any Qigong practitioner, we see many "miracles" in our practice, some remarkable. A "miracle", however, may be as ordinary as a smile or a teardrop. Once again, the miracles of Qigong are freely available to all. Your job as a healer is to serve as a facilitator, or catalyst, for your patients, to help them awaken to wisdom within, the healer within, and to the healing possible with Qi.

More definitive rigorous clinical studies are certainly needed, as are accredited, clinical medical Qigong teaching programs for health professionals. Although the research and accreditation of Qigong is a work in process, Qigong has had such a profound impact in my life and in my practice of medicine that I am thankful to share these simple yet profound tools with you now. What words can express the tremendous difference Qigong can make in your life, your practice, and in the lives of your patients?

We invite you to give yourself a minute to take a deep breath, go within, be still, feel into your heart, and see for yourself.

ACKNOWLEDGMENTS AND THANKS

My special thanks to my children Ben, Fred, Tara, and Christopher. Thanks to my parents Dr. Chi-Chao Chiu, MD and Dr. Yung-Tsing Wong, MD and to the following people for their support, teachings, wisdom, and interviews for this chapter:

- Qigong Master Stephen Aung, MD, FAAFP, Faculty, University of Alberta Medical School and President Canadian Medical Acupuncture Society
- Qigong Grandmaster Effie Pow Yew Chow, PhD LAc, founder of East West Academy of Healing Arts, World Qigong Federation & American Qigong Association
- Qigong Master Roger Estes, Qigong Master
- Robert Ibriham Jaffe MD, founder of Jaffe Institute
- Richard Lee, founder of China Healthways Institute
- Carole and Charles McGee, MD, co-author with Dr Effie Chow of *Miracle Healing from China*
- Qigong Master Stephen Kong, PhD, Qigong Master and Chairman Sino-American Communications
- Kahuna Lokahi Ku, native Hawaiian healer and holy man
- Michael Mayer, PhD of Body Mind Healing
- Charles McGee MD, co-author with Dr. Effie Chow of *Qigong Miracle Healing from China*
- Qigong Master Dr. Yoshiaki Omura, MD, Director of Medical Research Heart Disease Research Foundation
- Ken Sancier, PhD, Founder and Director Qigong Institute
- Jim Self and Roxanne Burnette, Directors of the Avalon Institute
- Sidi, UN Peace Talk speaker and holy man
- Katherine and Richard Weiner, PhD, founders of the American Academy of Pain Management

REFERENCES

Please note that many of the references cited were made available for this publication thanks to Ken Sancier, PhD, Director of the Qigong Institute, in abstract form by the Qigong Institute's computerized Qigong database.

1. Dossey L: Reinventing medicine: beyond mind body to a new era of healing, New York, 1999, Harper Collins.
2. Chow E: The miracles of medical qigong: directed energy for healing of self, The Second World Congress on Qigong and the 1st American Qigong Association Conference, San Francisco, 37, 1998.
2a. Chow E: Chow Qigong: an antidote for modern day stress, The Second World Congress on Qigong and the 1st American Qigong Association Conference San Francisco, 37, 1998.
3. Hayashi S: Qigong and mental health, Fourth International Congress on Qigong, 26-27, 1995.
4. Wang J: Role of Qigong on mental health, Second World Conf Acad Exch Med Qigong, 93, 1993.
5. McGee C, Chow EPY: Qigong miracle healing from China, Coeur d'Alene, ID, 1994, Medipress.
6. Sancier KM: Therapeutic benefits of qigong exercises in combination with drugs, Int Soc Life Inf Sci 5(4):383-389, 1999.
7. Van Collie S: While they sleep, Pacific Sun, April 23, 1997.
8. Ornish D: Dr. Dean Ornish's program for reversing heart disease, New York, 1990, Random House.
9. Ornish D, Brown SE, Scherwitz LW et al: Can lifestyle changes reverse coronary arteriosclerosis? Lancet 336:129-133, 1990.
10. Lee R: Scientific investigation into Chinese Qigong, San Clemente, Calif, 1999, China Healthways Institute.
11. Chow EPY, Hole LCN: Report on the 2002 Fifth World Congress on Qigong, American Holistic Medical Association Newsletter VII:1, Winter 2003.
12. Eisenberg D: Encounters with Qi: exploring Chinese medicine, New York, 1985, WW Norton.
13. Wu H: Chinese super power meditation: the experiment, healing effort, and theory of a new technique for training qi-energy, Second International Conference on Qigong, 267, 1989.
14. Xin Yan: Basics of Qigong, Version 1.4, 2003, International Yan Xin Qigong Association, Berkeley, CA.
15. Sancier, K: San Francisco Qigong database, Menlo Park, Calif, 2002, Qigong Institute of San Francisco.
16. Mayer MH: Qigong clinical studies. In Jonas WB, editor: Healing, intention, and energy medicine, New York, 2003, Churchill Livingston.
17. Kuang A, Wang C, Xu D, Qian Y: Research on antiaging effect of qigong, J Tradit Chin Med 11(2):153-158 and 11(3):224-227, 1991.
18. Li Z, Zhang B: Group observation and experimental research on the prevention and treatment of hypertension by qigong, Proc First World Conf Acad Exch Med Qiqong, Beijing, China, 113-114, 1988.

19. Wu R, Liu Z: Study of qigong on hypertension and reduction of hypotension, Second World Conf Acad Exch Med Qigong, Beijing, China, 125, 1993.

20. Jing G: Observations on the curative effects of qigong self adjustment therapy in hypertension. Proc First World Conf Acad Exch Med Qigong, Beijing, China, 115-117, 1988.

21. Shih TK, Zucker P, Ohrenstein N: The effects of qigong on resting systemic BP and quality of life in hypertensive adults, Qi: J Tradit East Health Fitness 8(2):31-33, 1997.

22. Chu C: Changes in blood viscosity and rheocardiogram in 44 cases with cardiovascular diseases after qigong, First World Conf Acad Exch Med Qigong, Beijing, China, 57, 1988.

23. Huang, X: Clinical observation of 204 patients with hypertension treated with qigong, Proc First Intl Conf, 101, 1990.

24. Liu S: Treatment and clinical research of hypertension, Fourth World Conf Acad Exch Med Qigong, 161-162, 1998.

25. Lim J: Qigong in Australia, an effective weapon against stress, First World Conf Acad Exch Med Qigong, 155, 1988.

26. Pan LB, Zhang ZF: Qigong treatment for hypertension caused by renal insufficiency, Third Natl Acad Conf Qigong Sci, Guangzhou, China, 90, 1990.

27. Huang Z: Effect of qigong on heart function, Second World Conf Acad Exch Med Qigong, Beijing, China, 1993.

28. Wen DE: Static qigong, cross-legged sitting posture and the blood redistribution, Fourth Conf Acad Exch Med Qigong, 201-202, 1998.

29. Sancier K: Medical applications of qigong, Altern Therap 2(1):40-46, 1996.

30. Chai Z, Wang B: Influence of qigong state on blood perfusion state of human microcirculation, Third Natl Acad Conf Qigong Sci, Guangzhou, China, 116, 1990.

31. Wang C, Xu D, Qian Y et al: The beneficial effects of qigong on the ventricular function and microcirculation of deficiency in heart energy hypertensive patience, Chin J Intern Med 1(1):21-23, 1995.

32. Sancier K: Anti-aging benefits of qigong, Third World Conf Acad Exch Med Qigong, 147, 1996.

33. Qu Z, Wang C, Xu D, Qian Y: Peripheral resistance variances and qigong therapy in hypertension of the heart-qi deficiency and blood stasis type, Seventh Intl Symp Qigong, Shanghai, 134, 1998.

34. Cheng K, Zhu R, Zhu J et al: Study of the Chinese ancient method for keeping in good health and longevity of the Taoist School: an analysis of 102 cases, Fourth Int Symp on Qigong, 57, 1992.

35. Guo Yangui: Scientific way of health preservation, Fourth World Conf Acad Exch Med Qigong, 224-225, 1998.

35a. Guo Yangui: Everyone preserving health scientifically, Fourth World Conf Acad Exch Med Qigong, 219-220, 1998b.

36. Jing Y, Liu X, Wang Z, Wang Q, Yao A: Effect of Hichugong on 31 cases of diabetes, Second World Conf Acad Exch Med Qigong, 135, 1993.

37. Xian BH. Clinical observation of 204 patients with hypertension treated with Chinese Qigong, Fifth Intl Cong Qigong, Berkeley, Calif, 1990.

38. Xu S: Effect of qigong exercise on high density lipoprotein content and subfractions in human serum, Third Nat Acad Conf on Qigong Science, 13, 1990.

39. Wang C, Xu D, Qian Y et al: Beneficial effect of qigong on improving the heart function and relieving multiple cardiovascular risk factors, First World Conf Acad Exch Med Qigong, 88, 1988.

40. Fu Q: Treatment and prevention of coronary heart disease by digital pressure, Third World Conf Acad Exch Med Qigong, 136, 1996.

41. Hu X, Zhang G: The effect of daoyin health qigong to improve the function of nerves and heart in aged women, Fourth World Conf Acad Exch Med Qigong, 118-120, 1998.

42. Jin KQ: Effect of qigong on electrocardiographic autopower spectrum function, Chung Kuo Chung Hsi I Chieh Ho Tsa Chih 12(7): 412-13, 1992.

43. Li S, Chen Z: 40 cases of coronary heart disease treated by qi operating method and its mechanism, Third World Conf Acad Exch Med Qigong, 134, 1996.

44. Lu L, Liu Y, Zhuang Y: The clinical study of coronary heart disease treated by qigong with music, Third World Conf Acad Exch Med Qigong, 135, 1996.

45. Liu J, Chen J, Jia S: Clinical observation of the effects on hypertension complicated by coronary heart disease treated by China Informative qigong, Fourth World Conf Acad Exch Med Qigong, 151-152, 1998.

46. Sun J, Yuan R, Yang C: Analysis of 51 cases with coronary heart disease treated by qigong, First World Conf Acad Exch Med Qigong, 135, 1988.

47. Xing ZH, Li W: Effect of qigong on blood pressure and life quality of essential hypertensive patients, Chung Kuo Chung His Chieh Ho Tsu Chih Institute of Combined TCM-WM, Hunan Medical University, Changsha, China, 7:413-414, 1991.

48. Xu D, Wang C: Recuperative function of qigong on hypertensive target impairment, Second World Conf Acad Exch Med Qigong, 124, 1993b.

49. Zhou S: Effects of qigong on the prostacyclin thromboxane balance in patients with coronary heart diseases, First World Conf Acad Exch Med Qigong, 117, 1988.

50. Zhuo P: Preliminary report of treating 32 cases of coronary heart disease by a system of deep breathing exercises, Second Int Conf on Qigong, 188, 1989.

51. Wang C, Xu D, Qian Y et al: The beneficial effect of qigong on the hypertension incorporated with coronary heart disease, Third Int Symp on Qigong, 40, 1990.

52. Wang Z, Zhou L, Li C et al: Experimental research on the values of cardiac function by Dao Yin Yang Sheng Gong, Second Int Conf on Qigong, 40, 1989.

53. Yang YG: A clinical study on qigong combined with medicine in the treatment of 30 rheumatic heart disease cases, The Second World

Congress on Qigong and the 1st American Qigong Association Conference, San Francisco, 52, 1998.

54. Johnson JA: Medical qigong therapy and surgery, Fourth World Conf Acad Exch Med Qigong, 163-164, 1998.

55. Lin H: Clinical and laboratory study of the effect of qigong anaesthesia on thyroidectomy, First World Conf Acad Exch Med Qigong, 84, 1988.

56. Inosuke Y: Fundamentals of qigong anesthesia and examples, Second World Conf Acad Exch Med Qigong, 117, 1993.

57. Machi Y, Chu WZ: Physiological measurement for qigong anesthesia, J Int Soc Life Inf Sci 14(2):129-145, 1996.

58. Seto A: Detection of extraordinarily large bio-magnetic field strength from human hand, Acupunc ElectroTherap Res Intl J 17:75-94, 1992.

59. Niu X, Liu G: Measurement and analysis of the infrasonic waves from the emitted qi, Proc First World Conf Acad Exch Med Qigong, Beijing, China, 1988.

60. Lee RH: Bioelectric vitality: exploring the science of human energy, San Clemente, Calif, China Healthways Institute, 1997.

61. Lin M: Observation on skin thermography during qigong needling, First World Conf Acad Exch Med Qigong, 147, 1988.

62. Nishimoto S: Report on the changing of the autonomic nervous system reducing pain of patients treated by external qi with alpha wave 1/F music, Third World Conf Acad Exch Med Qigong, 147, 1996.

62a. Wang Y: Miraculous qigong for slimming down, Fourth Intl Conf on Qigong, 30-31, 1995.

63. Omura Y: Storing of qigong energy in various materials and drugs (qigongization), Acupunct Electrotherap Res Intl J 15(2):137-57, 1990.

64. Lim J: Healing with qi magnetic tape: a new development in qigong healing, Second World Conf Acad Exch Med Qigong, 143, 1993.

64a. Liu H: Mastering miracles, New York, 1997, Warner Books.

65. Liu B, Jiao K, Chne Q et al: Effect of qigong exercise on the content of monoamine neurotransmitters in blood, First World Conf Acad Exch Med Qigong, 67, 1988.

66. Wang C, Xu D, Qian Y et al: Effects of qigong on preventing stroke and alleviating the multiple cerebro-cardiovascular risk factors: a follow-up report on 242 hypertensive cases over 30 years, Proc Second World Conf Acad Exch Med Qigong, Beijing, China, 123-124, 1993.

67. Wang CX, Xu DH, Qian YC: Effect of qigong on heart-qi deficiency and blood stasis type of hypertension and its mechanism, Chung Kuo Chung Hsi I Chieh Ho Tsa Chih 15(8):454-8, 1995.

68. Lee MS, Huh HJ, Kim BG et al: Effects of Qi-training on heart rate variability, Am J Chinese Med 30(4):463, 2002.

69. Higuchi Y: Endocrine and immune response during guolin new Qigong, J Int Soc Life Inf Sci 15(1):138, 1997.

70. Yang K, Xu H, Guo Z et al: Analgesic effect of emitted qi on white rats, First World Conf Acad Exch Med Qigong, 45, 1988.

71. Zhang J, Chen Y, He J et al: Analgesic effect of emitted qi and the preliminary study of its mechanism, Third Nat Acad Conf on Qigong Science, 37, 1990.

72. Omura Y. Bidigital O-ring test for diagnosis, treatment and evaluation of therapeutic effects and localization of meridians and acupuncture points. 1st Int Cong of Qigong, 97, 1990.

73. Kuang AK, Chen JL, Lu YR. Changes of the sex hormones in female type II diabetics, coronary heart disease, essential hypertension and its relations with kidney deficiency, cardiovascular complications and efficacy of traditional Chinese medicine or qigong treatment, Chung Hsi I Chieh Ho Tsa Chih 9(6):331-34, 1989.

74. Lu H, Zhen J, Luo J et al: Effect of emitted qi on testosterone and estradiol in rats, Third Nat Acad Conf on Qigong Science, 63, 1990.

75. Sancier K: Anti-aging benefits of qigong, J Intl Soc Life Inf Sci 14(1):12-21, 1996.

76. Wang C, Xu D, Qian Y et al: Research on anti aging effect of qigong, First World Conf Acad Exch Med Qigong, 85, 1988.

77. Wu T, Wu J: Increase the immune system naturally, The Second World Congress on Qigong and the 1st American Qigong Association Conference, San Francisco, 51, 1998.

78. Jang J: A brief review of Kong Jim Qigong's influence on immunologic function, Second Intl Conf on Qigong, 131, 1989.

79. Sancier KM: The effect of qigong on therapeutic balancing measured by electroacupuncture according to voll (EAV): a preliminary study, Acupunct Electrother Res Int J 9 (2/3):119-127, 1994.

80. Omura Y: Simple method for evaluating qigong state; reversible changes in qigong master and subject; effect of qigong on bacteria, viruses, and acupressure points, First Int Cong of Qigong, 129, 1990.

81. Sun C, Liu C, Shen Z et al: Effect of Xiantian-ziran qigong on red blood cells, Third Nat Acad Conf on Qigong Science, 48, 1990.

82. Sha, ZG: *Power Healing*, San Francisco, 2002, Harper.

83. Johnson JA: Chinese medical Qigong therapy, Pacific Grove, Calif, 2000, International Institute of Medical Qigong.

84. He J: Qigong acupuncture therapy, Second Int Conf on Qigong, 196, 1989.

85. Hole LC: Qigong miracle healing for the new millennium and Koryo hand therapy: acupuncture to go. In Weintraub M, editor: Alternative and complementary treatment in neurologic illness, New York, 2001, Elsevier.

86. National Institute of Health Technology Assessment Panel: Integration of behavioral and relaxational approaches into the treatment of chronic pain and insomnia, JAMA 276(4):313-318. 1996.

87. Jaffe RI: An Interview with Dr. Jaffe (audiocassette), Pope Valley, Calif, Jaffe Institute, 2004.

88. Hole LC: Qigong: a paradigm shift tool for pain management, and Qi-KHT Koryo hand therapy for pain relief. In Wiener R, editor: Pain management: a practical guide for clinicians, ed 6, Boca Raton, FL, 2002, CRC Press.

CHAPTER 11

Qigong and Tai Chi: Traditional Chinese Health Promotion Practices in the Prevention and Treatment of Cardiovascular Disease

Roger Jahnke, OMD

Although morbidity and mortality from cardiovascular disease in the United States have declined with concurrent biomedical advances, these conditions claim the lives of more men and women each year than the next five leading causes of death combined. The 2003 expenditures for cardiovascular disease are estimated at $351.8 billion, including the direct costs of physician, hospital, and nursing home services; the cost of medications; home healthcare costs; and loss of productivity. Nonetheless cardiovascular disease is well known to be preventable through behavioral change.[1]

Patients' incorporating complementary and alternative therapeutic modalities into their healthcare activities, including the traditional components of Chinese medicine—even at their own expense—is a clear trend.[2,3] In the area of cardiovascular diseases, the National Center for Complementary and Alternative Medicine (NCCAM) at the National Institutes of Health (NIH) are supporting clinical trials, specialized centers, research training, and investigator-initiated projects. Two of the strategies that are generating a wider research audience are the combination of exercise and meditation that have evolved as the self-care components of Traditional Chinese Medicine (TCM): Qigong (Chi Kung) and Tai Chi (Taiji).[4]

A recent review of research on the physical and psychological effects of Tai Chi on various chronic medical conditions in the *Archives of Internal Medicine* reported that this gentle mind-body practice has been found to have a positive effect for prevention and treatment of a wide array of chronic disorders, including cardiovascular diseases.[5]

Qigong and Tai Chi provide powerful, easy-to-implement, cost-effective strategies for the prevention and treatment of cardiovascular disease. Along with acupuncture, herbal medicine, and traditional Chinese physical therapy (Tui Na, acupressure), TCM emphasizes the importance of teaching the patient how to remain well through Qigong and Tai Chi. Combining gentle exercise and meditation cultivates inner strength, calms the mind and nervous system, and helps the body to regain its natural state of health by activating and maximizing natural self-regulatory function. In the written medical literature of several millennia ago, the Chinese proclaimed that the human body naturally produces an inner elixir, an internally produced medicine, "the healer within." Because healthy individuals, as well as the severely ill, can use Qigong and Tai Chi, they represent two of the most broadly applicable systems of holistic self-care.

WHAT ARE QIGONG AND TAI CHI?

Qigong and Tai Chi combine gentle body movement, postural correction, mental focus, visualization, and breath regulation to enhance overall physiological and psychological function (Fig. 11-1). These practices—moving meditation, dynamic meditation, or meditation in motion—are suited for all populations.

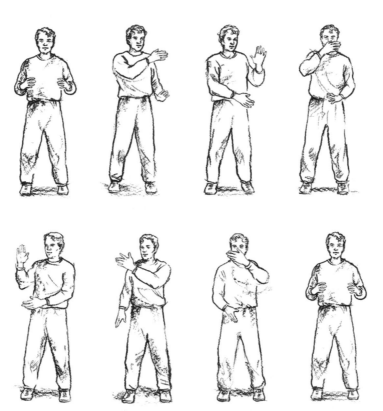

Fig 11-1. Qigong and Tai Chi are easy to learn and practice methods of self-care that are cost effective and can be modified for each patient's clinical needs. (*From Jahnke R: The healing promise of Qi: creating extraordinary wellness through Qigong and Tai Chi, New York, 2002, McGraw-Hill. Illustration by Susan Spellman. Copyright © 2002 by Roger Jahnke.*)

They are perfect representatives of what has come to be called *mind-body therapies* or *methodologies* and are sometimes called *Chinese Yoga*. It is often said that Qigong and Tai Chi activate effects similar to acupuncture in a self-implemented context and without the needles.

Long before written language, shamans and priests developed Qigong-like practices for both healing and spiritual ritual, as well as martial arts and athletic applications. The original Chinese concept of Qigong is that the practices promote a natural balancing and harmonization of inner and outer forces or vital energy flow to improve blood circulation, enhance organ and immune function, and to heal disease. Qi cultivation—Qigong—according to Chinese medical texts, stimulates and balances the flow of Qi, or vital life energy, along the acupuncture channels (energy pathways in the body) (Box 11-1).

Tai Chi, also known as Tai Chi *Chuan (Taijiquan)* was developed between the 12th and 14th centuries and has become one of the best-known and most highly choreographed forms of Qigong. Roughly translated, Tai Chi *chuan* means *grand ultimate fighting art* and is part martial art, part moving meditation. Interestingly, Tai Chi without *chuan* means just "grand ultimate". It is a way of describing the universe in its natural state of dynamic change.

It is easiest to say that Tai Chi, the exercise, is a kind of Qigong. Qigong is the overarching, more ancient discipline. Tai Chi is one form or approach to Qigong from a much more recent era. To clarify, Qigong is not a kind of Tai Chi. It is estimated that there are 10,000 forms of Qigong, including the numerous long and short forms of Tai Chi. Dynamic meditation and meditation in motion, in the therapeutic or rehabilitation context, are actually better referred to and perhaps best discussed as various forms of Qigong.

Research from Asia over millennia and recent medical studies in the United States and Europe have shown that Qigong and Tai Chi have a wide array of benefits, including fall prevention, stress and blood pressure reduction, pain control, immune function enhancement, and increased circulation without stressing the heart. These findings suggest that Qigong and Tai Chi may hold significant promise in reducing some of the key contributing risk factors for cardiovascular disease and could be suited as complementary practices in cardiac disease prevention and rehabilitation.

Box 11-1   Definition of Qi

Qi (pronounced *chee*) is the central concept of Chinese medicine that is variously translated to mean *vital energy, essence of life,* and *living force*. In Chinese medicine, the proper flow of Qi along energy channels (meridians) within the body is crucial to a person's health and vitality. The many types of Qi are classified according to source, location, and function: nutrient Qi, defense Qi, source Qi. Within the body, Qi and blood are closely linked because each is considered to flow along with the other. The manipulation and readjustment of Qi to treat disease and ensure maximum health benefit is the basic principle of acupuncture, remedies (herbal), body therapies (massage and other physiotherapies) and both Qigong and Tai Chi.

DYNAMIC MEDITATION AND CARDIOVASCULAR HEALTH

Of the conventional risk factors for cardiovascular disease, age, gender, and heredity are considered to be nonmodifiable; tobacco smoking, high blood cholesterol, hypertension, physical inactivity, obesity, and diabetes mellitus are considered to be modifiable through behavioral change.[1] Many sources agree that emotional stress, anxiety, and depression are also secondary risk factors for cardiovascular disease.[6-8]

The rationale for the medical/therapeutic application of regular Qigong and Tai Chi practice in cardiovascular health care can directly and indirectly address all of the conventional modifiable risks for cardiovascular disease. Qigong and Tai Chi may lower blood pressure, increase the size of occluded arteries, and decrease the negative effects of inactivity and obesity. Indirectly, Qigong and Tai Chi have an effect on an individual's capacity to curtail negative habits and alter dietary intake. In the research literature, as well as in the traditional wisdom of the Chinese culture, Qigong and Tai Chi also create tranquility, patience, and inner calm, thus reducing the adverse effects of emotional stress.

Dynamic or moving meditation, in a comprehensive or holistic program in which the benefits of combined gentle exercise and meditation are accompanied by group support, is an approach both to fitness and meditation that is more widely accessible and easier to implement than either traditional exercise or traditional sitting forms of meditation. Several studies that used the lifestyle modification program for the reversal of coronary heart disease developed by Dean Ornish and colleagues have demonstrated this.[9,10] In the Ornish program, Yoga, the Qigong of India, is combined with nutritional guidelines and group support. Their findings suggest that a mind-body program that includes a moving meditation practice, dietary change, and support group could literally reverse coronary disease. In a number of cases this program has resulted in patients who were listed for heart transplants actually recovering healthy cardiac function.

HOW QIGONG (CHI KUNG) AND TAI CHI (TAIJI) WORK

Qigong and Tai Chi practice can range from simple calisthenic movements with breath coordination to more complex methods in which the practitioner intentionally alters brain-wave frequency, heart rate, and other organ functions. When practiced regularly, the combination of movement, deep relaxation, and breathing common to both Qigong and Tai Chi can improve strength and flexibility, reverse damage caused by prior injuries and disease, and promote relaxation, awareness, and healing.

TCM holds that Qigong and Tai Chi stimulate and nourish the internal tissues, organs, and glands by circulating Qi (also Chi, see Box 11-1). With regular practice, these techniques can break down energy blocks and facilitate the free flow of energy throughout the body, thus promoting blood and lymph flow and the even flow of nerve impulses necessary for proper health maintenance.

Because these moving meditation practices are easy to learn and practice, when modified and adapted for the therapeutic context, they have even a wider range of effects. The effects on balance, well-being, and healing operate in collaboration with economic and social benefits. The literature on costs for proactive lifestyle enhancement including exercise and meditation demonstrates that it is more cost effective to prevent disease than to treat it.[11] The literature on the benefits of social interactivity in chronic and life-threatening disease has rapidly proven that any sort of social interactivity or support has significant health benefits. Qigong and Tai Chi are generally learned in a context of weekly training and practice with a group. One recent study found that supportive group activity not only assists in moderating risk for future cardiac events but also fosters self-efficacy in sustaining an exercise program.[12]

THE EFFECTS OF REGULAR QIGONG OR TAI CHI PRACTICE

Qigong and Tai Chi are holistic practices that can affect simultaneously many functions of the body and mind. TCM theory suggests that this is mediated through the Qi. The concept of Qi has several equivalents in the Western scientific view, including the following:[13]

- **Physiologic:** Equivalent to physiological functionality
- **Bioenergetic:** Equivalent to the activity of ions in the body
- **Biofield:** Equivalent to the magnetic field throughout and near the body, generated by ion flow
- **Quantum:** Equivalent to the effects of Quantum Dynamics in the human system

Many scientists are working toward a deeper understanding of the full range of Qi and its equivalents in an emerging new science of bioenergetics and biofield research.[13,14] Conventional Western science is well versed in the first of these equivalents of Qi—the physiologic mechanism. Research in the near future may clarify that the bioenergetic, biofield, and quantum mechanisms are actually primary and the physiological mechanisms, secondary effects.

Until then, however, the following are some of the key physiological mechanisms that are well documented by conventional science and triggered by regular Qigong or Tai Chi practice:

- Initiate the "relaxation response" triggered by any form of mental focus that frees the mind from its many distractions and decreases the sympathetic function of the autonomic nervous system. This effect would serve to decrease heart rate and blood pressure, dilate the blood capillaries, and optimize the delivery of oxygen and nutrition to the tissues.
- Alter the neurochemistry profile (the balance of neurotransmitters, brain chemicals that bond with receptor sites on tissue, enzyme, immune, and other cells to excite or inhibit their function), moderating pain, depression, and addictive cravings, as well as optimizing immune capability.
- Increase the rate and volume of the flow of the fluid in lymphatic system, enhancing the elimination of toxic by-products from the interstitial spaces in the tissues, organs, and glands and accelerating the propulsion of immune cells to their target sites.

- Gently increase the rate of cell metabolism and tissue regeneration through increased circulation of oxygen and nutrient-rich blood to the brain, organs, and tissues.
- Coordinate right/left brain hemisphere activity, promoting deeper sleep, reduced anxiety, and mental clarity.
- Induce alpha and, in some cases, theta brain waves, which accompany reduced heart rate and blood pressure, thus facilitating relaxation, mental focus, and natural self-regulation (healing).
- Moderate the function of the hypothalamus, pituitary, and pineal glands as well as the cerebrospinal fluid system of the brain and spinal cord, which mediates pain and mood and accelerates immune function.[15]

Simply stated, the physiological mechanisms of self-regulative repair are triggered by the three traditional aspects of Qigong, Tai Chi (and Yoga)—regulation of body movement and posture, regulation of the breath, and specifically focusing the mind and awareness.

As further research is conducted on Qigong and Tai Chi, the list of effects will evolve to better explain the wide spectrum of benefits from the practices. For example, recent research on one form of Qigong (called a modified form of Tai Chi) was found to alter immune function.[16] Moreover, a form of "walking" Qigong was found to alter cytokine productivity.[17] As the research progresses, more subtle aspects of the moving meditations will be uncovered.

Research on mind-body practices like Qigong and Tai Chi, along with their sister from India (Yoga), may revolutionize medicine as it is further substantiated that the most important and least expensive medicine is actually produced within the human body, as the ancients described thousands of years ago.

WHAT IS THE DIFFERENCE BETWEEN QIGONG AND TAI CHI?

Essentially there is no difference in the three primary features of Qigong and Tai Chi: body posture and movement, breath regulation, and mental focus. These are known as the three intentful corrections. These basic characteristics are also common to Yoga, which the Chinese call *Indian Qigong*. As mentioned previously, original forms of Qigong, called *Dao Yin (Tao Yin)* have been traced to tomb records from the Han Dynasty (200 BCE) and earlier. Tai Chi is an ancient concept (universal harmony); however, it does not appear historically as a health cultivation or martial arts practice until the Ming Dynasty (1368-1644).

Although Tai Chi is currently better known in the popular culture, the healthcare applications of Qigong are actually more accessible because it is easier for most people to learn and practice its more simple forms. In the United States, qualified instructors are now teaching both Tai Chi (usually highly modified from the original, as in Tai Chi Easy™, Integral Tai Chi™, etc) and Qigong in innovative complementary and integrative medicine programs in hospitals, adult education centers, schools and universities, community fitness programs, and in numerous social service agencies. Applicable to young and old alike, and for people in any state of health, these Asian mind-body fitness programs are unique because they can be performed standing, walking, sitting, or lying down. Dynamic meditation exercises can even be performed by those confined to wheelchairs or hospital beds and have tremendous merit in hospice and palliative care for both patients and families.

The biggest difference between the two is that Tai Chi has a wider exposure (in name only), whereas Qigong is currently less visible to the public. Most Tai Chi in the news—and even in research—is modified to the extent that it is more a form of Qigong that is being called Tai Chi. However, this is rapidly changing because Qigong is actually the larger, more ancient, more medically focused body of information and practice. The traditional styles of Tai Chi with 108 movements are much more complex to learn than many Qigong forms. Adaptive Qigong including Tai Chi Easy™ and other therapeutic forms of Tai Chi would be considered by most experts to be more Qigong than Tai Chi.

CHINESE MEDICINE AND WESTERN MEDICINE: SIMILARITIES AND DIFFERENCES

Although conventional Western medicine and TCM have many obvious differences, it is interesting to note that they are also based on a number of shared principles. In a way, Chinese medicine, including Qigong and Tai Chi, is perfectly suited to complement conventional medicine because of the following shared principles:
• The mind and body interact
• The body is a functionally integrated whole
• The human system has inherent self-regulatory, self-repair capacity
• When normal adaptability is disrupted, dysfunction ensues
• Normal adaptability can be fostered, sustained, and rehabilitated
• The state of functionality can be enhanced or optimized
• Healthy function is in large part sustained or optimized by maximum delivery of metabolic factors to the body parts and the maximum elimination of metabolic byproducts

Interestingly, without the need to understand or believe in the Chinese concept of Qi, it is possible to understand Qigong and Tai Chi in terms of these shared principles. Therefore given that Western medical tradition has not created a specific self-care system or even, until recently, understood the relevance of purposeful health maintenance, the ancient self-care systems of Asia are perfect candidates for implementation as complements to Western clinical practices.

With this commonality in mind, it is interesting to note briefly one of the major differences between Asian and Western medicine. In cardiology, for example, the range of Chinese diagnoses is vastly different than that in the West. Several of the diagnostic categories (syndromes) from TCM (Box 11-2) parallel conventional cardiovascular disease, and some are associated with the traditional Chinese concept of the HeartMind (*Xin* or *Hsin*), that is the interface of the psyche and the nervous system.

A significant difference between Chinese and Western medicine, in cardiology, is that in the most recent era of conventional medicine, the heart and cardiovascular system are typically perceived as a set of purely physiological parts

> ### *Box* **11-2**   Traditional Chinese Medicine Heart Diagnoses
>
> - Heart Qi Deficient
> - Heart Yang Deficient
> - Heart Blood Deficient
> - Heart Yin Deficient
> - Heart Blood Stagnant
> - Heart Fire Blazing
> - Phlegm Mist the Heart
> - Phlegm Fire Agitating the Heart

and interactions. The ancient Chinese view is that the physical heart and the mental/emotional heart are one.

As Western medicine continues to uncover the economic and clinical rationale for prevention, health promotion, wellness, performance enhancement in addition to disease intervention, the implementation of programs including Qigong and Tai Chi will likely increase, regardless of whether the Chinese paradigm and language of diagnosis is fully understood. The information on the benefits of Qigong and Tai Chi tend to transcend the boundaries of language and scientific bias.

RESEARCH ON QIGONG AND TAI CHI

In China and the rest of Asia, research on the benefits of Qigong and Tai Chi is common. However, the literature is neither accessible nor particularly rigorous in all but a few cases. Since 1980 in the United States and Europe a landslide of research on Tai Chi and Qigong has been reported in the peer-reviewed literature. The findings of numerous clinical trials reflect that Qigong and Tai Chi are beneficial in a wide array of diagnostic areas, including the prevention and integrative treatment of cardiovascular disease. In addition, much can be done to improve research methodologies and more directly target studies to enhance findings on clinical outcomes and the mechanisms of action.

Dynamic or moving meditations, including Tai Chi and Qigong, are beneficial in a broad spectrum of health improvement contexts from wellness and risk pool management to healing a wide range of diagnoses and even for perisurgical programming. The need for a clear and widely agreed upon research framework has become essential. Because of functional compromise in most populations that are experiencing disease or are at risk for disease, the forms of Qigong and Tai Chi documented in research are usually simplified, modified, and adapted. Forms common in traditional Chinese practice, whether martial, sports related, or from esoteric roots, are generally not prevalent in the medical or therapeutic context, particularly outside of Asia.

Given this, therapeutic or medical Tai Chi is almost always adapted or modified significantly from the traditional 108 movements and their martial arts applications. Therapeutic or medical Qigong practices are typically developed with the limitations posed by many health challenges in mind. Therefore except for in rare cases, a study naming Tai Chi is almost never traditional Tai Chi but instead is almost always an adaptive form, which is actually more a kind of therapeutic or medical Qigong. Such practices may be called Tai Chi, but they are probably more what the Chinese call *Tai Chi Qigong* (also Taiji Qigong), movements from Tai Chi adapted in a Qigong type format. Typically Qigong for the health promotion and therapeutic contexts is extremely easy to practice and can be significantly modified for use by patients in wheelchairs or hospital beds.

It is therefore reasonable to think of both Qigong and Tai Chi as a single body of practice in the medical, therapeutic, and functional enhancement context. Tai Chi is a kind of Qigong. However, much of the literature has separated them, as if they are completely different methods.

For the purposes of this chapter it was determined to review Tai Chi and Qigong studies separately but only in the context of an overview of clinical trials since 1980. This review revealed a number of interesting things, including the fact that both Qigong and Tai Chi were found to be particularly useful in the cardiovascular field. Qigong citations (for clinical trials only, which included studies on "breathing practices") addressed predominantly the cardiovascular area (15 citations), followed by COPD/asthma (14 citations). Tai Chi citations for clinical trials addressed primarily falls prevention and balance (11 citations), followed by cardiovascular studies (4 citations). Both Qigong and Tai Chi are clearly very suited for application in the prevention, treatment, and rehabilitation of cardiovascular health. It is reasonable to consider the bodies of available research on Qigong and Tai Chi as one, single, inclusive body of information because they are both forms of moving meditation that trigger the activity of identical physiological mechanisms. When taken as a single body of research, their strength in cardiovascular health care becomes even more convincing—with 19 clinical trials since 1980.

A search of literature reviews yielded seven studies that explore Qigong and Tai Chi in preventive health care as well as integrative medical treatment (Table 11-1).[18-24] Four of these seven reviews had a cardiovascular focus. The recent review from Wang points to significant effects of Tai Chi (implying Qigong *and* Tai Chi, as they are so nearly identical in the therapeutic context) specifically for the prevention, treatment, and rehabilitation of cardiovascular disease.

RANDOMIZED CONTROLLED TRIALS ON TAI CHI AND QIGONG AND CARDIOVASCULAR DISEASE

The randomized controlled trial is considered to be the most highly refined research method in the Western sciences. Studies in this context tend to be more credible than less rigorous clinical trails. A search of randomized controlled trials (Table 11-2) found only three that specifically explored Qigong and Tai Chi in the cardiovascular context.[25-27]

The few randomized controlled trials that are available reveal a number of important findings in both cardiovascular disorders and chronic disease in general.[25-27] It appears that Qigong and Tai Chi can lower blood pressure, stabi-

Table **11-1**   LITERATURE REVIEWS OF QIGONG AND TAI CHI RESEARCH

Author/Year	Topic	Comments
Wang et al[18] 2004	Tai Chi and chronic disease	High quality, specific diseases
Wayne et al[19] 2004	Tai Chi and postural control	Several studies, general benefits
Chen & Yeung[20] 2002	Qigong and cancer	Chinese literature
Taylor-Piliae[21] 2003	Tai Chi and cardiac rehabilitation	Cost-effective, behavioral modification
Kreitzer & Snyder[22] 2004	Complementary therapies, cardiac	Mentions Tai Chi
Mayer[23] 1999	Qigong and hypertension	Critique of research methods
Luskin et al[24] 1998	Mind-body, cardiovascular	Mentions Tai Chi

Table **11-2**   RANDOMIZED CONTROLLED TRIALS

Author/Year	Topic	Comments
Lee et al[25] 2003	Qigong and hypertension	Qigong effective in lowering blood pressure
Lee et al[26] 2003	Qigong and hypertension	Qigong stabilized sympathetic nervous system
Channer et al[27] (1996)	Tai Chi and myocardial infarction	Tai Chi effective after infarction

lize the sympathetic nervous system, and reduce the presence of stress neurohormones.

In medical and therapeutic terms, Qigong and Tai Chi trigger the same inner mechanisms of physiological, energetic, and emotional self-repair and self-regulation, thus suggesting that they be considered slightly similar aspects on one area of research. Eventually, a lexicon of terms will emerge to more efficiently define a framework for research in this field. For now, both Tai Chi and Qigong are best defined as personally applied practices that focus simultaneously on posture enhancement, gentle movement, breath regulation, and meditative or relaxation methods and are modified for use in specific therapeutic settings.

Favorable effects have also been reported on balance and muscular strength, flexibility, symptoms of arthritis, and psychological symptoms.[5]

Hypertension

Short-term studies using Tai Chi training (Table 11-3) have revealed sustained reductions in blood pressure that are comparable to those seen with aerobic exercise.[27-30] The reductions in both systolic and diastolic blood pressure are modest; however, no long-term follow up data are available. Many of these studies have specific design flaws with less than conventional statistical analyses of the data. Much of the benefit in hypertension may relate to favorable effects on mood, stress, and anxiety.[5] Other studies confirm that Qigong and

Table 11-3   EFFECTS OF TAI CHI ON HYPERTENSION[5]

Source	Country	# Subjects*	Mean Age or Range (y)	Study Design	Practice Duration and Style	Outcome Measured	Main Conclusion
Young et al[28] 1999	US	62	69-80	RCT	12 weeks (1 hour, 2 times/week) Yang style	BP, MVO2, physical activity, cardiorespiratory fitness	↓ BP in both Tai Chi and aerobic groups
Channer et al[27] 1996	US	126	56	RCT	8 weeks (1 hour, 2 times/week for 3 weeks, then 1 time/ week for 5 weeks) Wu style short form	BP[†], cardiorespiratory fitness[†]	↓ BP in both Tai Chi and aerobic groups in patients recovering from acute MI
Chou and Li[29] 1995	China	143	54	NRS	3 years (every morning) No data for style	BP[†], cardiorespiratory fitness[†]	↓ BP
Fang and Wang[30] 1985	China	70	40-70	NRS	12 weeks (40 minute, 2 times/week) simplified 24 forms	BP[†]	↓ BP

BP, Blood pressure; MI, myocardial infarction; NRS, nonrandomized controlled trial; RCT, randomized controlled trial; ↓decreased.
* Includes control group.
† Outcomes were not well defined in the original article.

Tai Chi have significant benefits in the area of the nervous system and mood modulation.

Other Cardiovascular Effects

Multiple studies have evaluated the effects of Tai Chi on cardiovascular function.[5] Investigators have documented a training effect in humans with increases in oxygen uptake. However, because Tai Chi is a low- to moderate-intensity form of exercise, some of the training effects are less than those seen with more intensive aerobic training. Given many cardiac patients are severely compromised, this allows access to a rehabilitative form of exercise for many patients who otherwise could not benefit from exercise for prevention or rehabilitation.

As with hypertension, significant design flaws complicate the studies that have evaluated cardiorespiratory function. The use of moving meditation practices as a post–myocardial infarction rehabilitation approach has been explored in a preliminary way; however, the trials to investigate the effects of this intervention have not been efficiently designed.

THE ASIAN RESEARCH LITERATURE

A very broad and diverse body of Qigong and Tai Chi research exists in Asia, almost completely in Chinese, Japanese, and Korean. Several challenges are inherent to the Asian research: language and translation, rigor, and conceptual framework. Much of the published research is out of reach because of the language barrier. Much of the research does not include significant numbers of participants, controls, or conventionally recognized methodologies. Much of the Asian research reflects a scientific worldview that is unfamiliar to Westerners. However, this unfamiliarity is changing. As noted earlier, heart Qi deficiency is not recognized in the Western clinical model and is only in part associated with the physiological heart.

The Qigong Institute (http://QigongInstitute.org) has developed a database of several thousand citations from the Asian literature, which includes any presentation on Qigong (and some Tai Chi) from a wide array of conferences in the United States and China. The primary criterion for inclusion is that an abstract be made available in English. Unfortunately, many of the citations are either based on fewer than five to ten participants or are philosophical reflections. However, many of the studies investigated important questions with robust numbers, reasonable controls, and parameters that are equivalent to the Western model. Currently, the Institute is releasing a new Version 7 that looks at Qigong and Tai Chi along with Yoga, meditation, and prayer.

A significant amount of research hopefully will be done in the West to explore the Chinese paradigm—Heart Qi, Heart Yin, Heart Yang, and so on. This would complement research that explores the conventional Western, physiological, and diagnostic aspects of cardiology and cardiopathology and will create a true integration. A bias in favor of the Western paradigm will constitute a tragic loss of very important and highly refined Chinese knowledge and wisdom.

THE CONTINUUM OF CLINICAL APPLICATION

Dynamic meditation can be adapted to any population of any age with any level of disability. Some forms of Qigong and simplified Tai Chi are so simple that new learners can use the practices after just a few moments of explanation.

Moving meditation has been found to be easy, interesting (linked to intriguing medical theories of the ancient Chinese), and fun. They can be taught by a wide range of practice facilitators/instructors: physical therapists, activities coordinators, rehabilitation therapists, occupational therapists, social service professionals, case managers, nurses, and lay people.

Because the classes or practice sessions are group based, the economics of implementation are compelling. Large numbers of customers/patients can be served, with a wide range of health challenges. The reach of Qigong and Tai Chi programming is wide, and the barriers are few.

PREVENTION, HEALTH PROMOTION, WELLNESS, PERFORMANCE ENHANCEMENT

In the late 1980s and throughout the 1990s startling breakthroughs occurred in the area of exercise for disease prevention—of all causes. It was found in a number of huge studies that mild to moderate exercise is more health-inducing and less health-compromising than more vigorous exercise.[31] This finding opened the door in the West, where "no pain no gain" had become the rule in exercise, to the gentler mind-body practices of exercise and meditation, including Qigong and Tai Chi. The practices of dynamic meditation are now used in wellness programs, prevention programs, social service agencies, churches, schools and universities, corporations, retreat centers, spas, and even correctional facilities.

COMPLEMENTARY TO MEDICAL TREATMENT

In the emerging new models of complementary and integrative medicine, many methods for modifying unhealthy behaviors and reducing disease risk are being combined with both conventional and alternative therapies. Qigong and Tai Chi are among the most easy and cost effective to implement. These behavioral or mind-body practices are much less expensive to implement than clinical treatments, especially since they are delivered in a group setting.

PERISURGICAL AND SURGICAL TREATMENTS

Complementary medicine programs have begun to use many natural healing methods in preparation for surgery, recovery after surgery, and even during surgery (see Chapter 27). The breath practice and relaxation learned with Qigong and Tai Chi are perfect tools for achieving these goals.

POSTSURGICAL RECOVERY AND REHABILITATION

Because the moving meditations are completely adaptive, a person can practice in bed, even in the recovery room. As soon as he or she can sit, the practice is modified to sitting. When the patient can stand with a walker or with a chair to stabilize himself or herself, the practice is modified again. This practice continues through free-standing exercises and the walking motions of Tai Chi.

ECONOMIC INCENTIVES FOR THE INCLUSION OF SELF-DIRECTED DYNAMIC MEDITATION

Numerous factors might predict a significant use of Qigong and Tai Chi (and other self-directed mind-body practices) in prevention, as a complementary therapy to medical treatment, in perisurgical programming, and in rehabilitation programs.

LOW COST

The cost of group Qigong and Tai Chi instruction for prevention or treatment, even at the highest fees, is far less than the cost of most one-to-one clinical interventions. A class in the moving meditations can easily accommodate 10 to 15 people. Self-practice is free. The classes or practice sessions are usually in groups.

PRACTICE AT HOME

Individuals can practice at home or at work, school, or church—or, as is done in China, in the park.

EASY ENTRY LEVEL

The entry level for adaptive Qigong and Tai Chi is unlimited because the practices can be modified, even for people who cannot move but still wish to participate in relaxation and breath exercises.

NO EQUIPMENT REQUIRED

Tai Chi and Qigong require no special equipment or clothing.

CONCLUSION

Preliminary investigation into the use of Qigong and Tai Chi for the prevention and treatment of cardiovascular disease has opened our awareness to an inexpensive and easy-to-implement complementary medicine intervention for potential heart health promotion and rehabilitation. These dynamic meditation practices could have nearly unlimited applications in a wide spectrum of disease risk populations and to the general public. However, from the available clinical data, it is not yet possible to ascertain the extent of the benefit in cardiovascular disease or the mechanism of action. More investigations, with rigorous study designs, will help to define the potential of Qigong and Tai Chi for both health promotion and clinical practice.

REFERENCES

1. American Heart Association: Heart Disease and Stroke Statistics: 2003 Update, Dallas, 2002, American Heart Association.
2. Eisenberg, DM, Kessler RC, Foster C et al: Unconventional Medicine in the United States: prevalence, costs, and patterns of use, N Engl J Med 328:246-252, 1993.
3. Eisenberg DM, Davis RB, Ettner SL et al: Trends in alternative medicine use in the United States, 1990-1997: results of a follow-up national survey, JAMA 280:1569-1575, 1998.
4. Wong SS, Nahin RL: National Center for Complementary and Alternative Medicine perspectives for complementary and alternative medicine research in cardiovascular diseases, Cardiol Rev 11(2):94-98, 2003.
5. Wang C, Collet JP, Lau J: The effect of Tai Chi on health outcomes in patients with chronic conditions: a systematic review, Arch Intern Med 164(5):493-501, 2004.
6. Denollet, J, Brutsaert, DL: Personality, disease severity, and the risk for long-term cardiac events in patients with a decreased ejection fraction after myocardial infarction, Circulation 97:167-173, 1998.
7. Denollet J, Brutsaert DL: Reducing emotional distress improves prognosis in coronary heart disease: 9-year mortality in a clinical trial of rehabilitation, Circulation 104(17):2018-23, 2001.
8. NHLBI Study Finds Hostility, Impatience Increase Hypertension Risk. http://www.nhlbi.nih.gov/new/press/03-10-21.htm
9. Ornish D, Scherwitz LW, Billings JH et al: Intensive lifestyle changes for reversal of coronary heart disease, JAMA 280(23):2001-07, 1998.
10. Ornish D, Brown SE, Scherwitz LW et al: Can lifestyle changes reverse coronary heart disease? The Lifestyle Heart Trial, Lancet 336(8708):129-33, 1990.
11. Fries JF, Koop CE, Beadle CE et al: Reducing health care costs by reducing the need and demand for medical service: the Health Project Consortium, N Engl J Med 329(5):321-325, 1993.
12. Carlson JJ, Norman GJ, Feltz DL et al: Self-efficacy, psychosocial factors, and exercise behavior in traditional versus modified cardiac rehabilitation, J Cardiopulm Rehabil 21(6):363-73, 2001.
13. Jahnke R: The light of science on Qi: the Healing Promise of Qi, New York, 2002, Contemporary Books.
14. Rubik B: The biofield hypothesis: its biophysical basis and role in medicine, J Altern Complement Med 8(6):703-17, 2002.
15. Guyton, AC: Textbook of Medical Physiology, ed 10, Philadelphia, 2002, WB Saunders.
16. Irwin MR, Pike JL, Cole JC, Oxman MN: Effects of a behavioral intervention, Tai Chi chih, on varicella-zoster virus specific immunity and health functioning in older adults, Psychosomatic Med Sep-Oct;65(5):824-30, 2003.

17. Jones BM: Changes in cytokine production in healthy subjects practicing Guolin Qigong: a pilot study, BMC Complement Altern Med 1(1):8. Epub 2001 Oct 18, 2001.

18. Wang C, Collet JP, Lau J: The effect of Tai Chi on health outcomes in patients with chronic conditions, Arch Intern Med 164:493-501, 2004.

19. Wayne PM, Krebs DE, Wolf SL et al: Can Tai Chi improve vestibulopathic postural control? Arch Phys Med Rehabil 85:142-52, 2004.

20. Chen K, Yeung R: Exploratory studies of Qigong therapy for cancer in China, Integr Cancer Ther 1:345-70, 2002.

21. Taylor-Piliae RE: Tai Chi as an adjunct to cardiac rehabilitation exercise training, J Cardiopulm Rehabil 23:90-96, 2003.

22. Kreitzer MJ, Snyder M: Healing the heart: integrating complementary therapies and healing practices into the care of cardiovascular patients, Prog Cardiovasc Nurs 17:73-80, 2002.

23. Mayer M: Qigong and hypertension: a critique of research, J Altern Complement Med 5:371-82, 1999.

24. Luskin FM, Newell KA, Griffith M et al: A review of mind-body therapies in the treatment of cardiovascular disease, part 1: implications for the elderly, Altern Ther Health Med 4:46-61, 1998.

25. Lee MS, Lee MS, Kim HJ, Moon SR: Qigong reduced blood pressure and catecholamine levels of patients with essential hypertension, Int J Neurosci 113(12):1691-701, 2003.

26. Lee MS, Lee MS, Choi ES, Chung HT: Effects of Qigong on blood pressure, blood pressure determinants and ventilatory function in middle-aged patients with essential hypertension, Am J Chin Med 31(3):489-97, 2003.

27. Channer KS, Barrow D, Barrow R et al: Changes in haemodynamic parameters following Tai Chi chuan and aerobic exercise in patients recovering from acute myocardial infarction, Postgrad Med J 72(848):349-51, 1996.

28. Young DR, Appel LJ, Jee S, Miller ER The effects of aerobic exercise and Tai Chi on blood pressure in older people: results of a randomized trial, J Am Geriatr Soc 47:277-84, 1999.

29. Chou WS, Li Z: The effect of Tai Chi chuan training on blood pressure, ECG and microcirculation in older people, Chin Sports Med 14:249, 1995.

30. Fang Z, Wang ZY: Clinical comparison of simplified Taichiquan, breathing exercise, and simple convalescence in treatment of hypertension, J Clin Phys 2:96-97, 1985.

31. Blair SN, Kohl HW III, Paffenbarger RS Jr et al: Physical fitness and all-cause mortality. A prospective study of healthy men and women, JAMA 262(17):2395-401, 1989.

CHAPTER 12

Native American Healing for the Heart

Ai Gvhdi Waya

Native Americans have a tradition of healing that is handed down verbally from one medicine person to another within each nation. There are no books written on healing ceremonies. Further, each nation has its own ceremonies or rituals to deal with disease. One perspective they hold in common is that all disease begins and ends in the spirit of the person. Therefore we work first with the spirit, and our primary concern and focus are placed on this level. If the spirit is made whole, the mental, emotional, and physical body will also heal as a result of this repair.

Every nation has ceremonies that are specific for healing of the spirit, and these ceremonies differ from nation to nation. I have not encountered one that is specific for cardiac symptoms. Instead, the holistic approach is taken: the spirit, mind, emotions, and physical body are seen as one and are approached on that level by a medicine person. We understand there is cause and effect.

Medicine people come in two categories. The first group are those who may use one or more of the following tools: medicinal herbs, singing of songs, dance, sand painting, quartz crystal, a feather, a rattle, a doctoring sweat lodge ceremony, and a vision quest or other ceremonies to effect healing for the patient. The second group includes a shaman, a trained individual who works directly with a person's spirit. A shaman can be of either gender. Shamanism is the ability of a healer, at will and under full control of this technique, to move into nonordinary reality and retrieve missing pieces of the patient's spirit and bring it back to him or her. Once the pieces are returned, the person regains his or her health.

No single way nor one right way exists for approaching a person who has a cardiac condition in our Native American culture. How the patient is treated depends upon the nation involved and the traditions of that nation that are handed down by word-of-mouth from one medicine family generation to the next.

CAUSES OF ILLNESS

A medicine person's main concern is understanding why a person's spirit is sick, out of balance, or in a state of disharmony. Again, depending upon the belief system of the nation involved, the reasons can vary widely. For example, the Navajo nation believes sickness can begin in the spirit from a curse placed on a person by a sorcerer or Skinwalker. The person could have encountered a snake or been struck by lightning. Either of these last two encounters are considered negative taboos by the Navajo people, and the unlucky person involved in seeing a snake or getting bit by one will have severe, negative repercussions with his or her family. In some cases, the person can be told to leave and never return to the family because they are seen as cursed.

The same holds true in the Navajo tradition for a person struck by lightning. The family and the clan may disown the person, and he or she must leave forever, left to wander the nation alone and without any familial or clan support thereafter. People who have been struck by lightning are seen as carrying bad energy, and Navajos do not want it to "rub off" on them.

Another reason for sickness of the spirit, in the Navajo tradition, is speaking of bad things that have happened to themselves or to others. That could mean speaking the name of a person who has died. In their tradition, after the person dies, their name is never mentioned again; if it is, the person who speaks it may be cursed. Bad things will happen to the speaker of the name as a consequence of uttering this deceased one's name. Usually, the bad thing comes in the form of physical, mental, or emotional sickness and may be either chronic or acute in nature.

Sickness is also brought on by talking about something bad that happened to someone else. The Navajos believe that by speaking of an evil, that energy is drawn to the individual speaking, who will be adversely affected as a result. The old adage "see no evil; speak no evil; and hear no evil," is a major part of Navajo cosmology. All these things can cause sickness to a person's spirit in reality.

Every nation has its belief system of what is bad and what can cause a person illness. An owl hooting may mean death or bad news coming to a person in the Apache nation, whereas in the Cherokee nation the owl seen or heard is considered the eagle of the night and is a protector of our sleep. The same bird is seen in two very different ways—negatively and positively.

Another major reason sickness of spirit may occur in many nations is a curse. An angry individual will pay a witch or sorcerer to put a curse on the party who has caused him or her grief. This is a common occurrence on reservations and certainly keeps medicine people employed fulltime to perform ceremonies to rid persons of a sorcerer's curse or nasty spirit who was sent to do them harm.

SHAMANIC INTERVENTION

The person who is sick visits a medicine person who is trained in the shamanic technique to bring back a lost piece or pieces of his or her spirit. The loss of spirit pieces by an individual may occur in many ways. The person could have been in an automobile accident, tripped and fallen, been involved in some kind of horrific event, suffered from shock due to trauma from a jolting experience, lost a loved one, been fired from a job, gone through a divorce, or been shamed or humiliated by another person. These experiences can cause "soul loss."

The pieces are lost as they are removed from the person's spirit. Without these energetic pieces of spirit in their rightful place, the individual becomes sick over time. The medicine person is paid to take a shamanic journey for the patient, with guides to retrieve the lost pieces of that sick person's spirit and bring them back to the patient. The ceremony around it varies with the nation involved, but the basic tenets are generally the same. There will more than likely be certain songs sung by the shaman before, during, or after the journey. A drum may be used and beat at a certain speed, the sound vibration and frequency allowing the shaman to move into nonordinary reality, a shift of consciousness in order to make the journey with ease.

In some cultures, hallucinogenic herbs may be used to help the shaman depart his or her body to make the journey on behalf of the patient. The family may or may not be involved in this process, although in most Native American nations, the family is a very strong support system that underlies the health or illness of an individual. More than likely, the family will be involved in it to some degree, either paying for the shamanic journey, bringing food after the ceremony is completed, or remaining in the room or area where the journey is taken on behalf of the patient.

If all goes well with the journey by the shaman, the pieces are brought back and given to the patient. If further work needs to be done, the shaman, still in a nonordinary state of consciousness, will kneel by the patient and perceive clairvoyantly what else is wrong. The shaman looks into the person's aura or energy fields that enclose each person like an onion (in layers). This is called internal and external extraction.

The centers of energy (known in Eastern medicine traditions as *chakras*) are found at the vertex (top of the head and known as the Crown Chakra), the center of the forehead (Brow Chakra), the throat (Throat Chakra), the heart (Heart Chakra), the stomach (Solar Plexus Chakra), the abdomen (Sacral Chakra), and the tailbone or coccyx area (Root Chakra). If the shaman sees damage to one, he or she will repair it through the aid of spirit guide helpers.

The shaman overlaps two different realities while in the shamanic state—that of the third dimensional, everyday reality that we all know and that of the multidimensional worlds, known as nonordinary reality. Simultaneously, the shaman is hearing his or her guides speak to him or her to reveal something about the patient or instruct how to facilitate healing for the patient. The shaman has one foot in the real world and one foot in the other worlds. To be able to hold this tension of opposites, a tenuous thread of consciousness between these different realities is both an art and a skill that takes decades to develop properly. For the shaman must not only do what his or her guides advise but also hold information that may be passed on to the patient after the shaman returns from the nonordinary state into third dimensional reality once again.

We can liken this situation to being in the air control tower of Chicago O'Hare International airport. Imagine being expected to keep a hundred departing and arriving planes in order, with clarity, and remembering each one of them and where each is going. Performing shamanic work like this requires 20 to 30 years of training.

WOUNDS TO THE HEART CHAKRA

EMOTIONAL BLOCKAGE/SLUDGE

A shaman in nonordinary reality who is visiting a person with a cardiac condition may clairvoyantly perceive a dark gray fuzzy or cottony-appearing cloud hanging above the person's chest where the real (physical) organ is located. This gray cloud indicates a block. A block of energy tells the shaman that the person has had some kind of heart trauma that has not yet been addressed; rather, the patient has repressed or suppressed it. The *emotion* of that heart trauma (usually connected with grief through someone they love who dies, a divorce, the loss of a child, loss of a beloved pet, having to move away from their family, or move to another state or country, or any other emotion that involves *love*) that is not discharged and worked through (vented emotionally) becomes a block that will surround the organ itself. Unexpressed emotions also include anger, humiliation, shame, jealousy, envy, or any other negative human emotion as well. The key here is that it is either unconscious in the patient so that he or she cannot process it or that the person knows about it, but jams it back down into himself or herself and suppresses it instead. Eventually this invisible (to most people) block will cause harm to the physical organ over time.

Ideally, if the person had worked through this heart shock event(s) and discharged the emotions in a healthy, positive manner (such as crying; talking it out with someone who cares; grieving; or going to a minister, therapist, or other trusted person), he or she would not have heart symptoms.

Shamans can see the dross or etheric debris that comprise this cloud of blocked energy around a person's heart. They can also feel it with their hands; in fact, anyone can. It is a very easy test to perform. Simply open up your left hand and gently place the palm downward, toward the person's chest region, with his or her permission. Ideally, you don't need to be any closer that 6 inches or farther away than 12 inches from the person's actual physical body. Never touch them at any time. Slowly move your palm from one side of the person's chest to the other. Then, move it from the bottom of the chin, down below the heart and back. If there is etheric dross or a block in the heart, the temperature will change where this block is located. The block may be cool or cold feeling, or it can be hot feeling. Sometimes, a texture difference can be felt as one slowly passes his or her palm across the patient's heart area. It is important to start above the heart and move downward. In this way, the person can actually feel the temperature or texture difference.

The examiner may also feel a tingle or some other sensation as he or she moves his or her palm across the patient's heart region. What is important is that a change is noted in the palm as it is passed across the damaged heart region. If the heart is injured, one will always feel this change. If there is no change, then there is no heart problem.

An examiner will usually feel this area as coldness or heat only where the injured heart resides. The temperature goes back to normal as his palm moves away (up or down, or from side to side) from the blocked region of the heart. As one moves his or her palm back toward and around the heart region, one will feel the temperature or sensation differential from the rest of the chest region.

It might take 10 or 20 times of trying this method before one is able to feel the difference. Remember that cool, cold, or hot indicates a block where the person has not released or expressed his or her emotions adequately (hasn't cried, hasn't screamed, hasn't grieved, for example, and has repressed/suppressed the emotions instead).

Sometimes, the area around the heart is hot; this signals a different situation to the shaman. Keep in mind that the root issue is about love (or not being loved or feeling unlovable). Heat is symbolic of anger, rage, humiliation, shame, and not being loved or lovable enough by the patient. The temperature differences are clues to the shaman as to how he or she will deal with the patient afterward, although the fixing of this energy wound is the same. It does tell the shaman the root cause of the person's heartache and after the ceremony he or she will speak of this event or trauma that was experienced earlier in the patient's life, in hopes of catalyzing further healing of this wound in them.

Giving voice to the patient's emotions that, on a subconscious level, signal that he or she is unlovable, has been shamed, or has been made to feel unimportant is an important aspect of the ongoing healing of this patient. These abhorrent, festering feelings and distorted reality attitudes of the patient build up the invisible (except to the shaman) etheric dross over time, and it becomes a gray, cottony, or fuzzy cloud around the heart.

Eventually, this negative energy begins to wear on the physical organ itself. The heart chakra that moves through the heart, front to back of the person, becomes, in simple terms, jammed with this debris that makes the physical heart work much harder. One can look at etheric dross as sludge. The heart is not receiving the pranic energy (consider this prana energy food and nutrition for the heart chakra, which in turn feeds the organ itself to keep it strong and vital) and it begins to wear out. When this process begins, the walls of the heart may become thin. The valves may become delicate, leak, or wear out. The heart has many parts, and one or more of them can be affected by this etheric sludge buildup. This can be likened to plaque or high levels of unhealthy cholesterol building up in the patient's arteries; however, etheric sludge is not seen by the physician but can certainly be seen by a shaman. Both do equal damage—seen or not.

A shaman may perceive a dark spot of energy around a vein or artery, as well. This usually indicates a cholesterol/plaque buildup that is preventing the even flow of blood or encouraging a clot to form that could eventually break off and cause more damage to the patient.

The healthy heart, when perceived by a shaman in nonordinary reality mode, is a clean red brick color, undiluted and vibrant appearing. However, when damage is done to the heart, it can turn to a lurid red, reddish-black, or a yellow-green color, instead. Only part of the heart (one side of it) may be involved with one of these unhealthy colors, and this tells the shaman where the damage is, so that he or she may effect a catalytic healing to remove the offending energy or etheric dross from that region.

The heart chakra can become so slowed down or stop because of etheric dross buildup that the shaman must remove this sludge so the heart chakra can again begin to spin. As it begins to spin once more, it will pull in the pranic energy to "feed" the heart organ once more. If this is done, the heart symptoms will improve or disappear over time (usually 3 months or less).

PAST LIFETIME INJURY

A reincarnated person who has brought in an old "wound" that involved the heart (a love-related issue or possibly a wound caused by warfare or actual heart damage) will be born into this lifetime with a heart defect as a result because the issue was not thoroughly worked through in that past life nor between the worlds, which is after death of our physical body and before we assume another body in which to be reborn. With this kind of scenario, the individual may be born with a congenital heart defect, or a hole may occur in a valve through contact with rheumatic fever, or show up as a mitral valve leak later in life (usually in the person's forties). It is also possible that this may not trip-lever until the appropriate moment, when the person experiences a cardiac arrest or some other life-threatening form of heart-related symptoms. These issues and wounds can reappear in the new body and new life until they are properly resolved by the soul by some sort of intervention (physical, mental, emotional, and/or spiritual in nature).

A shaman can take a nonordinary journey to retrieve those pieces from that past life and bring them into the present lifetime and give the pieces back to the patient. The heart will heal itself (understanding that the heart is a muscle and can never be revived, the heart will heal to the optimum, despite this situation). Nothing short of a miracle can replace damaged heart muscle and make it whole. Native American medicine people are not miracle workers, but energy workers.

Several physical heart symptoms can disappear after this experience of bringing pieces back to the patient. For example, the organ may stop deteriorating at that point. Extra heartbeats disappear. Blood pressure may drop. Whatever the symptoms, the patient may improve markedly, although not completely, depending upon the irreversible damage to the heart before the shaman is called in to work on behalf of this individual.

RAGE

Medicine people recognize that rage that has sat for decades and never been expressed by a patient may reside in either the heart or kidneys, or both of these organs. The kidneys very often are involved with anger; the heart is not always the core focus. In these cases, the patient should be asked about his or her anger or the latent rage that he or she is carrying and thereby damaging the spirit, which, in turn, affects the kidneys and possibly the heart, later on.

People also have high blood-pressure symptoms because of abuse issues present in their lives. The adrenal glands sit just above the kidneys. The release of too many of the 'fight or flight' adrenal hormones make the person jumpy and easily stressed, easily irritated, and quick to explode into violent emotions or defensive postures; they are in a constant "combat mode" of protecting themselves unconsciously. As a result, their blood pressure rises. Most people are not consciously aware of this trip-lever situation unless the medical doctor, medicine person, or therapist brings it to their attention.

HEALING TOOLS

The tools used by a medicine person are diverse and unique to each. Each nation has its own protocols. Each medicine person is instructed—usually by spiritual teachers—to use certain items from nature or the natural world to help create catalyzation in his or her patient. Employing these tools gives the patient permission (consciously and unconsciously) to begin to heal.

Medicine people fully recognize that they are not the healer. Instead, they understand intrinsically that all sickness and health possibilities reside within the patients themselves. The shaman sees himself or herself only as a catalyst who creates an energy opening (a door to possible healing) and uses the trust between himself or herself and the patient to create this energy paradigm shift on the patient's behalf. Medicine people also recognize that the patient puts great faith and trust in the tools that we use; just as a person going to a surgeon in traditional medicine feels better that the surgeon uses certain tools in his or her work and that he or she will be better off for it. It is no different in the Native American world.

The healing tools that are part of our catalytic ceremony to support patients in allowing them to give permission to heal their heart-related wounds are many and diverse. I'll cover some (but certainly not all) of them. Again, each nation has particular tools, based upon thousands of years of knowledge and application, and each Nation knows from experience passed down to each succeeding generation how they work best for the patient's healing.

FEATHER

This can be the feather of any bird, although the medicine person or shaman will be working with a specific bird spirit (or perhaps, more than one). The feather that the medicine person uses symbolizes the person on all levels.

As an example, a woodpecker feather is often used when the medicine person is going to use the point of the feather to dig out an energy block from the heart; much like the bird pecks into the bark of a tree, boring a small, focused hole to get the insect hiding within the wood. This technique holographically mirrors the same dynamic between the medicine person and patient. When the block of energy is perceived around or in the patient's heart, a woodpecker feather is used. The spirit of the bird is invoked first and asked to help to remove the debris from around that person's heart. Everything is done in concert with whatever tool is used; in this case, the spirit of the bird may also tell the medicine person what to do, how to use the feather, and how to guide his or her fingers as they work the block loose from around the physical organ.

RATTLE

Most people think Indians use rattles as musical instruments or to keep time to music. Nothing could be further from the truth. Certain items, such as seeds, anthill stones, dried leaves, or other articles derived from nature are placed within the dried gourd. First, the spirit of each item used in the rattle is asked permission to be taken and used. We never take anything from nature without asking first or without receiving permission from the spirit to do so. The gourd rattle, once dried and with the unique contents placed within it, may or may not be painted. If it is, the colors and symbols have great significance and meaning to the medicine person. The energy from the Great Spirit flows through the mandala.

The medicine person is aided and assisted by the spirits of those items who helped create this gourd, and all of this willing, healing energy is sent to the patient. Perceiving a block of energy around a patient's heart, the medicine person will ask the spirits of the rattle to participate in breaking up that block. On an energetic level, the rattle may be likened to a 16-pound sledge hammer being aimed at a crystal glass (the block around the heart). Once the power of that rattle is aimed and focused, the block will break up. Once the block is shattered, the heart is freed and allowed to fully function once again.

HANDS

The medicine person can ground himself or herself and ask the energy of Mother Earth to come up through him or her and out of his of her hands and then transfer it to the patient, with the intent of allowing the block of energy to be removed or dissolved from around the patient's heart. The medicine person may or may not physically touch the patient. They may work only out in the auric energy field. The block is then picked up with one or both hands and removed.

Another technique used by a medicine person is to hold his or her hand, palm opened, about 6 inches above the heart of the patient and literally, like a vacuum cleaner, "suck" up the energy of the block and take it into his or her own body. Medicine people are trained on how to pull energy off people and run it through themselves and then release it back to Mother Earth so that they are not harmed or impacted by taking on patients' energy. Once this is done, the person's heart will begin to function correctly.

DRUMMING

The sound of a drum mirrors Mother Earth's heartbeat. The planet's heartbeat pulses at 8 hz. A drum used by a medicine person is usually an alto or bass and is beat in rhythm with Mother Earth's heart pulse. This in turn creates a very healing resonance where the patient gives permission (usually subconsciously) and the block of energy around the heart will dissolve beneath this sound and frequency.

This said, special drums have great, resounding power because of the wood and skin of the animal used to create it. Not every drum can break a block around the heart. The spirit of the tree and the spirit of the animal work in concert with the medicine person who is beating the drum. It can be a potent combination, especially to people who like drum music; they respond well to this type of therapy.

SINGING

The power of song is greatly underestimated in the medical world. Native Americans have ceremonial songs that can, quite literally, remove blocks of energy around a person's heart (or wherever the block resides in the patient's body). Music consists of tones and frequencies, and all people are responsive to certain sounds. When the sound creates an energetic bridge connection to the patient (like cures like here), harmony and balance are achieved and the energy block around the heart will dissolve.

CEREMONY

This tool in our arsenal is highly undervalued by allopathic medicine. Within the Native American world, however, there is great power, healing, and release for the patient through a ceremony, whether simple or intricate. A ceremony can be likened to a safe that has a combination. What is inside the safe is the Great Spirit's energy, which is boundless and healing and filled with pure love. The ceremony can be viewed symbolically as the medicine person having the numbers or secret combination in which to open this door of powerful and positive energy on the patient's behalf.

The medicine person then acts as a hollow tube through which this healing energy is harnessed and focused to flow directly to the patient. A heart patient who believes in such a ceremony may experience a great healing effect. The medicine person is key in a ceremony. He or she is the fulcrum point, the catalyst who knows how to open the door to that energy and has the training and spiritual strength to allow it to course through his or her physical body to embrace the patient. He or she also is trained to know how to shut off this energy and close that door once more. The ceremony has a beginning, middle, and end. The cardiac patient can experience a powerful healing in such a ceremony.

I am aware of no single specific ceremony for a cardiac patient. Each nation has their own ceremony that would assist the patient in getting well. These ceremonies are as diverse as the nations.

HERBS

Again, depending upon where the nation lives, a particular herb or herbs may be used for someone having cardiac symptoms. Native Americans have an old saying: "Everything you need to heal you is within walking distance of where you were born." In other words, the Great Spirit has provided plants, bushes, and trees that can assist us with whatever symptoms we have. There is a plant nearby that can help cure us.

SWEAT LODGE

A "doctoring" sweat is one of our most powerful tools; however, not all medicine persons are able to conduct one. They usually can, but this depends upon the nation and extent of training involved for the medicine person or shaman. The ceremony before, during, and after a sweat lodge is thousands of years old in each nation's tradition. These sweats quite literally can turn a dying person into a living one. There is darkness, high humidity, and heat. A heart patient may not do well in such a situation because it may raise their blood pressure, and a physician must evaluate this idea beforehand. However, a cooler sweat can be managed, depending upon the medicine person in charge of the sweat, so that the patient can successfully participate in one.

The sweat lodge ceremony is conducted in four steps, or rounds. Each round is designed to help catalyze the patient into surrendering over to a higher power. Once that is accomplished, the person will get well. The energy is invoked from Mother Earth, the four major directions, and Father Sky in most traditions, although this can vary. The sweat lodge ceremony remains one of the most consistent tools of healing to Native Americans to this day. It is deeply spiritual at its roots, and because all sickness begins in spirit, this tool is considered primary to any healing because it invokes and uses Mother Earth's own healing energy for her child (the patient).

IMPACT ON HEART DISEASE

From our perspective, a heart patient is hurting emotionally from issues about love. It is usually a wound from loved ones that sets this person on the path to cardiac-related symptoms later in life. Typically, heart patients do not like to be touched, hugged, held, or embraced, and yet because they have not been nurtured and loved properly as infants and children, they now feel alone and unloved in the world around them.

Heart symptoms are related to problems regarding love: being lovable or unlovable. It is about a person shutting down his or her heart chakra, which directly injures the physical organ over time because it hurts too much for the patient to feel that serrating emotional pain. Another type of person refuses to tap into his rich emotional world and tries to keep everything rational and logical in his mind only. We say that these people are alive only from the neck up. In other words, they have failed to connect their hearts and heads, which in the Native American paradigm is essential for being in harmony or balance with oneself. We cannot live our life only in our head. We also must feel, or we are said to be out of balance or out of harmony.

What can result from any of these scenarios is injury and damage to the heart itself. If that person could give himself or herself permission to feel, he or she wouldn't get heart problems in the first place. Unfortunately, in this society, men have been taught that it is not all right to cry, to feel their feelings or, indeed, to emote them. No wonder men have so many heart attacks. They are being asked to remain out of balance (be mental, rational, and logical but don't feel and don't emote).

When a gender is out of balance like this, heart problems are going to be widespread. Society should give men permission to connect with their emotions once again. I will revel in the day that men can cry openly as women do. There will be far fewer cardiac arrests in men when that happens.

Women who have cardiac problems have a different societal ball and chain to drag around with them when it comes to cardiac symptoms. Modern-day society has denigrated all women and made them feel like second-class citizens. Most Native American nations were matriarchal before the Puritans landed on the shores of North America. It meant that women were seen and respected as equals to men. They could and did hold positions as chiefs, leaders, hunters, and warriors. Each person in the matriarchal society was valued for his or her skills and talents–not his or her gender. Nowadays, our society is a patriarchal or male-dominated one. The Puritans unfortunately brought those European values with them. As a consequence, all women were made to feel worthless, helpless, or unworthy, and certainly never equal to a man. The toxic message sent by the patriarchal society is sent very clearly and consistently to women: "You are not lovable. You are not worthy like we men are." On the unconscious level of a woman's psyche, that can be heartbreaking.

Consequently, some women whose spirits are not as strong as others absorb this message of being unlovable and unworthy of mutual respect by everyone around them, and heart damage follows. A woman who has been suppressed as a human being and individual often makes a break for her personal freedom around age 40, or menopause. Those who have been thirsting for decades for this type of freedom (the children are gone, usually, at age 40), pour an intense amount of emotional energy into this break for individuation and freedom as a human and into being able to express all of oneself without the constraints of our patriarchal society.

Mitral valve leakage often occurs around this time. It is akin to a thoroughbred who is bred to run, but who is left at the gate until the rest of the field is half a mile ahead, and then the horse is loosed to run. In trying to catch up , the thoroughbred's heart can burst; this is a symbolic parallel to a woman's situation. Cardiac problems manifest as she struggles to cease being dominated and strikes out for individuation as a human being instead. As we can see, the reasons that cardiac symptoms occur in men and women are completely different.

The bottom line of cardiac disease and symptoms is about love. The issues surrounding love (or the lack of it) need to be investigated by the medical doctor who is caring for this heart patient. A link will always be found.

The medicine person sits and listens to the patient and allows him or her to talk out his or her story. Often, just having someone sit and listen without looking at a watch or looking like he or she needs to move to the next patient can provide powerful foundational building blocks of healing for that patient. Medicine people don't wear watches—and for good reason. They understand the value of "giving voice" to what ails the person. In bearing witness to the patient's story, the injustices, the lack of love, nurturance or support, the medicine person becomes a catalytic mirror to this person–and healing begins. The medical doctor can do the same thing. Sometimes, spending a few more minutes with a patient, being a compassionate witness to that person's suffering, will create a miracle of cure in and of itself. It should be tried before it is dismissed. Medicine people have known for thousands of years that spending time with someone who is ill and listening is more than placebo at work. It is the act of compassion between two people that creates healing for the patient, and isn't that what medicine is really all about?

SUGGESTED READINGS

Ingerman S: Soul retrieval: mending the fragmented self, San Francisco, 1991, Harper Publishing.

McGaa E (Eagleman): Mother Earth spirituality: native American paths to healing ourselves and our world, San Francisco, 1990, Harper Publishing.

McGaa E (Eagleman): Rainbow tribe: ordinary people journeying on the red road, San Francisco, 1992, Harper Publishing.

Myss C: Why people don't heal and how they can, New York, 1997, Harmony Books.

Myss C: Anatomy of the spirit: the seven stages of power and healing, New York, 1996, Harmony Books.

Perera SB: The scapegoat complex: toward a mythology of shadow and guilt, Toronto, 1986, Inner City Book.

Smith MC: Jung and shamanism in dialogue: retrieving the soul/retrieving the sacred, Rahway, NJ, 1997, Paulist Press.

Talbot M: The holographic universe, New York, 1991, Harper Collins.

Waya AG: Soul recovery and extraction, ed 3, Cottonwood, Arizona, 1998, Blue Turtle Publishing.

Waya AG: Path of the mystic, Sedona, Arizona, 1997, Light Technology Publishing.

Whitmont EC: The alchemy of healing psyche and soma, Berkeley, 1993, North Atlantic Books.

Wolf FA: The eagles' quest, New York, 1991, Touchstone Books.

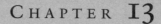

CHAPTER 13

Homeopathy With a Special Focus on Treatment of Cardiovascular Diseases

Ronald D. Whitmont, MD, DABIM, DABHM
Ravinder Mamtani, MBBS, MD, M Sc, FACPM

HOMEOPATHY AND HOMEOPATHIC PHILOSOPHY

WHAT IS HOMEOPATHY?

Homeopathic principles may have been used before the 18th century, but the German physician Samuel Christian Hahnemann (1755-1843) was responsible for the first thorough scientific study and systematic investigation of its effects. Hahnemann's work led to the consolidation of homeopathy as an organized medical specialty. The roots of homeopathy can be traced back through the writings of Paracelsus and other alchemical physicians of the Middle Ages and as far back as the ancient medical writings of Hippocrates.[1]

Homeo or *homoeo* is derived from the Greek and means similar. *Pathos* means suffering. Homeopathy is the medical specialty that treats illness by using agents capable of producing a similar state in a healthy host. Homeopathy is based on observed clinical phenomena that lead to the general theory of healing known as The Law of Similars. In other words, an illness with symptoms could be treated with a substance that produces similar symptoms in a healthy person. Homeopathic medicines consisting of such substances are given in diluted form to avoid any toxicity associated with these substances. Treatments are patient-specific and individualized.

Homeopathy is rooted in the Hippocratic method of medicine, which stresses the following: (1) rational principles of observation; (2) the study of the patient who is sick rather than the disease; and (3) assisting the natural process of healing by strengthening the individual's resistance to illness. Homeopathy is practiced upon a foundation of careful history taking, objective observation, and thorough physical examination. Homeopathy does not rely upon extensive diagnostic testing, radiographic imaging, or blood chemistry analysis. Homeopathic medicines are prescribed on the basis of directly observed and subjectively reported symptoms of the individual patient.

Homeopathy is a holistic system. It treats the whole person in terms of the mind, body, and spirit to create balance to optimize health and well-being.

Homeopathy has been used to treat a wide variety of medical conditions in nearly every branch of human and veterinary medicine, and it has also been used to support the agricultural practices of biodynamic farming, a system of organic farming.

This chapter briefly describes homeopathy and examines the scientific evidence concerning its usefulness in the treatments of various health problems with a special focus on cardiovascular diseases. It is beyond the scope of this review to examine the details of the art and practice of homeopathy. The discussions on various topics are brief and focused to give the reader an overview of the subject material to stimulate their clinical interest in what remains a largely unexplored field of complementary medicine.

EARLY TRIALS OF HOMEOPATHY AND THE PREVALENCE OF ITS USE

Samuel Hahnemann was one of the first physicians to devise and apply the concept of a drug trial to study the effects of medicines in healthy hosts. As part of his investigations, he used "quantitative and systematic procedures, clinical trials with control groups, and ... statistics in medicine."[2]

Modern homeopathy started in 1789 when Hahnemann became interested in the Peruvian bark called *china*, or *cinchona* (which contains quinine). Refuting the current dogma of the time, which asserted that the drug was effective because of its bitter taste, Hahnemann devised a plan to take the medicine himself so that he could observe its effects. When he ingested this drug, he developed symptoms of intermittent fevers with malaise. He noted that the "paroxysm lasted from two to three hours every time, and recurred when I repeated the dose and not otherwise. I discontinued the medicine and I was once again in good health."[3]

Hahnemann knew enough to realize that he had stumbled upon a basic relationship between medicine and illness. His hypothesis, which was born out, was that the curative power of a medicine lay in its ability to produce a similar state of suffering, not in its taste. Before this time, Hippocrates, Paracelsus, and others had suggested that this relationship might exist, but none had taken to time to actually test the theory.

The Law of Similars describes the fundamental healing law of homeopathy, but homeopathy would be difficult to practice without knowledge of other basic tenets set down by Hahnemann in his text *The Organon of Medicine: The Rational Art of Healing*. This text outlines the essential components of homeopathic prescribing, the principles of treatment, and the nature of healing within a homeopathic system. Review and study of this text is essential for any serious student of homeopathy.[4]

With painstaking effort, Hahnemann proceeded to carry out the process of retesting this theory on other drugs. Over the next decade he conducted many drug trials, which were later called "provings" (a corruption of the German word *pruefing*, which means "to test"). Hahnemann's intent was to test the action of drugs on the healthy and to study the pure effects of medicines—not to "prove" anything. He carried these drug tests out on himself, family members, friends, and colleagues and observed and recorded the findings. Over his lifetime he conducted studies and cataloged the results of more than 100 medicinal substances. The results of these studies were organized in meticulous detail as the *Materia Medica Pura* and published in six volumes, beginning in 1830.[5]

Soon others confirmed Hahnemann's work, and his reputation quickly spread until the practice of homeopathy was carried from Germany throughout Europe, Asia, Australia, and into the Americas. In 1844 the American Institute of Homeopathy was formed, marking the acceptance of homeopathy in the United States. Homeopathy gained a wide following as it spread; homeopathic medical kits accompanied early American settlers in their migrations across the continent, and it gained substantial footing through its success in the major epidemic outbreaks of influenza and cholera of the last century. At the turn of the 20th century 8% of U.S. physicians used homeopathy, there were 20 homeopathic medical schools and over 140 homeopathic hospitals in the United States alone.[6]

Although the use of homeopathy has declined in the United States, its use around the world is again widespread and growing. Many reports indicate a high level of patient satisfaction and improvement with homeopathy. In one questionnaire-based study, performed at Royal London Homeopathic Hospital, 81% of patients reported an improvement in their well being and 90% expressed that they were satisfied with the care they had received.[7] The use of homeopathy among medical doctors is also widespread in areas like Latin America, where there are over 10,000 medical doctors trained in homeopathy and using it in their practices.[8]

Homeopathic Treatment Approach

After Hahnemann completed the "provings" of drugs in his early pharmacopoeia, he administered them to the sick by matching the "proven" symptoms of the drugs with the symptoms belonging to the patient; selecting those drugs capable of producing pictures that were most similar to the state of the patient. Hahnemann chose to focus on the characteristic symptoms that differentiated individuals suffering from the same diagnosable illnesses. He used the differences between individual experiences of illness as a basis for differentiating between closely comparable treatments. Hahnemann considered the subjective experience of illness to be paramount in the correct application of medicinal treatment to bring about a cure. Using this approach, many individuals with the same diagnosis could conceivably receive different treatments if their symptoms varied from one another even to a subtle degree.

Hahnemann elevated the characteristic symptoms of a particular individual's illness over the common symptoms that were shared by all those suffering from the same diagnosis. In this manner, homeopathic treatment relies upon individualizing treatments to fit the subjective diseased individual instead of basing treatment upon objective, universally applied diagnostic criteria over large populations of patients.

Hahnemann believed that the health of the individual was ultimately under the jurisdiction of an energy that he called the "vital force." He considered the observable, pathological state of illness to be a secondary condition that developed after an individual had already been sick at a deeper, more energetic level. The physical manifestations of illness were relatively late effects of disease that had started with a disturbance of the vital force.

This energy system, or "vital force," was believed to act as a governor or central directing agency in the balance between health and illness. If this state of energy was disturbed, then the physical body became susceptible to illness from infection, and other environmental factors. These physical illnesses were clearly understood to be secondary events that took place after the vital force was disturbed. Hahnemann believed that homeopathic medicines (because of the manner in which they were prepared) were capable of acting at the energetic level of the vital force to simulate and redirect it to balance health.

He felt that the orthodox, or "old school" approach to medicine, which he called "allopathic," acted to suppress the symptoms of illness and worked against the body energetically, thus causing more illness to develop. Homeopathy acts by working with the body to assist it in throwing off the disease process to restore health.

THE HOMEOPATHIC PRESCRIPTION

The process of selecting a homeopathic medicine begins with the patient interview. Once the key symptoms and characteristics of the diseased patient are determined, the homeopathic practitioner refers to the text of a homeopathic medical *repertory*. The *repertory* is a catalog of symptoms (organized as *rubrics*) divided into sections corresponding to each organ system of the body, including the mind. Each *rubric* is listed with a reference to the corresponding medicines, which have been shown to evoke those particular symptoms in clinical drug *provings*, toxicity studies or, sometimes as a result of experience with prior cured cases.*

The process of medicine selection involves performing a series of cross-referencing analyses that use the key symptoms of an individual case. When this cross-referencing of rubrics is complete, the field of potential medicines has usually been narrowed from many to just a few medicines. Once a short list is formed, each potential medicine is reviewed in a homeopathic textbook of *materia medica*. The *materia medica* contains more detailed information about each medicine derived from its proving as well as symptoms gathered by experience with cured cases and records of its toxicity. When the characteristic symptoms of the patient are compared with the symptoms elicited from the medicine, the closest match is sought. This match is called the *simillimum*. This *simillimum* medicine is then administered to the patient in the desired potency, usually as a single dose.

HOMEOPATHIC MEDICINES

The drugs in the homeopathic pharmacopoeia of the United States are derived from all three kingdoms of nature: plant, mineral, and animal. Some are derived from diseased tissues, some from conventional medicines, and a few even from

---

*Homeopathic medicines are typically prescribed on the basis of what is called the psychosomatic totality of symptoms. This refers to the equal weighting that an experienced homeopathic physician places on physical and emotional symptoms during the prescription process.

nonphysical sources (i.e., magnetic fields, electrical currents). Homeopathic remedies are often confused with herbal products.[9] Homeopathic medicines can come from virtually any source, but the pharmacopoeia specifies the way in which these medicines must be prepared and tested before use.*

Hahnemann believed that many substances that could be poisonous in crude form could be highly beneficial for healing when administered in less toxic concentrations. To test this theory, he experimented with the administration of smaller and smaller quantities of drugs in his test *provings*. In this manner he developed a unique method of medicine preparation that involved diluting and shaking (termed "succussing") a substance according to a very specific protocol. This method of production is still in use today.

Hahnemann developed this unique method of medicine preparation when he observed that as larger amounts of many substances (i.e., arsenic, mercury, lead, etc.) often produced symptoms of toxicity, overdose, and poisoning, the administration of highly diluted forms of the same medicinal substances not only lacked the toxic reactions but also appeared to possess a unique power to heal.

Preparation of a homeopathic medicine begins by taking one part of a crude amount of a particular substance, pulverizing and grinding it (if it is a solid) or dissolving it (if it is liquid), then diluting it in a solvent of either alcohol, water, or sugar. In the second step, the substance is diluted again in the same solvent. This process proceeds in serial steps of dilution until the desired attenuation ("potency") is obtained. This dilution process reduces the amount of material substance in a homeopathic medicine up to and beyond the point where one might not expect to find even a trace of the original chemical substance. In other words, homeopathic medicines are so diluted that they often contain none or almost none of the original medicinal substance.*

When medicines are prepared according to the guidelines set down by Hahnemann: "the properties of crude medicinal substances gain . . . [by repeated succussion or trituration] . . . such an increase of medicinal power, that when these processes are carried very far, even substances in which for centuries no

---

*Homeopathic medicines are derived from many sources. Before they are accepted into the homeopathic pharmacopoeia of the United States they must be tested ("proven") on healthy individuals and their characteristic symptoms must be clearly identified. Because almost any substance can be made into a homeopathic medicine, the determining factor that makes a medicine homeopathic is the manner in which it is prescribed for use. If this prescription process follows the principles of the Law of Similars, it may be considered homeopathic to the case (regardless of the source of the medicine). If these medicines are selected randomly, by a machine, or on some basis other than the law of similars, they are not, by definition, homeopathic.

*The dilutional process (termed "potentization") involves taking one part of the raw medicinal substance and diluting it in either 9 or 99 parts of diluent to produce a 1X or 1C (from the system of Roman numerals designating the total number of parts X = 10 and C = 100); taking one part of the new concentration (1X or 1C) and adding one part of it to another 9 or 99 more parts of fresh diluent to produce a 2X or 2C dilution. This process is repeated serially as many times as desired to create 3X or 3C; 4X or 4C; 5X or 5C etc., etc., *ad infinitum*. This process of dilution often goes on into the hundreds and even thousands of steps of dilutions! After this process of dilution is carried out with a specified number of shakes (termed "succussions") at each level, the vial containing the new mixture is called a "potentized" homeopathic medicine. The potency is assigned a number depending upon the number of steps of dilution used (i.e., 30 make 30X or 30C, etc).

medicinal power has been observed in their crude state, display under this manipulation a power of acting on the health of man that is quite astonishing."[10]

This process of homeopathic medicine production is known as "potentization." When potentization is taken beyond a few dilutional steps, almost no chance of detecting a single molecule of the original chemical medicinal compound exists. This dilutional process produces what is known as the "infinitesimal dose."

The "infinitesimal dose" often has been the subject of ridicule and arguments pertaining to the credibility of homeopathy. Nevertheless, this discovery enabled Hahnemann to use the medicinal action of many drugs that were heretofore considered either too toxic to use safely or too inert to produce any beneficial effect. During the treatment phase of his trials, Hahnemann found that by using these infinitesimal doses, his treatments were more easily tolerated and more effective, accomplishing a swifter cure than the medicines given in crude form did.

THE HOMEOPATHIC DILEMMA

Homeopathic practice has been the object of ridicule, skepticism, and vehement resistance since its inception. The use of "potentized" homeopathic medicines of infinitesimal doses, which possess no material substance beyond the solvent, has raised serious ideological and scientific questions. Reasonable scientific explanations of how homeopathy could possibly work are missing.

Over two centuries of clinical experience in the field of homeopathy has generated a voluminous amount of anecdotal information on homeopathy's effectiveness in a wide range of medical conditions. Only recently have good double-blinded, placebo-controlled studies been performed and show that homeopathy is effective above and beyond a placebo response.

SCIENTIFIC APPRAISAL

DOES HOMEOPATHY WORK?

The question concerning the effectiveness of homeopathy relies on two types of research studies: (1) studies aimed at determining whether homeopathy is any different from placebo; and (2) studies that have examined the role of homeopathy for particular conditions.

The question dealing with the biomedical plausible mechanisms of homeopathy presents many challenges, given the ultra–high-dilutional nature of the homeopathic treatments.

Comparing Homeopathy with Placebos

A vast majority of mainstream research and clinical communities attribute any health benefits of homeopathy to placebo effects. However, many health care practitioners and researchers disagree with those observations. Therefore the question "Is homeopathy a placebo response?" requires a closer scrutiny.

In three randomized, controlled trial studies involving the use of homeopathy immunotherapy in the treatment of asthma and hay fever, researchers determined that the effect of homeopathy was not a placebo response.[11,12] Subsequently, a meta-analysis of the three trials published in the *Lancet* "strengthened the evidence that homeopathy does more than placebo (p= 0.0004)." The authors concluded that "homeopathy differs from placebo in an inexplicable but reproducible way."[12]

Subsequently, several independent reviews or meta-analyses of randomized controlled trials have shown positive results in favor of homeopathy (Table 13-1). A review of 17 trials by Cucherat et al demonstrated a low level of positive evidence for homeopathy.[13] Linde and Melchart, in their review of 32 trials, suggested that homeopathy has effects over placebo.[14] However, they noted methodological problems with several studies. The systematic review by Linde et al, involving a total of 2588 patients, determined that their findings are incompatible with the hypothesis that all of homeopathy is a placebo.[15]

Some reviews have failed to demonstrate the superiority of homeopathy to placebo interventions.[16] Despite these negative findings, some evidence suggests that homeopathy offers more than placebo.[11,12,15,17]

Homeopathy for Cardiovascular and Other Clinical Conditions

Based on many randomized controlled trials, sufficient evidence suggests that homeopathy is useful in the treatment of influenza, allergic conditions, child-

Table **13-1**   SELECT SYSTEMATIC REVIEWS AND META-ANALYSES COMPARING HOMEOPATHY WITH PLACEBO

Author	Trials/ Number of Patients	Results	Conclusions
Cucherat[13]	17 RCTs comparing homeopathy and placebo	Combined p value <0.0001 in favor of placebo	Evidence in favor of homeopathy; evidence of low level for best trials
Linde and Melchart[14]	32 RCTs comparing homeopathy and placebo, conventional	RR homeopathy versus placebo, 1.62 (CI, 1.17-2.23); for better quality trials, 1.12 (CI of 0.87-1.44)	Some evidence; not convincing for better quality results
Linde et al[15]	89 RCTs comparing homeopathy and placebo	OR for all trials 2.45 in favor of homeopathy (CI, 2.05-2.93); for good trials OR 1.66 (CI, 1.33-2.08)	"Clinical effects of homeopathy are not completely due to placebo."
Kleijnen et al[18]	107 nonrandomized trials	81 trials reported positive results	Definitive conclusions could not be drawn.

Modified with permission from Ernst E: A systematic review of systematic reviews of homeopathy, Brit J Clin Pharmacol 54:577-582, 2002; Jonas BJ, Kapchuk TJ, Linde K: A critical overview of homeopathy, Ann Intern Med 138:393-399, 2003. CI, Confidence intervals; OR, odds ratio; RCT, randomized controlled trial; RR, relative risk.

hood diarrhea, and postoperative ileus.[17,18] A summary of systematic reviews of homeopathy for these conditions appears in Table 13-2.

The number of randomized trials reported in the literature concerning the role of homeopathy in the treatment of cardiovascular disease is very small. In a detailed comprehensive review, Kleijnen and colleagues examined the role of homeopathy in the treatment of various conditions.[18] Their review included 107 controlled trials involving a wide range of problems including diseases of respiratory, cardiovascular, nervous, and musculoskeletal systems. For cardiovascular problems such as hypertension and stroke, the results are mixed (Table 13-3). Overall, the evidence of the trials is positive but "not sufficient to draw definitive conclusions."[18]

Based on the available evidence, the effectiveness of homeopathy in the treatment of cardiovascular problems and its associated symptoms can be neither confirmed nor ruled out.*[19] Additional research studies are warranted to better understand its role in cardiology.

Biological Plausible Mechanisms of Homeopathy

In this section, an attempt is made to explain the two essential principles of homeopathy from a biomedical standpoint. These principles, as previously mentioned, are the Principle of Similars, or "treating like with like" (*similia similibus curentur*), and the principle of infinitesimal dose, according to which homeopaths prescribe medicines in extremely high dilutions in which not a single molecule of the original starting substance is present.

Table **13-2**   CLINICAL TRIALS OF HOMEOPATHY FOR CARDIOVASCULAR DISEASES

Author/Year	Indication	Result
Bignamini, 1887	Hypertension	Negative
Wiesenauer et al, 1987	Hypertension	Positive
Savage, 1977	Stroke	Negative
Hitzenberger, 1982	Hypertension	Negative
Master, 1987	Hypertension	Positive
Dorfman et al, 1988	Venous perfusion	Positive
Savage and Roe, 1978	Stroke	Negative

Modified with permission from Kleijnen J, Knipschild P, ter Riet G. Clinical trials of homeopathy, BMJ 302:316-23, 1991.

---

*A homeopathic medical repertory of heart disease symptoms lists a large range of symptoms based upon subjective descriptions. These descriptions are from drug "provings," case reports of toxic reactions, and reports from cured cases. The descriptions of cardiac symptoms are quite diverse and colorful. A sample from the cardiology section of Murphy's Medical Repertory includes the following rubrics: aching, alive sensation, angina, anguish, anxiety, apprehension, boring, bruised, bursting, buzzing, cold, congestion, constriction, cramps, crushing, darting, dragging, emptiness, fluttering, griping, gurgling, hanging, heat, heaviness, jerks, looseness, movement, neuralgia, oppression, palpitation, piercing, pinching, pressing, prickling, pulsation, purring, qualmishness, quivering, restlessness, rigidity, shocks, shooting, smothered, sore, spasm, squeezing, stabbing, sticking, stinging, suspended, swollen, tearing, throbbing, tired, trembling, turned, twisted, twitching, unsteady, weak.[20]

Table 13-3   REVIEWS OF SELECT CLINICAL TRIALS OF HOMEOPATHY FOR SPECIFIC CONDITIONS

Author/Year	Indication	Studies Numbers	Results
Linde et al, 1998	Asthma	Three RCTs	Two trials with positive results; evidence inconclusive
Ernst, 1999	Headache prophylaxis	Four RCTs	One trial positive, one partially positive and two negative
Ludtke and Wilkens, 1999	All trauma and postoperative	23 RCTs and 14 nonrandomized trials	Evidence suggests that *Arnica* homeopathic medication can be useful.
Vickers and Smith, 2000	Influenza-like syndrome	Seven RCTs	*Oscillococcinum* reduces duration of the syndrome.
Wiesenauer and Ludtke, 1997	Pollinosis	Seven RCTs, one controlled trial	*Galphimia glauca* is more effective than placebo.
Barnes, 1997	Postoperative ileus	Four RCTs, four uncontrolled trials	Evidence weak
Taylor, 2000	Allergic conditions	Four RCTs	Pooled results in favor of homeopathy
Jacobs, 1993	Childhood diahrrea	Four RCTs	Homeopathy reduces duration of diarrhea.

Modified with permission from Jonas BJ, Kapchuk TJ, Linde K: A critical overview of homeopathy, Ann Intern Med 138:393-399, 2003.
RCT, Randomized controlled trial.
Several trials have suggested that homeopathy is ineffective for migraine, delayed onset muscle soreness, and influenza prevention.

That a chemical medicinal substance can have one action (inhibition, toxicity) at a high dose and an opposite action (stimulation, healing) at a low dose has been known to mankind for many years. Reports, for example, have claimed that microdilutions of antibiotics and insecticides actually enhance the growth of bacteria and crickets respectively.[8] This mechanism of "paradoxical opposite action of pharmacological substances above and below their threshold concentrations or threshold signal strengths" is called *hormesis*.[8]

Conventional treatments of oral immunotherapy and allergen desensitization are considered to be forms of applied hormesis. Therefore homeopathy, by providing an obnoxious stimulus at a low dose, similar to vaccines, may provoke a kind of immune and defensive response so as to strengthen the host to fight disease and its symptoms.

The real resistance of the medical community at large to the acceptance of homeopathy comes from its principle of infinitesimal dose. In terms of basic conventional principles of pharmacology, biochemistry, and physics, it is impossible to explain that ultramolecular dilutions of homeopathic medicines can actually have clinical effects. In fact, this suggestion makes homeopathy appear to be an "absurdity and a foolish science."

If it is not the infinitesimal molecules of medicine in the treatments that cause the clinical effects observed in research studies, perhaps it is something else. Several thoughts have been put forward to solve this question. Do homeopathic medicines possess a special form of energy, or biophysical type of information with healing properties, which cannot be measured with the available tools of medical technology? Does the use of alcohol, water, and other solvents or the process of rigorous shaking required in the preparation of homeopathic medicines generate a biophysically different molecule with encoded biological information?

David Reilly, a world-renowned physician researcher writes, "Physicists seem more at ease with such ideas than pharmacologists, considering the possibilities of isotopic stereodiversity, clathrates, or resonance and coherence within water as possible modes of transmission, while other workers are exploring the idea of electromagnetic changes."[8]

Homeopathy does appear to work, but the final answer on how homeopathy works will have to wait until further research is done.

ADVERSE EFFECTS AND SAFETY

Homeopathic medicines are recognized and regulated by the U.S. Food and Drug Administration. The medicines are manufactured under strict guidelines, and many can be purchased over the counter from specialty and nutrition stores. Homeopathy is considered to be safe and lacks the potential for life-threatening side effects, although minor side effects have been reported.

Any reported adverse effects are usually mild and transient in nature. Examples of such side effects include headaches, skin rashes, dizziness, diarrhea, and sometimes exacerbation of existing symptoms. The incidence of aggravation of existing symptoms is estimated to occur in 20% cases.[7,20] It should be mentioned that similar side effects are also observed with placebo interventions.[7] Additional studies are warranted to better understand the direct and indirect risks of homeopathy.

HOMEOPATHY RESEARCH: PROBLEMS AND DIFFICULTIES

A lack of funding and the lack of an academic infrastructure are common problems facing research in homeopathy. There are methodological problems as well.

Homeopathy, like other alternative medicine treatments such as Ayurveda and acupuncture, are not only disease-specific but also person-specific. Two persons with similar disease patterns could receive two entirely different treatments. Such a treatment approach cannot lend itself to a randomized controlled trial (RCT). This is because in a RCT all patients in the treatment group must receive the same treatment while those in the control group must receive an indistinguishable placebo. This makes homeopathy incompatible with the RCT methodology. This has restricted the extent of research in homeopathy; as a result, most of the information on its efficacy comes from anecdotal reports of day-to-day practice.

PRACTICAL CONSIDERATIONS

Although abundant empirical data from over 2 centuries of homeopathic practice from around the world support the use of homeopathy in the treatment of a variety of cardiovascular conditions (Box 13-1), essentially no data have come

---

Box 13-1   A Partial Listing of Conditions for Which Homeopathy Has Been Used Worldwide*

- Alcoholic cardiomyopathy
- Angina pectoris
- Arrhythmia
- Atrial fibrillation
- Bradycardia
- Cardiac disorders of menopause
- Cardiac disorders of puberty
- Cardiac disorders of systemic lupus erythematosus (SLE)
- Cardiac dyspnea
- Cardiac syncope
- Congestive heart failure
- Coronary artery disease
- Hypertension
- Hypertrophic cardiomyopathy
- Hypotension
- Palpitations
- Paroxysmal nocturnal dyspnea
- Tachycardia

*A huge amount of cardiac pathology has been managed effectively in the more than 2 centuries of homeopathic practice worldwide, although because of a number of problems no objective data on efficacy exist.

---

from any controlled studies that evaluate its use objectively. The evidence of homeopathy's effectiveness in these conditions is entirely anecdotal; however, the case reports are voluminous and compelling.

Empirical data from homeopathic texts demonstrate a wide spectrum of uses of homeopathic medicines (Box 13-2). What these texts do not offer are scientific explanations of how and why homeopathy works, nor do they offer any insight into statistical analysis of homeopathic treatment in comparison to conventional approaches or placebo.

Although homeopathic materials are inexpensive, the delivery of homeopathic care may be both time and manpower intensive. Each medicine demands a thorough clinical proving in a double-blinded setting before its acceptance into the homeopathic pharmacopoeia of the United States. The practice of homeopathy requires a thorough knowledge of its principles and methods. Homeopathic practitioners must also be thoroughly versed in the fundamentals of medicine and have expert training in differential diagnosis and referral, and the principles of informed consent must be observed at all times.

Practitioners of homeopathy can be licensed in four states (Arizona, Connecticut, Nevada, and Washington). Certification for physicians is offered by the American Board of Homeotherapeutics and involves course training, 3 years of practice treating cases, preparation of case reports on patients, and written and oral exams.[21]

Box 13-2   A Partial List of Commonly Used Homeopathic Medicines and Their Indications

It should be reemphasized that although many homeopathic medicines have been used to treat cardiovascular pathology, they have only been found to be effective when selected on the basis of the Law of Similars.

Ammonium Carbonicum

Carbonate of ammonia: congestive heart failure, paroxysmal nocturnal dyspnea, palpitations, and angina.

Arnica Montana

Leopard's Bane: palpitations after exertion, angina, congestive heart failure, fatty heart, hypertrophic cardiomyopathy.

Arsenicum Album

White oxide of arsenic: palpitations with anguish, cardiac dilatation, fatty degeneration, angina into neck, cardiac syncope, pericardial effusion.

Aurum Metallicum

Gold: hypertension, coronary artery disease, palpitations, tachycardia, hypertrophic cardiomyopathy, angina.

Digitalis

Foxglove: angina, palpitations on movement, congestive heart failure, slow atrial fibrillation, dilated cardiomyopathy, hypertrophic cardiomyopathy, pericarditis.

Kalmia

Mountain laurel: palpitations with anxiety, angina, tachycardia, bradyarrhythmia, hypertrophic cardiomyopathy, subaortic stenosis.

Lachesis Muta

Bushmaster snake: palpitations, cardiac syncope, coronary artery disease, carditis, bradyarrhythmia.

Lycopodium Clavatum

Club moss: aneurysm, aortitis, palpitations, hypertrophic cardiomyopathy.

Oxalic Acid

Sorrel Acid: palpitations worse lying down, cardiac dyspnea, angina, aortic insufficiency.

Phosphorus

Elemental phosphorus: palpitations, fatty degeneration, dilated cardiomyopathy, endocarditis, right ventricular hypertrophy.

Sulphur

Sublimated sulphur: palpitations, pericarditis, pericardial effusion, angina, tachycardia.

Each patient under the care of a homeopathic physician requires an intensive and sometimes lengthy interview process to determine the exact nature of his or her ailment. The recent introduction of the computer database into homeopathic case taking and repertorization has greatly simplified this procedure.

Homeopathy relies on defense and self-regulatory responses, unlike the conventional approaches of symptom suppression, replacing deficiencies or blocking body reactions. What homeopathy cannot do is correct a dysfunction beyond the healing potential of the body. It will not help deficiencies or irreversible breakdowns of body functions. However, for patients with chronic cardiovascular conditions who wish to be treated homeopathically, the adjunctive and supportive use of homeopathic treatments in certain situations is worth exploring. Examples of situations in which homeopathy could be explored include the following situations: (a) conventional treatments for the condition being treated do not exist; (b) conventional treatments have produced maximal benefit; and (c) patients are unwilling to accept side effects of the conventional treatments. It is imperative that physicians explain the benefits, limitations, and risks associated with homeopathy before making any recommendation concerning its use. Practicing homeopathy within the framework of evidence-based medicine, and informed consent is essential.

CONCLUSION

The practice of homeopathy is worldwide. It has a demonstrated favorable safety profile. The practice of homeopathy lends itself to an integrated approach so long as the standards of care and homeopathic guidelines are appropriately observed.

Homeopathy is currently being used by over 3% of the United States population and is practiced by 2500 physicians and 4000 nonphysician practitioners. Sales of homeopathic remedies have increased by 1000% over the past 20 years and now total over 1 billion dollars.

The homeopathic medicines, which are mostly based on vegetable or mineral and sometimes are of animal origin, are manufactured under strict guidelines. Mild and transient side effects with these treatments have been reported. The most dangerous side effect of homeopathy is its use in place of proven conventional treatments and other life-saving measures.

Many survey studies have documented the usefulness of homeopathy in ameliorating troublesome symptoms associated with allergic asthma, hay fever, allergic rhinitis, postoperative ileus, migraine headaches, and some arthritic conditions. However, no good scientific explanation for the mechanism of action of homeopathy currently exists. However, current evidence would suggest that the beneficial effects of homeopathy may not be entirely due to placebo actions.

Based on the available evidence, the effectiveness of homeopathy in the treatment of cardiovascular problems and its associated symptoms can be neither confirmed nor ruled out. However, the absence of evidence supporting homeopathy is not the same as lack of its effectiveness in day-to-day clinical situations.

"Rather than stressing its implausibility and the notion that its practice fits the definition of quackery or represents a cult, . . . the best way forward is clearly to do rigorous research until the truth is found.... We ought to keep an open mind and remember that a treatment might work even if we fail to understand why."[2]

Homeopathy appears to provide a unique and a refreshing approach to disease management and its role in the treatment of cardiovascular diseases merits further investigation.

The authors would like to express their thanks to Julian Winston for his many helpful editorial comments in the preparation of this manuscript.

HOMEOPATHIC RESOURCES

The following is a list of professional homeopathic organizations currently active in the United States.

American Institute of Homeopathy
801 North Fairfax Street
Alexandria, VA 22314-1757
(888) 445-9988
www.homeopathyusa.org

National Center for Homeopathy
801 North Fairfax Street, Suite 306
Alexandria, VA 22314
(703) 548-7790
www.homeopathic.org

Homeopathic Medical Society of the State of New York
6250 Route 9
Rhinebeck, NY 12572
(845) 876-6323
www.hmssny.org

Homeopathic Medical Society of the State of Pennsylvania
637 West Lincoln Highway
Exton, PA 19341
(610) 269-0255

The Ohio State Homeopathic Medical Society
5779 Wooster Pike
Medina, OH 44256
(330) 784-4493

The California State Homeopathic Medical Society
169 East El Roblar Drive
Ojai, CA 93023
(805) 646-1495

The Illinois Homeopathic Medical Association
400 East 22nd St., Suite F
Lombard, IL 60148
(630) 792-9311

The Southern Homeopathic Medical Association
10418 Whitehead Street
Fairfax, VA 22030
(703) 273-5250

American Board of Homeotherapeutics
1913 Gladstone Drive
Wheaton, IL 60187
(630) 668-5595
www.homeopathyusa.org/ABHt

The Homeopathic Pharmacopoeia Convention of the U.S. (publisher of the "Homeopathic Pharmacopoeia")
P.O. Box 2221
Southeastern, PA 19399-2221
(610) 783-0987
www.HPCUS.com

REFERENCES

1. Lyons AS, Petrucelli RJ: Medicine, an illustrated history, New York, 1987, Harry N. Abrams, Inc.
2. Ernst E, Kaptchuk TJ: Homeopathy revisited, Arch Intern Med 156:2162-2164, 1996.
3. Haehl R: Samuel Hahnemann: his life and work, 1922, Homeopathic Publishing Co. (quoted in Jonas WB, Jacobs J: Healing with homeopathy: the doctors' guide, New York 1996, Warner Books).
4. Hahnemann S, Boericke W: Translation organon of medicine, ed 6, Philadelphia, 1922, Boericke & Tafel.
5. Hahnemann HCF: *Materia medica pura*, Dresden, Germany, 1830, Arnoldischen Buchhandlung.
6. Rothstein WG: American physicians in the 19th Century, Baltimore, 1992, Johns Hopkins University Press.
7. The evidence base of complementary medicine, ed 2, London, 1999, The Royal London Homeopathic Hospital.
8. Reilly DT: The puzzle of homeopathy, J Altern Comp Med 7(2):S 2103-09, 2001.
9. Frye JC: Herbal and homeopathic medicine: understanding the difference, Sem Integrat Med 1:158-66, 2003.
10. Tyler ML: Homoeopathic drug pictures, Saffron Walden, Essex, England, 1982, Fifth Impression: The C.W. Daniel Company, Ltd.

11. Reilly DT, Taylor MA, McSahrry C, Aitchison T: Is homeopathy placebo response? Controlled trial of homeopathic potency, with pollen in hay fever as model, Lancet ii:881-86, 1986.
12. Reilly DT, Taylor MA, Beatle N et al: Is evidence for homeopathy reproducible? Lancet 344:1601-06, 1994.
13. Cucherat M, Haugh MC, Gooch M, Boissel JP: Evidence of clinical efficacy of homeopathy: a meta-analysis of clinical trials, Homeopathic Medicines Research Advisory Group (HMRAG), Eur J Clin Pharmacol 56:27-33, 2000.
14. Linde K, Melchart D: Randomized controlled trials of individualized homeopathy: a state of the art review, J Altern Comp Med 4:371-88, 1998.
15. Linde K, Clausius N, Ramirez G et al: Are the clinical effects of homeopathy placebo effects? a meta-analysis of placebo controlled trials, Lancet 350:834-43, 1997.
16. Ernst E: A systematic review of systematic reviews of homeopathy, Brit J Clin Pharmacol 54:577-582, 2002.
17. Jonas BJ, Kapchuk TJ, Linde K: A critical overview of homeopathy, Ann Intern Med 138:393-399, 2003.
18. Kleijnen J, Knipschild P, ter Riet G. Clinical trials of homeopathy, BMJ 302:316-23, 1991.
19. Murphy R: Homeopathic medical repertory, Pagosa Springs, 1993, Hahnemann Academy of North America.
20. Ernst E, editor: The desktop guide to complementary and alternative medicine. an evidence based approach, St Louis, 2001, Mosby.
21. Milan F: An overview of complementary and alternative medicine for the primary care provider, Primary Care Rep 7:17-28, 2001.

CHAPTER 14

Osteopathic Manipulative Medicine in the Treatment of Hypertension*

Adam J. Spiegel, DO
John D. Capobianco, DO

Elevated systemic blood pressure is one of the most prevalent and important public health concerns in Westernized and developing countries alike. Nearly 50 million hypertensive patients live in the United States alone.[1] Our basic understanding of the etiology and pathophysiology of elevated arterial pressure has improved over the years. However, in 90% to 95% of existing cases the etiology and thus the potential means of prevention or cure is still largely unknown.[2] As a consequence, most cases of hypertension are treated nonspecifically, thus resulting in a large number of minor side effects from treatment and a relatively high (50% to 60%) noncompliance rate.[2] Several studies have demonstrated that improved control of blood pressure in hypertensive patients has a significant impact on morbidity and mortality from cardiovascular disease and stroke.[3-6] However, the third National Health and Nutrition Examination Survey (NHANES III) trial demonstrated that only 53% of patients treated for hypertension had blood pressure actually controlled to less than or equal to 140/90 mm Hg.[1] Given these data and the seriousness of the effects of hypertension on the individual and society as a whole both economically and socially, the physician must look for more effective ways to approach the hypertensive patient. Osteopathic medicine appears to offer an approach to more effectively combat hypertension.

The intellectual roots of osteopathic medicine were conceived in the middle to late 1800s by Andrew Taylor Still, MD, who believed the medical practices of the day often caused more harm than good. Still focused on developing a system

*Modified from Spiegel AJ, Capobianco JD, Kruger A, Spinner WD: Heart Disease 5:272-278, 2003, Lippincott Williams & Wilkins, with permission.

of medical care that would promote the body's innate ability to heal itself. Osteopathic medicine is an established and recognized system of diagnosis and treatment that emphasizes the structural and functional integrity of the musculoskeletal and other organ systems of the body.[7] Osteopathic physicians use their hands to diagnose and treat somatic dysfunction. A somatic dysfunction is defined as an impaired or altered functional state of related components of the soma.[7] Somatic dysfunction is a very broad term that involves disharmony of the connective tissue, muscle, bone, joint, nerve, and/or fluid, including lymph. The diagnosis of a somatic dysfunction is based upon physician's palpatory skills. Through years of experience, physicians who practice osteopathic manipulation learn how to discern subtle changes in tissue texture. For example, soft tissue may take on a boggy feel because of small amounts of edema. Chronic alterations of tissue have a more ropy texture.

The osteopathic manipulative techniques are categorized according to the physician's findings, such as generalized muscle spasm, bony alterations, or even somatic responses to visceral disease. Patient participation in these techniques is also considered.[7] For example, in a patient who has spasm of the myofascia the physician may use isometric contractions to activate the Golgi tendon reflex in order to inhibit neuronal impulses at the spinal level. This will help to relax extrafusal fibers of the main muscle mass. Thrusting techniques ("joint-popping") are sometimes used to increase the motion of small or large caliber joints. Operator-generated rhythmic motions may propel lymphatic fluids. Other more subtle approaches may involve spontaneous release of soft tissue strain by turning down gamma gain to the involved pathology and thus providing for a more normal relationship of the length of the extrafusal to intrafusal muscle fibers. Osteopathic considerations also include the articulations, membranes, fluctuation of the cerebrospinal fluid, motility of the central nervous system, and the connective tissue attachments of the cranium to a mobile pelvis. Also, the operator may create a manual fulcrum and observe the unfolding of the body's inherent biodynamic healing forces. The endpoint of one or a combination of the above approaches may allow for a normalization of imbalances between the sympathetic and parasympathetic nervous systems and improved vascular motion which would result in a more balanced homeostatic mechanism.

A review of the literature reveals that osteopathic manipulative medicine (OMM) has been demonstrated to be of benefit to some patients with a wide variety of cardiovascular diseases.[8-14] The majority of this literature examines the effect of OMM on hypertension.

EARLY STUDIES ON OSTEOPATHIC MANIPULATIVE MEDICINE UTILITY

As early as 1914, John Downing concluded that osteopathic treatment offered one of the best methods of normalizing abnormal blood pressure.[8] Downing found that OMM helped decrease blood pressure, presumably by improving cardiovascular circulation and relaxing the musculoskeletal system. Confirming the results of Downing almost 50 years later, Thomas Northup in 1961 offered OMM as a method to relax tense tissue and lower blood pressure.[9] Several cases in which OMM was helpful in reducing both systolic and diastolic blood pressure were outlined. Northup found that the most effective of such techniques involved cranial manipulation, which, for example, involves gentle mobilization of the temporal bones. Osteopathy in the cranial field may facilitate better central venous drainage by alleviating dural tension and restriction of the bones that compromise the jugular foramen. The relationship of the cardiorespiratory centers of the medulla to the fourth ventricle are also appreciated and cradled by the osteopathic physician. In addition, Northup employed techniques to rotate specific vertebrae while providing mild traction to the cervical spine. In 1964, Harold Blood described several OMM approaches that he used to successfully treat hypertension.[10] Several patients with moderate hypertension were kept normotensive via manipulation. Patients with higher blood pressures were adequately treated with a combination of manipulation and pharmacotherapeutics.

RECENT STUDIES ON OSTEOPATHIC MANIPULATIVE MEDICINE UTILITY

In the late 1960s Celander et al and Fichera et al described alleviation of hypertension through the use of soft tissue manipulation of the upper thoracic and cervical vertebrae in both humans and dogs.[15,16] This study noted a cumulative synergism of multiple simultaneous treatments accomplishing a greater blood pressure reduction than a single treatment. In addition, Celander et al examined the effect of OMM on the autonomic nervous system by studying the fibrinolytic enzyme system and fibrinogen levels. The application of soft tissue manipulation therapy caused a decrease in plasma fibrinogen and total fibrinolytic activity consistent with an increased parasympathetic tone and decreased sympathetic tone. By making these observations, the authors may have supplied the first basic scientific justification for the effects of OMM on hypertension and autonomic nervous function.

Brown and colleagues in 1970 conducted the first published larger scale study on the effectiveness of soft tissue manipulation applied to the cervical and thoracic paraspinal muscles in reducing blood pressure.[17] With a patient pool of 86 individuals (44 hypertensive and 42 normotensive controls) significant reductions in both systolic and diastolic pressures were observed with OMM alone. The authors concluded that OMM should be considered in combination with various pharmacologic agents as an effective treatment modality for mild to moderate hypertension.

A year later in 1971 Bayer reported on the application of OMM to treat hypertensive vascular disease of unclear origin.[18] In the report, Bayer put forth several hypotheses to explain the positive effects of OMM on elevated blood pressure. OMM was viewed as an agent of skeletal muscle relaxation and an anxiolytic, thus causing a decrease in mean arterial pressure and was likened in this regard to a "physical placebo." Bayer went on to specifically describe a technique to relax the plantar fascia, which produced a resultant decrease in systolic blood pressure. Primary musculoskeletal disorders were believed to be aggravators of hypertension in certain patients because of the mental and/or physical discomfort induced by these illnesses. OMM served to correct these dysfunctions, thereby reducing pain and improving mobility of the musculoskeletal system. Consequent reductions in blood pressure were attributed to reflex actions of the autonomic nervous system; reduction of the sympathetic and amplification of the parasympathetic nervous systems serving to decrease heart rate and lessen vasoconstriction. Soft tissue myofascial techniques applied to the thoracic and lumbar spine were found to lower systolic pressure, and to a lesser extent, diastolic pressure. The rationale was that treating the thoracic and lumbar spine would lead to decreases in sympathetic tone to organs, tissues, and blood vessels of the body, thereby decreasing blood pressure. The intimate relation of the sympathetic division of the autonomic nervous system with the thoracic and upper lumbar spine, as mentioned by Bayer, could be taken advantage of to normalize these areas of the spine through osteopathic manipulation. Bayer concluded that although OMM was not a cure for essential hypertension, it did represent a valuable adjuvant to the medical regimen.

Gerber reported on the workup and office management of hypertensive patients in 1976.[11] In support of previous studies, Gerber alluded to OMM as a beneficial treatment for hypertension and peripheral vascular disease. He hypothesized that techniques of manipulation might act to release vasodilative prostaglandins, either locally or in distant segmentally related vascular beds, thus leading to a decrease in blood pressure. In addition, Gerber saw manipulation as a method to decrease the state of excitability of the sympathetic nervous system, thus encouraging peripheral vasodilation and blood pressure reduction. In addition, OMM was offered as a way to promote the relaxation of tense muscles and increase flexibility, thus helping to reduce blood pressure.

In 1977 Stiles examined the osteopathic approach to treating hypertension. He observed that specifically designed and appropriately administered osteopathic care promoted a patients' emotional and musculoskeletal relaxation.[12] Stiles noted that the upper thoracic areas of the spine are the location for sympathetic ganglia that distribute postganglionic sympathetic outflow to the cardiac plexus. Stiles postulated that somatic dysfunction in the upper thoracic region could lead to facilitation (a lowering of the synaptic threshold of the dorsal horn of the spinal cord) of motor supply to the cardiac plexus which may lead to tachycardia and/or increased stroke volume. Stiles additionally noted that sympathetic output from the thoracolumbar area sends vasomotor supply to both the adrenal glands and the kidneys. He noted that increased vasomotor tone to the kidney could increase peripheral resistance within the kidney, thereby decreasing glomerular flow. Secondary increases in the secretion of antidiuretic hormone (ADH) from the pituitary gland, and aldosterone from the adrenal glands, could lead to retention of fluid and electrolytes. In addition, facilitation of sympathetic supply to the adrenals could cause increased production and secretion of catecholamines. Stiles observed that all of these factors could collectively contribute to a hypertensive state. Finally, Stiles described the role of poor lymphatic return on the total body physiology. Inefficient lymphatic flow produces an inability of protein substances to be adequately returned to the vascular system. Thus the patient with poor lymphatic return could develop a rapid hypoproteinemia that could affect fluid and electrolyte balance, thus encouraging shifts of fluid from the intravascular to the extravascular compartments. The decreased intravascular volume would trigger the aldosterone and ADH compensatory mechanism, thus further complicating the hypertensive state. Stiles' report clearly supports a role for appropriately tailored and administered OMM in the management of hypertension.

Mannino performed a crossover study to ascertain the effect of osteopathic manipulation on serum aldosterone levels in hypertensive patients.[19] The study used Chapman's neurological reflex techniques to treat the adrenal glands. These neurologic reflexes are mediated by excess sympathetic tone on the vasculature, including the arterioles, venules, and lymphatics. The response of the tissues may involve congestion and tension of the myofascia. The treatment involves a rotatory motion to points that are situated along the dermatomal lines of embryological development (Figures 14-1, 14-2, and 14-3)[20-22] and, in the case of the adrenal glands, along the lower thoracic region. Significant declines in aldosterone levels were observed within 36 hours of manipulation. However, no significant reduction of systemic blood pressure was demonstrated. Mannino hypothesized that manipulation-associated aldosterone reductions may have resulted from an interruption or dampening of a positive feedback loop to the adrenal medulla from the sympathetic nervous system. A dampening of the circulating catecholamine concentrations would diminish the effects on the cardiovascular reflex, which in turn exerts its influence on the renin-angiotensin-aldosterone axis. Mannino also questioned why the decrease in serum aldosterone did not lead to a significant alteration in blood pressure. He pointed out that each patient in the study did have a significant drop in blood pressure after the administration of spironolactone before the study. Mannino hypothesized that perhaps not enough time was allocated for an eventual decrease in blood pressure to develop. He noted that spironolactone typically takes 5 to 7 days to exert its maximal effect on blood pressure.

Morgan and coworkers studied the effects of osteopathic manipulative treatment on hypertension.[23] This controlled trial included 29 subjects who were randomly assigned to two treatment groups. The patients in group I received weekly spinal manipulation of the occipitoatlantal joint, T1 (the first thoracic vertebrae) through T5, and T11 through L1 (the first lumbar vertebrae). Those in group II received sham manipulation in the form of soft-tissue massage of T6 through T10 and from L4 to the sacrum. The regions to be manipulated were chosen because a literature review indicated that manipulative treatment of these regions was routinely used in the management of patients with hypertension, and because major autonomic outflows are present at each location.

Contrary to some of the previous studies, the results of Morgan et al failed to demonstrate a reduction or control of systemic blood pressure after either of the two manipulative treatments. Morgan et al noted the possibility that a different manipulative protocol effective at lowering systemic blood pressure might be found. He added that such an effective manipulative protocol could represent a

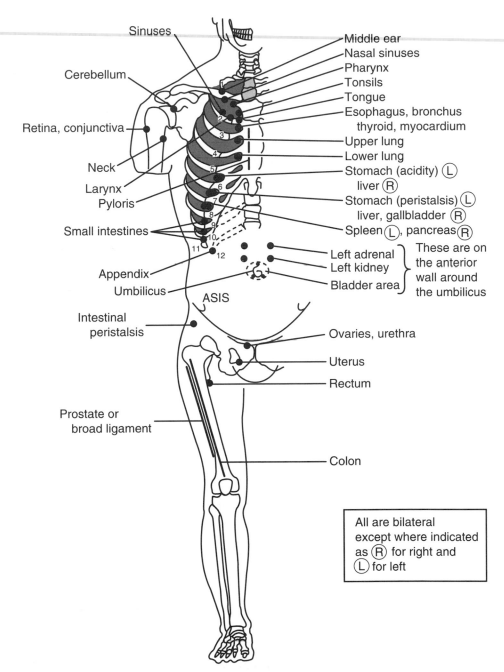

Fig 14-1. Chapman reflexes: anterior points. (*From Kuchera ML, Kuchera WA: Osteopathic considerations in systemic dysfunction, ed 2, Columbus, OH, 1994, Greyden Press.*)

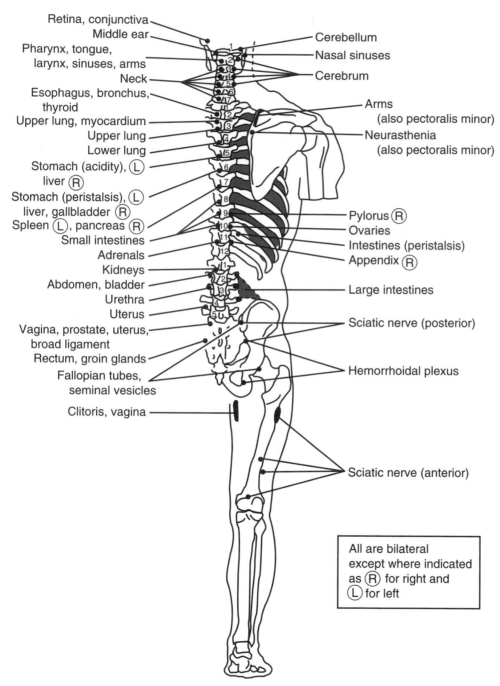

Fig 14-2. Chapman reflexes: posterior points. *(From Kuchera ML, Kuchera WA: Osteopathic considerations in systemic dysfunction, ed 2, Columbus, OH, 1994, Greyden Press.)*

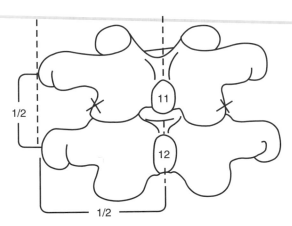

Fig 14-3. Rotatory stimulation of the posterior Chapman's points (T11-12) depicted above have been shown to effectively lower blood pressure and decrease serum aldosterone levels. (*From Kuchera ML, Kuchera WA: Osteopathic considerations in systemic dysfunction, ed 2, Columbus, OH, 1994, Greyden Press.*)

safe and economical adjunct to drug therapy and lifestyle modifications in the treatment of hypertension. Morgan called for future studies to investigate manipulative treatment protocols effective at lowering systemic blood pressure, and toward determining if certain types of hypertensive patients respond favorably to manipulative treatment.

MECHANISMS OF BENEFIT

From a physiologic perspective, the explanation for why OMM might work to lower blood pressure is understandable. Most individuals with essential hypertension demonstrate vascular and cardiac hyperreactivity to sympathetic stimuli.[20] A prolonged sympathetic stimulus to the kidney creates a functional retention of water and salt, thereby increasing arterial pressure.[20] Increased sympathetic tone produces an increased catecholamine secretion. Catecholamines stimulate vasoconstriction in the subcutaneous, mucosal, splanchnic, and renal vascular beds by alpha-receptor–mediated mechanisms. Catecholamines increase myocardial contractility, heart rate, and cardiac output. Sympathetic stimulation also increases renin release by a direct beta-adrenergic receptor-mediated effect. Because renin secretion activates the angiotensin-aldosterone system, angiotensin-induced vasoconstriction supports the direct effects of catecholamines on blood vessels. Aldosterone-mediated sodium reabsorption complements the direct increase in sodium reabsorption induced by sympathetic stimulation.[19] These factors promote a hypertensive state. Therefore using OMM to decrease sympathetic tone can be theorized to reduce elevated blood pressure.

From an anatomic perspective, the preganglionic neurons of the sympathetic nervous system exit the spinal cord in the region of the thoracolumbar spine.[21]

The preganglionic neurons of the parasympathetic nervous system leave the central nervous system in the third, seventh, ninth, and tenth cranial nerves and in the second through fourth sacral nerves.[21] In addition, the relationship of the sympathetic chains to the ribs is important.[21] The sympathetic chains lie immediately anterior to the heads and necks of the ribs in the thorax. The sympathetic ganglia lie inferior to the junction between the head and neck of the ribs but posterior to the pleura. OMM seeks to take advantage of these anatomic and physiologic relationships in the treatment of hypertension. Osteopathic manipulation of the thoracic spine and ribs offers a method to modulate the sympathetic tone to the heart, kidneys, adrenal glands, and peripheral vasculature. A reduction of sympathetic tone can lead to a decrease in blood pressure, whereas an increase of parasympathetic tone can also lead to a reduction in blood pressure.

CONCLUSION

Although OMM alone may effectively decrease blood pressure, the reduction may be more dramatic and long-lasting if OMM is combined with lifestyle modifications and drug therapy. In this regard, OMM represents a method by which pharmaceutical dosages may be safely reduced while normotensive blood pressure is maintained. In addition, the burden of expensive drug therapy may be mitigated by use of less medication in smaller dosages. OMM represents a potential method to promote a more cost-effective approach to the treatment of hypertension. The doctor-patient relationship will also benefit from the hands-on contact that OMM provides to patients. Additionally, the reduction of debilitating pain via OMM will allow a patient to more easily relax and engage in exercise and physical activity, which may further reduce blood pressure in hypertensive patients.

Further studies are needed to determine the effectiveness of osteopathic manipulative medicine on blood pressure reduction. Clinical outcome studies may support and broaden the usage of OMM. Double-blind placebo-controlled trials involving the use of OMM in a treatment group, and sham manipulation in a control group, would bring into question whether the concept of osteopathic manipulation involves more than external force. The effect of OMM in combination with other approaches, such as lifestyle modification and drug treatment, should also be explored. Because OMM is considered a medical procedure, continuing medical education in hands-on diagnosis and treatment is available to the allopathic (MD) as well as the osteopathic (DO) physician. Because of its nature as a philosophy of medical science, a conventionally trained physician may consider osteopathy an alternative approach.[24] Ultimately, it is the patient who will most benefit from the incorporation of OMM into the overall treatment armamentarium for treating hypertension.

REFERENCES

1. Burt VL, Whelton P, Roccella EJ et al: Prevalence of hypertension in the US adult population: results from the third National Health and Nutrition Examination Survey, 1988-1991, Hypertension 25:305-313, 1995.

2. Williams GH. Hypertensive vascular disease. In Braunwald E, Fauci AS, Kasper DL et al, editors: Harrison's principles of internal medicine, ed 15, New York, 2001, McGraw-Hill, 1414.

3. Collins R, Peto R, MacMahon S et al: Blood pressure, stroke, and coronary heart disease: part 2, short-term reductions in blood pressure: overview of randomized drug trials in their epidemiological context, Lancet 335:827-838, 1990.

4. Levy D, Larson MG, Vasan RS et al: The progression from hypertension to congestive heart failure, JAMA 275:1557-1562, 1996.

5. Gueyffier F, Froment A, Gouton M: New meta-analysis of treatment trials of hypertension: improving the estimate of therapeutic benefit, J Hum Hypertens 10:1-8, 1996.

6. Chobanian AV, Bakris GL, Black HR et al: The Seventh Report of the Joint National Committee on Prevention, Detection, Evaluation, and Treatment of High Blood Pressure: the JNC 7 Report, JAMA 289: 2560-2572, 2003.

7. DiGiovanna EL, Marinke DJ, Dowling DJ: Introduction to osteopathic medicine. In DiGiovanna EL, Schiowitz S editors: An osteopathic approach to diagnosis and treatment, ed 2, New York, 1997, Lippincott-Raven, 2-13.

8. Downing JT: Observations on effect of osteopathic treatment on blood pressure, J Am Osteopath Assoc 13:257-259, 1914.

9. Northup TL: Manipulative management of hypertension, J Am Osteopath Assoc 60:973-978, 1961.

10. Blood HA. Manipulative management of hypertension, Year Book Acad Appl Osteopath 189-195, 1964.

11. Gerber S: Workup and office management of the hypertensive patient, Osteopathic Ann 4:234-241, 1976.

12. Stiles EG: Osteopathic approach to the hypertensive patient, Osteopathic Med 2:41-46, 1977.

13. Rogers JT, Rogers JC: The role of osteopathic manipulative therapy in the treatment of coronary heart disease, J Am Osteopath Assoc 76:21-31, 1976.

14. Frymann VM: The osteopathic approach to cardiac and pulmonary problems, J Am Osteopath Assoc 77:668-673, 1978.

15. Celander E, Koenig AJ, Celander DR. Effect of osteopathic manipulative therapy on autonomic tone as evidenced by blood pressure changes and activity of the fibrinolytic system, J Am Osteopath Assoc 67:1037-1038, 1968.

16. Fichera AP, Celander DR. Effect of osteopathic manipulative therapy on autonomic tone as evidenced by blood pressure changes and activity of the fibrinolytic system, J Am Osteopath Assoc 68:1036-1038, 1969.

17. Brown T, Celander E, Celander DR: A proposed mechanism for osteopathic manipulative therapy effects on blood pressure, J Am Osteopath Assoc 69:1035-1036, 1970.

18. Bayer JD: An osteopathic approach to the management of hypertension, The DO 11:143-151, 1971.

19. Mannino JR: The application of neurologic reflexes to the treatment of hypertension, J Am Osteopath Assoc 79:225-230, 1979.

20. Kuchera ML, Kuchera WA: Osteopathic considerations in systemic dysfunction, ed 2, Columbus, OH, 1994, Greyden Press.

21. Williard FH: Autonomic nervous system. In Ward RC, Hruby RJ, Kuchera WA et al, editors. Foundations for osteopathic medicine, ed 2, Philadelphia, 2003, Lippincott Williams & Wilkins, 93-95.

22. Patriquin DA: Chapman reflexes. In Ward RC, Hruby RJ, Kuchera WA et al, editors: Foundations for osteopathic medicine, ed 2, Philadelphia, 2003, Lippincott Williams & Wilkins, 1053-1054.

23. Morgan JP, Dickey JL, Hunt HH et al: A controlled trial of spinal manipulation in the management of hypertension, J Am Osteopath Assoc 85:308-313, 1985.

24. Spiegel AJ, Capobianco JD, Kruger A, Spinner WD: Osteopathic manipulative medicine in the treatment of hypertension: an alternative, conventional approach, Heart Dis 5:272-279, 2003.

PART V

Specific Approaches

CHAPTER 15

Acupuncture in Cardiovascular Diseases

Ravinder Mamtani, MBBS, MD, M Sc, FACPM
William H. Frishman, MD

A s developed by the Chinese, acupuncture is performed by stimulating designated points of the body. This is done through the insertion of thin flexible needles, finger pressure, application of heat or electricity, or a combination of these modalities. The procedure is based on the theory that a network of energy flows through the body through channels called *meridians*. These channels are related to internal functions. Any imbalance in the flow of energy creates a disease process, and the application of acupuncture can correct this imbalance. At its first encounter with acupuncture, Western medicine was understandably suspicious because explanations of how the procedure might work are bound up with mysterious concepts formulated 3000 years ago. However, in light of advances in our understanding of the neurophysiology of acupuncture, suspicion is giving way to tolerance and acceptance.

Acupuncture is one of the most widely used of the complementary medicine procedures.[1] Research studies have validated its beneficial clinical effect on chronic pain, nausea associated with anesthesia and chemotherapy, and drug addiction. Investigators have implicated therapeutic mechanisms involving the gate control theory of pain and the release of endogenous opioids. The effectiveness of acupuncture and similar complementary methods in the management of common cardiovascular problems such as heart disease and hypertension has not been studied extensively. This chapter reviews the traditional Chinese medicine (TCM) aspects of acupuncture and its neurophysiological mechanisms. The available published acupuncture research experiences and their relevance in the management of cardiovascular diseases are also reviewed.

TRADITIONAL ACUPUNCTURE

From the Latin *acus* (needle) and *punctura* (pricking), the term *acupuncture* was coined by Jesuit missionaries who returned from China reporting on the use of slender needles for medical treatment.[2] One of the most popular fields of TCM, acupuncture accounts for approximately 10 million treatments given annually in the United States.[3]

TCM is based primarily on two theories. The first is *tao*, or the natural law described by fifth century B.C. philosopher Laotse. According to this theory, energy fields known as *yin* and *yang* are in antagonistic—but balancing—interdependent forces in natural phenomena. The *yin* and *yang* can also apply to various organs; grouped under *yin* are the heart, lungs, spleen, liver, kidney, and pericardium. The second theory is based on the five elements—wood, fire, earth, metal, and water. Each one of the major organs of the body belongs to one of the five elements. Like the former theory, these five forces are also dynamically interactive; thus the organs are also interdependent with each other.[4]

When these forces are in balance, Qi flows without obstruction through the meridians of the body. Qi is the energy that nourishes the organs and the body as a whole. This energy is divided into congenital (which is inherited and present since birth) and acquired (which is received from food). The meridians are longitudinal lines that connect a yin organ to its corresponding yang organ. Transversely running collateral lines further interconnect these meridians. This system is comprised of 12 principal channels/meridians, eight minor (extraordinary) meridians, 15 collateral connections, 12 divergent meridians, and 12 channel sinews associated with body musculature. Principal meridians are associated and named after various organs of the body. These include urinary bladder (UB), kidney (Ki), heart (He), stomach (St), spleen (Sp), lung (Lu), large intestine (LI), liver (Lv), gall bladder (GB), pericardium (PC; also called *the master of heart*), and *san jiao* (SJ; also called *the triple heater*). The *san jiao* is the only channel that is not associated with any organ. Along the principal meridians and two of the minor meridians exist 361 acupuncture points.[4] Acupuncture diagnosis is based on the measurement of Qi energy flow through this system, and the goal of treatment is to maintain this flow by keeping the forces in balance.[2] The heart channel, one of the pathways involved in angina pain, is shown in Figure 15-1.

Being a ubiquitous term that refers to needling procedures explained by metaphysical concepts of TCM, acupuncture in its broadest sense also includes acupressure, laser acupuncture, scalp acupuncture, auriculotherapy (or otopuncture) (see Chapter 16), electroacupuncture, moxibustion, Korean hand acupuncture, and others.[3] In traditional Chinese acupuncture, a diagnosis is formulated from patient history and physical examination (appearance, speech quality, odor, local tenderness, and pulse quality). The acupuncturist then determines appropriate acupuncture points.

French energetic acupuncture focuses on bioenergetics and views the body as a circulating electrolytic environment that requires needling to correct the blockage of flow. Korean hand acupuncture emphasizes the hands and feet,

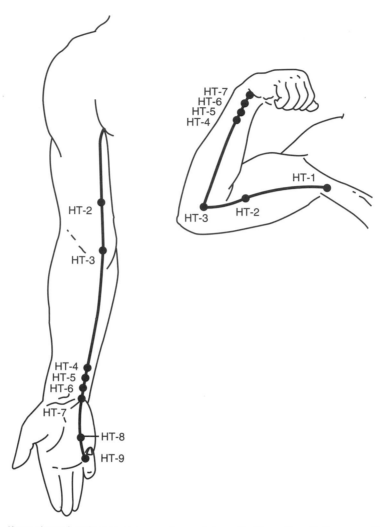

Fig 15-1. Heart channel pathway and acupuncture points on it. *(From Stux G, Pomeranz B: Basics of acupuncture, ed 2, New York, 1991, Springer-Verlag and Xinnong C: Chinese acupuncture and moxibustion, ed 5, Beijing, 1997, Foreign Language Press.)*

which are believed to be the origin of all the body's circulating energy (see Chapter 20). Auricular acupuncture correlates a somatotopic map on the ear with other anatomic regions, but this modality is often considered less effective and is usually employed in conjunction with other acupuncture techniques. Myofascial-based acupuncture involves the assessment of meridians and the needling of carefully palpated tender points that represent areas of excessive neural activity and unbalanced energy.[2]

The points used in the treatment of cardiovascular diseases are, for the most part, situated on the He, PC, and UB channels. Points from two minor channels—namely, the governing vessel (GV) and conception vessel (CV)—are also used. Depending upon the TCM diagnosis, points situated on other channels may also be used. Box 15-1 lists some commonly used points in the treatment of various cardiovascular diseases.

NEUROPHYSIOLOGICAL MECHANISMS OF ACUPUNCTURE

Western medicine was understandably suspicious of acupuncture because explanations of how the procedure might work are bound up with mysterious concepts formulated 3000 years ago. However, in light of advances in understanding of the neurophysiology of pain and scientific explanations of how acupuncture relieves pain, acupuncture is becoming an accepted practice.

Over the past 3 decades, increasing interest and scientific research have focused on the mechanism and use of acupuncture in pain control. Pain can be categorized as nociceptive and neurogenic. Nociceptive pain involves the activation of myelinated (A-delta) and unmyelinated (C-fiber axon) fibers present in the innervation to the skin and deep somatic and visceral structures. In normal, healthy tissue, both types of axons are insensitive to pain; however, in chronic pathologic processes, such as cancer, these axons become the source of extreme pain. Neurogenic pain is due to insults of the central or peripheral nervous system, thus resulting in altered pain sensation. Sympathetic pain is a type of neuropathic pain that involves peripheral nerve injury, which results in severe burning, or causalgia of the region of the nerve. Nociceptive pain is more responsive to acupuncture analgesia than neurogenic pain. However, disorders such as stroke or herpes zoster should not be assumed to be completely a neurogenic entity and refractory to acupuncture analgesia because these disorders concurrently cause nociceptive pain.[5]

Somatosensory afferent nerves have been demonstrated to be essential for acupuncture pain relief. Procaine infiltration of acupuncture points, which abolished afferent transmission from the stimulation site, resulted in a lack of analgesia from needling.[6,7] This phenomenon is often explained by the *gate control theory*, which states that nociceptive pain signals carried by small axons are blocked by acupuncture-induced impulses transmitted by large nerve fibers of the same spinal segment.[8] Afferent activity from both the heart and particular acupoints have been shown in experimental models to converge at the preoptic area of the anterior hypothalamus, posterior hypothalamus, the solitary nucleus, and the amygdala.[9]

Box 15-1   Common Acupuncture Points Used in the Treatment of Various Cardiovascular Diseases

Angina pectoris: GV 20, CV 14, CV 17, PC 6, and He 7
Hypertension: GV 20, UB 15, GB 20, UB 23, He 7, Lv 3, St 36, and Ki 3
Peripheral vascular supply problems: GV 20, UB 15, CV 17, Lu 9, LI 11, He 3, and Lv 3

CV, Conception vessel; GB, gallbladder; GV, governing vessel; He, heart; Ki, kidney; LI, large intestine; Lu, lung; Lv, liver; PC, pericardial; St, stomach; UB, urinary bladder.

An extensive review of acupuncture and its efficacy has shown that acupuncture is effective in treating chronic pain.[10] Neurologic mechanisms of acupuncture analgesia are rapidly becoming apparent. Acupuncture activates small myelinated nerve fibers (A-delta or Group III) in skin and muscle, which transmit impulses to the spinal cord and activate centers in the spinal cord, midbrain, and pituitary hypothalamus. At the spinal cord level, the neurotransmitters involved in blocking incoming painful stimuli, by inhibiting the substantia gelatinosa (SG) cells, include enkephalins and dynorphins. At the level of the midbrain, two descending mechanisms are involved: the serotoninergic mechanism, which involves the raphe magnus, and the noradrenergic mechanism, which involves the paragigantocellular nucleus. The serotoninergic system releases serotonin that activates cells at the junction of lamina I and II in the spinal cord, thus releasing enkephalin, which in turn inhibits the SG cells. The noradrenergic mechanism, on the other hand, releases noradrenaline throughout the dorsal horn of the spinal cord, thus inhibiting the SG cells. Finally, at the level of hypopituitary axis, a generalized hormonal mechanism is involved, which causes release of β-endorphin and adreno-corticotrophic hormone (ACTH).[10] The various mechanisms and or neurotransmitters involved in acupuncture are listed in Table 15-1.

The role of endorphins in acupuncture analgesia is supported by the finding that naloxone, the opioid antagonist, blocks the effect and may cause hyperalgesia.[11,12] Similarly, lesions of the arcuate nucleus of the hypothalamus, the site of β-endorphin release, block analgesia.[13] In regard to monoamines, lesions of the nucleus raphe magnus, a site of serotonin and norepinephrine secretion, also abolish the analgesic effect of acupuncture.[7]

Acupuncture affects the cardiovascular system in a variety of ways, and these effects are explained by both central and peripheral effects. It stimulates the β-endorphinergic system, which influences vasomotor areas in the brainstem, thereby regulating sympathetic tone. Acupuncture may also increase vagal (parasympathetic) activity, and may also exert peripheral effects by increasing the release of neuropeptides, such as calcitonin gene-related peptide (CGRP).

CLINICAL USEFULNESS OF ACUPUNCTURE

Acupuncture has benefited many patients in the relief of both acute and chronic pain. Common applications include the following conditions: rheumatoid arthritis, osteoporosis, osteoarthritis, fibromyalgia, myofascial pain syndrome, low back pain, headaches/migraine, and reflex sympathetic dystrophy.[5,14,15] The Consensus Development Conference Panel on Acupuncture sponsored by the National Institute of Health acknowledges the proven efficacy of acupuncture for postoperative and chemotherapy-induced nausea and vomiting, the nausea of pregnancy, and postoperative dental pain.[14] In addition, acupuncture has been concluded to be an effective adjuvant treatment for many other conditions. These include but are not limited to addiction, headache, stroke rehabilitation, menstrual cramps, carpal tunnel syndrome, and asthma. Electroacupuncture has been shown to have positive results in treating depression and posttraumatic

Table **15-1** NEUROTRANSMITTERS/MECHANISMS INVOLVED IN ACUPUNCTURE

Neurotransmitter/Mechanism	Effects
Needling causes A–delta fiber stimulation relaying information to spinal cord, midbrain, and hypopituitary axis.	Segmental and heterosegmental generalized effects. Segmental effects occur at the same spinal segment as the needle. The heterosegmental effects occur through the brainstem and higher centers and descending inhibition serotoninergic and adrenergic mechanisms.
Opioids—enkaphalin, dynorphins, β-endorphins.	Analgesia. Type of neurotransmitters released vary with the type of acupuncture used. For example, dynorphins release is predominant with high-frequency acupuncture.
Gamma-amino butyric acid (GABA)	Pain relief. GABA is released with high-frequency electrical acupuncture.
Serotonin	Analgesia and mood-enhancing effect.
Oxytocin	Analgesia and sedation.
Autonomic effects	Increases blood flow by vasodilatation, increases feeling of warmth, lowers blood pressure, and normalizes gastrointestinal motility.
Adrenocorticotrophic hormone	Antiinflammatory, immunomodulatory effect.
Nerve growth factor	Trophic effect on sensory and autonomic nerves.
Cholecystokinin	Antiepileptic and may contribute to acupuncture. Tolerance.

Modified from Filshie J: Acupuncture in palliative care, Eur J Palliative Care 7:41-44, 2000; Ernst E: Clinical effectiveness of acupuncture: an overview of systematic review. In Ernst E, White A, editors: Acupuncture: a scientific appraisal, Woburn, MA, 2000, Butterworth-Heinemann Publishers, 107-127.

stress disorder. Beneficial results have been reported for osteoarthritis and some intestinal problems as well (Table 15-2).[3]

ACUPUNCTURE IN CARDIOVASCULAR DISEASES

PERIPHERAL BLOOD FLOW

Various studies have shown that acupuncture causes vasodilatation.[16] In one study, various forms of acupuncture (manual stimulation, low-frequency, and high-frequency electrical acupuncture groups) were compared with superficial needling (control group).[17] Blood flow was measured from 20 minutes before

Table **15-2**   CLINICAL EVIDENCE FOR ACUPUNCTURE UTILITY

Conclusively Positive	Useful as an Adjunct	Inconclusive Evidence	Conclusively Negative
Dental pain	Neck pain	Angina	Weight loss
Nausea/vomiting	Headache/migraine	Hypertension	Smoking cessation
Low back pain	Osteoarthritis		
	Addiction		
	Asthma		
	Stroke		
	Carpal tunnel syndrome		
	Tennis elbow		
	Menstrual cramps		

Data from Ernst E: *Clinical effectiveness of acupuncture: an overview of systematic review*. In Ernst E, White A, editors: *Acupuncture: a scientific appraisal*, Woburn, MA, 2000, Butterworth-Heinemann Publishers, 107-127; Meyer DJ: *Acupuncture: an evidence-based review of the clinical literature*, Annu Rev Med 51:49-63, 2000; and Luundeberg T: *Peripheral effects of sensory stimulation (acupuncture) in inflammation and ischemia*, Scand J Rehab Med S 29:61-86, 1993.

the initiation of treatment until 20 minutes after the removal of the needles. Increased blood flow was observed in the groups that received manual stimulation and low-frequency electrical acupuncture. In another randomized, controlled trial involving Raynaud's syndrome patients, Moehrle and colleagues observed a significant reduction of symptom attacks and an increase in blood flow in the group receiving active acupuncture treatment in comparison to the sham control group.[18] Using thermography, Ernst and Lee were able to show that acupuncture causes an initial vasoconstriction due to an increase in sympathetic tone followed by a sustained decrease in sympathetic tone, thus resulting in vasodilatation.[19] It is possible that the initial feeling of coldness experienced by a small number of patients could be attributable to initial transient vasoconstriction. A feeling of warmth follows. The feeling of warmth that is felt by most patients undergoing acupuncture is attributable to vasodilatation.

The effect of transcutaneous electrical nerve stimulation (TENS), a variant of acupuncture, has also been studied. Studies involving the TENS have suggested that vasodilatation effects observed in low-frequency (2 Hz) and high-frequency (80 Hz) are due to the release of a vasodilator neuropeptide, vasoactive intestinal polypeptide (VIP), and CGRP, respectively.[17]

HYPERTENSION

Research in animals has shown that weak or lower intensity electrical acupuncture stimulus has a depressor response on arterial pressure, and higher stimulus strength has a depressor response.[15] In an experiment performed on rats, Yao and colleagues compared the effect of acupuncture-like stimulation on blood pressure in normotensive and hypertensive rats.[20] The pressure reduction was more marked in the hypertensive group. Reduced sympathetic tone, as measured by the rate of firing in the splanchnic nerve, was also observed, and this effect was reversed by naloxone. Similar results have been reported in human patients. In a study on patients with essential hypertension, acupuncture resulted in 5 to 10 mm Hg decline in diastolic pressure.[15] Temporary reduction in blood pressure has also been seen with auricular acupuncture.[21]

Acupuncture's ability to alter sympathetic activity seems to be the main mechanism underlying its blood pressure-lowering effect. Interestingly, an opposite effect with acupuncture (i.e, increasing blood pressure) has also been observed in hypotensive states. This could be possibly related to the baroreceptor sensitivities in hypotension and hypertension.[15] If this observation is true, acupuncture will have displayed a homeostatic phenomenon, acting to regulate blood pressure toward normal. All these findings are encouraging and merit further investigation.

ANGINA PECTORIS

Angina pectoris (chest pain) has not been studied rigorously with regard to acupuncture analgesia.[22] Moreover, because of the difficulty in blinding both patients and healthcare providers in acupuncture, most reported studies have been open and unblinded, which is deemed less credible by the standards of Western medicine. However, this remains an important area of research because cardiac disease is a major cause of death and disability in the United States, and many patients with angina pectoris are refractory to standard therapies.

Ballegaard et al published one of the first randomized trials to compare the effectiveness of acupuncture and sham acupuncture in patients with severe, stable angina pectoris resistant to medical treatment.[23] The active treatment group received acupuncture at bilateral points: PC 6, St 36, and UB 14. Sham acupuncture involved needling the patient in the same spinal segment as the active treatment—but outside the Chinese meridian system. The trial was single-blind in design because the acupuncturist could not be blinded. The evaluation of effectiveness was based on data collected from patient daily diaries (stating frequency of anginal attacks, activity during the attack, and nitroglycerin consumption), exercise tests (stepwise incrementing bicycle workload and 12-lead ECG), and a subjective global evaluation by the patient at the end of the trial. From the exercise tests, the following variables were assessed: exercise tolerance (cumulative work during exercise), difference in pressure-rate-product between rest and maximum exercise (dPRP) and maximal PRP during exercise, maximum ECG ST segment depression, and length of time until maximum ST segment depression. The study failed to find a significant reduction in pain between the treatment and control groups. However, in comparison to the sham group, the active treatment group had a significantly higher dPRP and higher maximal PRP, which was interpreted as an increase in cardiac functional capacity. This increase would be easily explained if the patient's pain had been relieved, but because that did not occur, other mechanisms to explain functional improvement were considered. The researchers postulated that the change was caused by a decreased workload secondary to systemic vasodilatation specific to the acupoints (not the spinal cord level). Additionally, six of the 12 patients in the active treatment group, whereas only one of 12 in the sham treatment group reported a subjective improvement of general well-being ($p = 0.10$).

In 1990, the same research group attempted to determine whether a clinical effect would be seen with acupuncture in less severely ill patients with less anatomical coronary artery disease and moderate, stable angina pectoris.[24] The active treatment patients demonstrated a significant increase in exercise tolerance and a significantly delayed time to pain onset compared to their pretreatment values, but this was not significant in comparison to the sham treatment group. Both groups showed a significant beneficial effect regarding nitroglycerin use, anginal attack frequency, and subjective overall well-being, thus contradicting the 1986 study. The researchers speculated that a noxious stimulus of the skin had an effect on the interior organs innervated by the same dermatome through a sympathetic cutaneous reflex and that a noxious stimulus to a trigger point of the heart dermatome had a beneficial effect on myocardial pain in both the sham and genuine treatment groups. The investigators also suggested an increased placebo effect was attributable to more extensive patient recruitment in this study.

Ballegaard et al subsequently investigated whether sham acupuncture could be regarded as an inactive control treatment and to distinguish responders from nonresponders to acupuncture by monitoring for skin temperature changes.[25] In the first trial, 49 patients with stable angina pectoris were randomized to receive genuine acupuncture (n = 24) or sham acupuncture (n = 25) for 10 treatments over a 3-week period. No significant differences between the groups were found in maximal PRP, dPRP, nitroglycerin consumption, anginal attack rate, and daily well-being self-assessment. In the second trial, electroacupuncture was performed at LI 4 bilaterally (between the first and second metacarpal bones) at 2 Hz, and skin temperature was recorded on the left hallux and index finger. The change of skin temperature on the index finger—but not the hallux—correlated with the clinical effect of acupuncture. Of the 33 patients, 14 were classified into Group 1 (increase in skin temperature, n = 12; no change in skin temperature, n = 2), while 19 were placed into Group 2 (decrease in skin temperature). Group 1 patients demonstrated a significant increase in exercise tolerance, an improved dPRP, decreased nitroglycerin use, a lower anginal attack rate, and an improvement in daily well-being in comparison to Group 2 patients. The investigators attributed the increase in skin temperature to a decrease in sympathetic tone leading to peripheral vasodilatation, and in these patients, acupuncture was more effective. However, the study did not address why acupuncture produced sympathetic inhibition in some patients and not others. A placebo effect was not likely because the skin temperature change was localized to the index finger and not the hallux (which would have implied a generalized effect of a placebo). The findings suggest some effect of acupuncture because of noxious stimulation of a dermatome.

Richter et al conducted a randomized, crossover study of 21 patients with stable angina pectoris, with at least five anginal attacks per week for 6 months despite intensive medical treatment.[26] Patients received two 4-week treatment periods of acupuncture or a placebo tablet (patients were under the impression they were using a new antianginal medication), with a 2-week wash-out period between treatment periods before crossover. Treatment was individualized, primarily using acupoints PC 6, He 5, UB 15, UB 20, and St 36, and using additional points at He 7, LI 4, LI 11, and Lv 3. The patients were evaluated using a bicycle ECG ergometer exercise test, blood pressure measurements, a chest pain scoring system between 0 (no pain) to 4 (maximal pain), and a self-rating quality of life survey. The exercise test evaluated heart rate, blood pressure, maximal and comparable workload, ST segment depression, maximal workload without pain, and maximal pain score. The average number of anginal attacks during acupuncture treatment were significantly decreased compared to both the run-in and placebo periods. The maximal workload until onset of chest pain was significantly increased and ST segment depression at maximal workload was significantly reduced. However, the study failed to find any significant difference in maximal physical performance on the bicycle ergometer at the end of the acupuncture period compared with placebo therapy. Furthermore, heart rate and systolic blood pressure showed no significant changes at both rest and maximal workload. Among 7 of the 21 patients with an unchanged number of anginal attacks, 6 showed a positive response in terms of ECG (less ST segment depression) or pain during exercise (higher maximal workloads until onset of chest pain). Finally, the quality of life survey showed significant improvement for chest pain, physical performance, peripheral coldness, pessimism, vertigo, and relaxation, but no difference was found for anxiety, tiredness, sleep disturbances, or gastrointestinal problems. The investigators concluded that in addition to the role of endorphins and monoamines in analgesia, acupuncture relieved myocardial ischemia, possibly by influencing coronary perfusion.

The role of otopuncture in angina pectoris has also been investigated (see Chapter 16). A study of reactive electropermeable points (REPP) focused on changes in electrical resistance in the skin.[27] When a body organ is diseased, the part of the auricle corresponding to the diseased part is believed to also undergo change, including pain, edema, hardening, and changes in resistance to electricity in the skin. The study looked at four groups of subjects: those with acute myocardial infarction (MI), old MI, angina pectoris, and healthy controls. The investigation correlated a higher electropermeability to electric current (a positive REPP) at He I and He II otopoints with acute MI, old MI, and angina pectoris compared to controls. The observations suggest a correlation with the functional anatomy of the heart, but the significance of these findings still warrant further investigation.

Juyun compared the effects of otopuncture of the He otopoint with that of the St otopoint (control) in 38 patients with symptomatic coronary heart disease.[28] Patients underwent pretreatment and posttreatment workups, which included ECG, blood lipid analysis, and blood viscosity determination. During the treatment, patients were assessed for the degree of angina pectoris and improvement of the clinical symptoms of cardiac disease (palpitation, shortness of breath). Known cardiac drugs were suspended during the treatment period, and only in cases of frequent angina pectoris or severe arrhythmia were drugs of the nitro-ester category temporarily used. The therapeutic effects for treatment of angina pectoris were significantly better in the treatment group. Of the treatment patients, 14 reported significant effects, five cases with improvement, and one with no effect. In the control group, nine patients reported significant effects, two cases with improvement, and six cases with no effect, and one patient reported aggravated angina pectoris ($p < 0.05$). The ECG in the treatment cases revealed three cases with significant effects, nine cases with improvement, and eight cases without effect, whereas the control group had only two cases of improvement, 15 without effect, and one with aggravation (p<0.05). Furthermore, treatment at the He otopoint also improved the symptoms of palpitation, oppressed feeling in the chest, and shortness of breath. There were also significant effects seen on blood rheology in the treatment group compared to the controls: decreases in whole blood viscosity, plasma viscosity, blood lipid, cholesterol, and hematocrit. Because of these changes, the investigator suggests that blood flow accelerates, blood pressure decreases, and blood volume to the coronary artery increases. This enhances recovery from ischemia and anoxia of the cardiac muscles.

In experimental studies, acupuncture has been shown to reduce ECG evidence of myocardial ischemia in animals, while improving regional wall motion.[29] The beneficial effects of acupuncture in humans may relate to an analgesic effect, an increase in coronary blood flow, and a reduction in myocardial oxygen demand. Li et al have demonstrated that acupuncture causes a reduction in stress-induced blood pressure.[29]

Transcutaneous Electrical Nerve Stimulation in Angina Pectoris

Other modalities have been found to have similar analgesic effects as acupuncture. TENS is one of these pain-relieving treatments. Commercially available TEN simulators are used to deliver constant current pulses at specific frequencies (70 Hz is standard). The intensity of the stimulation is adjustable to a level below that producing pain (15 to 50 mA). Electrodes are placed on the patient's chest over the site of the greatest pain. Three TENS sessions of at least 1 hour are self-administered by the patient during the day (morning, noon, and evening), with additional short treatments of less than 10 minutes given for anginal pain.[30]

In comparison to controls, patients with angina pectoris (New York Heart Association functional class II) have demonstrated a beneficial effect with TENS treatments in terms of less frequent anginal attacks, increased work capacity, decreased ST segment depression, and decreased use of nitroglycerin. The study relates the beneficial effects of TENS to the gate control theory of Melzack and Wall.[8] The pain production of TENS may block sympathetic outflow, or the electrical stimulation may be responsible for the sympathetic blockade. The researchers also implicate the role of the endogenous opioid system in inhibiting the transmission of noxious stimuli.[30]

Spinal Cord Stimulation in Angina Pectoris

Spinal cord stimulation (SCS), or epidural spinal electrical stimulation, is another treatment modality that has been shown to have both antianginal and antiischemic effects in patients with severe angina pectoris (see Chapter 26).

ACUPUNCTURE SAFETY

Acupuncture is done with extremely thin, steel metal alloy needles with a view to stimulate specific points in the body. The needle is merely a tool used to correct the energy imbalance in the body and to release neurotransmitters. A brief discomfort or a pricking sensation often occurs when the needle passes through the skin. As the effects begin to occur, the patient may feel numbness, heat, dull aching, or a tingling sensation at the site or in the vicinity of the needle insertion. Generally, the needles are left in place for about 15 to 30 minutes. They may be rotated by the practitioner or stimulated by electricity. Most side effects associated with acupuncture are minor and transient. They include occasional dizziness, light-headedness, and very slight bleeding after needles are withdrawn. Infection and other serious side effects such as lung puncture are rare. Needles used in the United States are sterile and disposable.

Contraindications to acupuncture might include a history of bleeding or the use of anticoagulant medication, a prosthetic or damaged heart valve, and—for electrical acupuncture—a pacemaker. Many practitioners consider pregnancy to be a relative contraindication. Caution should be exercised when needles are placed in the thorax.

PROBLEMS WITH ACUPUNCTURE RESEARCH

Despite some encouraging results, problems exist with the performance of quality studies of acupuncture. One reason for this may be the difficult nature of conducting Western medicine's gold-standard randomized, a double-blind trial on a treatment modality that is not based on the same empiric system. Specific methodological research problems with regard to acupuncture include the following: (a) constructing an inert placebo that parallels the insertion of a needle 2 to 4 cm into the skin is virtually impossible; (b) ascribing relief to acupuncture is not always certain because of the mediation of some nonspecific effects by endogenous opiates; (c) because the location of the insertion and manipulation of the needle are essential to successful acupuncture, the acupuncturist relies in individualizing treatment of each patient, two subjects with the same diagnosis may be prescribed different puncture sites, thus confounding the evaluation results.

CONCLUSION

Although acupuncture is used relatively little in this country today, it is likely to see substantial growth in the future. Acupuncture shows promise as one of several options. Its role has been well documented as an effective modality for pain relief and for a variety of musculoskeletal problems, headache/migraine, addiction, and nausea associated with chemotherapy and anesthesia. Few studies, however, have examined the role of acupuncture in the management of cardiac and vascular diseases. At the present time, the role of acupuncture in the management of cardiovascular diseases can be neither confirmed nor ruled out.[31] Nevertheless, the studies reviewed in this chapter have shown there may be validity to acupuncture in some patients with hypertension and angina pectoris. Additional research to examine acupuncture and its variants as primary and/or complementary therapies in patients with cardiac disease is greatly needed.

REFERENCES

1. Longhurst JC: Acupuncture's beneficial effects on the cardiovascular system, Prev Cardiol 4:21-33, 1998.
2. Ceniceros S, Brown GR: Acupuncture: a review of its history, theories, and indications, South Med J 91:1121-25, 1998.
3. Ulett GA, Han J, Han S: Traditional and evidence-based acupuncture: history, mechanism, and present status, South Med J 91:1115-20, 1998.
4. Hsu DT: Acupuncture: a review, Reg Anesth 21:361-70, 1996.
5. Mamtani R: Acupuncture for chronic pain management in the elderly, Longterm Care Forum 5:9-12, 1995.
6. Nathan PW: Acupuncture analgesia, Trends Neurosci 7:21-23, 1978.
7. Hans JS, Terenius L: Neurochemical basis of acupuncture analgesia, Ann Rev Pharmacol Toxicol 22:193-220, 1982.
8. Melzac R, Wall P: Pain mechanisms: a new theory, Science 150:971-73, 1965.
9. Wu D-Z: Acupuncture and neurophysiology, Clin Neurol Neurosurg 92:13-30, 1990.
10. Pomeranz B, Berman B: Scientific basis of acupuncture. In Stux G, Berman B, Pomeranz B, editors: Basics of acupuncture, ed 5, New York, 2003, Springer Verlag, 7-86.
11. Pomeranz B, Chiu D: Naloxone blocks acupuncture analgesia and causes hyperalgesia: endorphin is implicated, Life Sci 19:1757-62, 1976.
12. Mayer DJ, Price DD, Raffi A: Antagonism of acupuncture analgesia in man by the narcotic antagonist naloxone, Brain Res 121:368-72, 1977.
13. Wang Q, Mao L, Han JS: The arcuate nucleus of hypothalamus mediates low but not high frequency electroacupuncture in rats, Brain Res 51:60-66, 1990.
14. National Institutes of Health Consensus Statement: Acupuncture. 15(5):1-34, 1997.
15. Ernst E: Clinical effectiveness of acupuncture: an overview of systematic review. In Ernst E, White A, editors: Acupuncture: a scientific appraisal, Woburn, MA, 2000, Butterworth-Heinemann Publishers, 107-127.
16. Meyer DJ: Acupuncture: an evidence-based review of the clinical literature, Annu Rev Med 51:49-63, 2000.
17. Luundeberg T: Peripheral effects of sensory stimulation (acupuncture) in inflammation and ischemia, Scand J Rehab Med S 29:61-86, 1993.
18. Moehrle M, Blum A, Lorenz F: Proceedings of the Second Asian Congress for Microcirculation, Beijing, China, 1995.
19. Ernst M, Lee MHM: Sympathetic effects of manual and electrical acupuncture of the Tsuanli knee point: comparison with Hoku hand point sympathetic effect, Exper Neurol 94:1-10, 1986.

20.   Yao T, Anderson S, Thoren P: Long lasting cardiovascular depression induced by acupuncture like stimulation on the sciatic nerve in unanesthetized spontaneously hypertensive rats, Brain Res 244, 295-303, 1982.

21.   Goponjuk PJ, Leonova MV: Clinical effectiveness of auricular acupuncture treatment of patients with hypertensive states, Acupuncture Res 11:29-31, 1993.

22.   Bueno EA, Mamtani R, Frishman WH: Alternative approaches to the medical management of angina pectoris: acupuncture, electrical nerve stimulation, and spinal cord stimulation, Heart Dis 3:236-41, 2001.

23.   Ballegaard S, Jensen G, Pedersen F et al: Acunpuncture in severe, stable angina pectoris: a randomized trial, Acta Med Scand 220:307-13, 1986.

24.   Ballegaard S, Pedersen F, Pietersen A et al: Effects of acupuncture in moderate stable angina pectoris: a controlled study, J Intern Med 227:25-30, 1990.

25.   Ballegaard S, Meyer CN, Trojaborg W: Acupuncture in angina pectoris: does acupuncture have a specific effect? J Intern Med 229:357-62, 1991.

26.   Richter A, Herlitz J, Hjalmarson A: Effect of acupuncture in patients with angina pectoris, Eur Heart J 12:175-78, 1991.

27.   Saku K, Mukaino Y, Ying H et al: Characteristics of reactive electropermeable points on the auricles of coronary heart disease patients, Clin Cardiol 16:415-19, 1993.

28.   Juyun D: A clinical observation in coronary heart disease treated by otopuncture at heart otopoint, J Trad Chinese Med 18:43-46, 1998.

29.   Li P, Pitsillides KF, Rendig SV et al: Reversal of reflex-induced myocardial ischemia by median nerve stimulation: a feline model of electroacupuncture, Circulation 97:1186-94, 1998.

30.   Mannheimer C, Carlsson CA, Emanuelsson H et al: The effects of transcutaneous electrical nerve stimulation in patients with severe angina pectoris, Circulation 71:308-16, 1985.

31.   Krucoff MW, Liebowitz R, Vogel JHK, Mark D: Complementary and alternative medical therapy in cardiovascular care. In Fuster V, Alexander RW, O'Rourke RA editors:: Hurst's the heart, 11th ed. New York 2004, McGraw Hill: 2463-2472.

CHAPTER **16**

Auriculotherapy for Cardiovascular Disorders

Terry Oleson, PhD

The field of alternative and complementary medicine includes many therapeutic modalities that are considered unconventional and controversial because they seem outside the domain of classical anatomy and physiology. One of the most intriguing features of traditional Chinese medicine (TCM) is that distal acupoints on the body can be needled to relieve pathological conditions in parts of the body far remote from the site of stimulation. The pattern of these distal acupoints does not seem to follow any known nerve root or dermatome. Even within the field of classical acupuncture, the therapeutic effectiveness of stimulating acupoints on the auricle of the external ear seems surprising because the auricle is not directly connected to any of the primary meridian channels that are said to carry qi energy. Nonetheless, some of the most definitive neurophysiological research in animals and clinical studies in humans have been conducted by the stimulation of small loci on the auricle. Similar to the better-known system of foot reflexology (see Chapter 20), each region of the ear is said to correspond to a particular part of the body in a somatotopic pattern. Many of these auricular acupuncture points are used to both diagnose and to treat cardiovascular conditions, which is the focus of this chapter.

HISTORICAL AND THEORETICAL PERSPECTIVES

The origins of classical acupuncture have been dated to the Han dynasty of China in the second century BC, whereas auricular acupuncture, as it is currently practiced, was initiated by a French physician in the 1950s.[1] Although ancient Chinese medical texts listed several acupoints located on the external ear,[2] the concept that the auricle can be viewed as an inverted fetus was first proposed by Dr. Paul Nogier[3] of Lyon, France. Representation of the upside down baby on the auricle and the somatotopic connections of the ear to the body are shown in Figure 16-1. The Chinese did not develop their modern ear acupuncture charts until after they had learned of the somatotopic correspondences that Nogier had discovered.[4] In the several decades since then, medical doctors throughout China have conducted hundreds of observational studies that have verified the existence of particular auricular acupoints related to specific internal organs. Further developments in research and clinical investigations of auriculotherapy took different directions in China and Europe, leading to two separate systems.[5]

In 1990, a working group of the World Health Organization[6,7] met in Lyon, France to standardize the localization of acupoints for both Chinese and European systems of ear acupuncture. An international consensus conference was held in the United States in 1999. It brought together professionals in the field of auriculotherapy and auricular medicine from Asia, Europe, and America to collaborate on an integrated approach to auricular acupuncture.[8] The majority of research articles on auricular acupuncture have focused on the application of auriculotherapy for pain management and the treatment of addictions, but a significant number have addressed the use of auricular acupuncture for cardiovascular disorders.

Two different theoretical approaches to auriculotherapy have been developed. One approach is Oriental, the other is Occidental.[9] The Oriental approach relies upon the concepts mentioned in classical acupuncture texts, such as the energetic forces of qi and of yin and yang (see Chapter 15).[10] According to the TCM perspective, the ear is a self-contained microsystem that holographically resonates

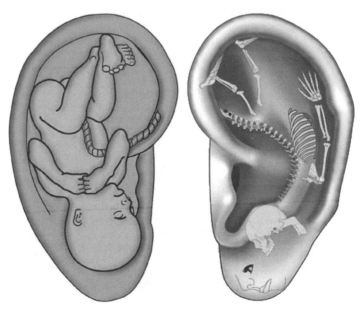

Fig 16-1. Depiction of an inverted fetus pattern represented on the external ear and the somatotopic relationships of the auricle to the body.

with the meridian macrosystem. Only the six yang meridians (the urinary bladder, gall bladder, stomach, small intestines, large intestines, and *san jiao* channels) extend to regions of the head that are near the external ear and thus are said to have direct connections to the auricular microsystem. A reactive ear acupoint is tender to applied pressure and exhibits low electrical skin resistance. It is called a *yang alarm point*. The yin meridians (the heart, lung, kidney, liver, spleen, and pericardium channels) are said to have indirect connections to the auricle through their corresponding yang channels. Health is said to be sustained by the harmonious flow of qi and blood throughout all the meridians, whereas pathology is due to the blockage, excess, or deficiency of qi or blood. Stimulation of acupoints on either the acupuncture channels or on the auricular microsystem are said to improve the circulation of qi and blood and thus to revitalize health.

The Western approach towards auriculotherapy rests upon the basic principles of anatomy and neurophysiology. The ear has both diagnostic and treatment properties because of its differential innervation by the vagus nerve, the trigeminal nerve, and the cervical plexus nerves.[11] The external ear contains cutaneous points of reduced electrical resistance that correspond to pathology or pain in specific body organs. Schematically, the external ear is like a computer keyboard, which acts on the whole organism through the intermediary of the central nervous system. This auricular system has two types of computer keys: a somatic set connected to the spinothalamic system that modulates pain perception and a visceral set that modifies internal organs. The American acupuncturist Ralph Alan Dale has described organocutaneous reflexes and cutaneoorganic reflexes that interconnect multiple microsystems with the central brain computer.[10,12] Dysfunction in an internal organ projects to specific points on the ear through the organocutaneous reflexes, whereas stimulation of an auricular acupoint relieves pathology in the correspondent organ. Research investigations in both animals[13] and humans[14] have shown that stimulation of specific auricular points selectively activates particular parts of the brain that are associated with the part of the body related to the correspondent organ. Both body acupuncture and auricular acupuncture are also related to the release of endorphins, thus providing a neurohumeral mechanism for their actions.[15-17]

The external ear is distinctive in the field of anatomy in that it is the only region of the body where the parasympathetic vagus nerve projects to the surface of the skin. The vagus nerve radiates throughout the central concha of the auricle, whereas the surrounding antihelix and antitragus regions of the external ear are innervated by the somatic trigeminal nerve and cervical sympathetic nerves.[18] These auricular regions of differential innervation are shown in Figure 16-2. In addition to the inverted fetus perspective, Nogier[19] proposed an embryological theory that the central concha represents endodermal internal organs; the surrounding antihelix and antitragus represent the mesodermal musculoskeletal system; and the lobe and tragus represent the endodermal nervous system. Localization of specific points for the cardiovascular system are represented in Figure 16-3. The correspondent ear points for the heart are found in the inferior concha in the Chinese auricular system, which makes sense because the heart is partially composed of endodermal tissue. In the European system, however, Nogier suggested

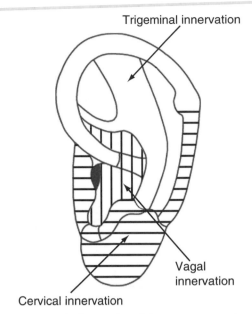

Fig 16-2. Indication of the differential innervation of the vagus nerve to the concha of the auricle, the trigeminal nerve to the antihelix, antitragus, scaphoid fossa, and triangular fossa regions of the auricle, and the cervical plexus nerves to the lobule, tragus, and helix tail.

that the heart is represented on the antihelix body as it is primarily mesodermal tissue. The Chinese have described a secondary heart point on the superior tragus of the ear and different ear points for the regulation of blood pressure.

It is not just theoretical differences that have led to the distinctions between the Chinese and European auricular microsystems. In both Asia and Europe, localization of ear acupoints has been based on repeated observations that patients with particular medical conditions exhibit distinct alterations of the ear at specific loci.[20] Moreover, stimulating those same points on the ear has led to clinical improvement of that condition. The basic science studies and clinical research on auricular acupuncture fall into two principal categories, those studies which have examined the diagnostic properties related to organocutaneous reflexes and those studies that have investigated the physiological and behavioral effects of auricular acupuncture stimulation. Only those research findings related to cardiovascular disorders will be examined in the present chapter. However, because TCM maintains that heart qi is related to mental well-being as well as cardiovascular disorders, the effect of stimulating the auricular heart point will also be examined as it relates to the treatment of anxiety.

DIAGNOSTIC ASSESSMENTS

Acupuncture points along the body are distinctive from neighboring regions of skin by their greater electrical conductivity.[21] Electrical differences and mor-

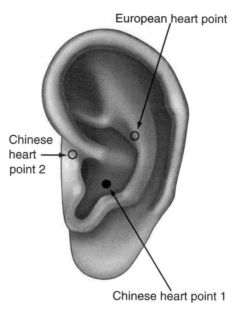

European heart point

Chinese heart point 2

Chinese heart point 1

Fig 16-3. Localization of specific anatomical regions of the external ear for representation of the heart according to Chinese and European auricular systems.

phological changes in auricular acupoints have also been detected when pathology exists in the corresponding area of the body.[22] The first double-blind assessment of auricular reflex points associated with musculoskeletal disorders was conducted by Oleson et al in 1980.[23] A positive correspondence with the parts of the body that experienced musculoskeletal pain was found between auricular points identified as reactive, tender to palpation, and exhibiting at least 50 microamps of electrical conductivity. Nonreactive ear points corresponded to parts of the body from which there was no reported musculoskeletal pain. The statistically significant correct detection rate was 75.2%.

Ear reflex points related to coronary disorders were examined by Saku et al in Japan.[24] They defined reactive electropermeable points as auricular areas that exhibited skin conductance current greater than 50 microamps. A significantly higher frequency of reactive ear points was found at the Chinese heart points in the inferior concha (84%) and on the tragus (59%) for patients with myocardial infarctions and angina pain than for a control group of healthy subjects (11%). No difference between the coronary heart disease group and the control group was found regarding the electrical reactivity of auricular points that did not represent the heart. The frequency of electropermeable auricular points for the kidney (5%), stomach (6%), liver (10%), elbow (11%), or eye (3%) was the same for coronary patients as it was for individuals without coronary problems, thus highlighting the specificity of this phenomenon.

Diagonal folds in the skin over the ear lobe have been associated with certain cardiovascular disorders. Lichstein et al[25] and Mehta and Homby[26] found a higher incidence of diagonal earlobe creases in patients with coronary problems. Their double-blind clinical studies showed that the presence of a crease running diagonally from the intertragic notch to the bottom of the lobe was more predictive of the occurrence of a coronary problem than knowing either the patient's blood pressure level or serum cholesterol level.

Guan Zunxin[27] reviewed the Chinese medical research on auricular points related to the heart. A 1988 study by Shizhang Zhou examined the auricular lobule of 76 patients with coronary heart disease in comparison to the auricle of persons without any coronary disorder. A distinctive crease on the lobule was found in 92% of the patients with coronary disorders and only 36% of the individuals without a cardiac problem. These observations in China were similar to those reported in a 1989 European study by Romoli et al.[28] The diagonal ear lobe crease is especially detectable after the age of 40. The Romoli group found that in 143 patients over 50 years of age, the patients with the earlobe crease also showed higher levels of anxiety than patients not having the crease.

Visual inspection of the external ear can reveal morphological changes of the skin surface in persons with cardiovascular disorders. After several decades of clinical observations at the Beijing General Hospital, Dr. Li-Chun Huang[29] documented specific characteristics that relate to different medical conditions. In persons with coronary artery disease, the heart area at the center of the inferior concha exhibits white edema after pressing on the point with a probe. Dr. Huang also found that the groove of coronary heart disease noted by other practitioners as a crease running diagonally across the center of the earlobe can be distinguished from a more medial groove of hypotension nearer the face.

According to Guan Zunxin, Peng Yingao found in 1987 that lesions induced in the hearts of rabbits by barium chloride led to low skin resistance points in the heart region of the auricle.[27] When that auricular point was needled, significant improvement in the cardiac lesion occurred. That same year, Wu Xinfa showed that the cardiac output of 18 rabbits exhibited significant increases 20 minutes after needling the auricular heart point. These animal studies support the existence of both organocutaneo and cutaneoorganic reflexes, which demonstrates the relationship between the heart and its correspondent representation on the auricle.

AURICULOTHERAPY OF CARDIAC DISORDERS

ARRHYTHMIAS

At a 1995 International Symposium on Auricular Medicine, which met in Beijing, China, clinical case observations were presented on the treatment outcomes with auricular acupuncture.[30] Wu Yiaolong and Xiao Wupi from the Hunan province reported on 100 cases of cardiac arrhythmia treated by auricular acupressure, as contrasted with another group of 30 cases treated by TCM and medical herbs. Of the 100 patients given auricular acupressure, 43 cases were reported as cured; in 24 cases treatment was obviously effective; in 25 cases treatment was effective; and in 8 cases treatment was ineffective. In the comparison

TCM group, only eight cases (26.7%) were reported as cured; 10 cases (33.3%) were reported obviously effective, five cases (16.7%) were reported effective; and seven cases (23.3%) were reported ineffective.

Angina Pectoris

Also at the 1995 International Symposium on Auricular Medicine, clinical observation on the auricular treatment of angina pain was presented by Peng Lihua.[30] Ear vaccarie seeds were taped onto the auricular heart and subcortex points as the main acupoints and then onto small intestines, sympathetic nerve, kidney, and endocrine auricular points as secondary acupoints. After 6 months of treatment, 18 patients (72%) with angina pectoris improved completely, four patients (16%) showed initial relief but did show subsequent reappearance of symptoms, and three patients (12%) received no benefit from treatment.

One of the primary contributors to cardiac dysfunction is stress and anxiety. The effect of auricular acupressure on perceived anxiety in patients who required ambulance transport to a hospital was examined in a randomized controlled trial by Kober et al.[31] Emergency transport patients were assessed for anxiety by a visual analog scale given at baseline and upon arrival at the hospital. Participants who received auricular acupressure at the relaxation point (n=17) reported significantly less anxiety than patients in a sham control group (n=19).

Hypertension

The most frequent use of auricular acupuncture for a cardiovascular disorder is for the treatment of essential hypertension. At the Beijing International Symposium, several studies examined the role of auriculotherapy for blood pressure disorders.[30] Luo Xingshong examined 124 cases of hypertension treated by pressing *otopoints*, a Chinese term for ear acupoints. Of the 124 cases treated, in 66 cases (53.2%) treatment was notably effective; in 51 cases (41.1%) treatment was effective; and in 7 cases (5.7%) treatment was ineffective. During the treatment, the patients reported no phenomenon of dizziness or tiredness, as distinguished from blood pressure medications. The auricular points were heart, small intestines, liver, spleen, kidney, shen men, endocrine, hypertension point, root of ear vagus, and two points identified as *jiogan* and *jiaowo*. In another 306 cases of hypertension, We Guangwei treated the patients with bloodletting at the ear apex point. Reduction in systolic and diastolic blood pressure was found in 282 cases (92.2%). These changes were most prominent 15 minutes after the ear apex bloodletting.

The effect of auriculotherapy on hypotension was examined by Norie Yoshimoto of Japan. Hypotension was defined as systolic pressure less than 90 mm Hg, and diastolic pressure less than 60 mm Hg, often accompanied by dizziness. Auricular press pellets were applied to four ear points selected from the following list: hypotension point (at the intertragic notch), adrenal gland, heart, occiput, and sympathetic. After 3 weeks to 3 months of treatment, blood pressure was increased, and symptoms of dizziness were reduced in 91 cases (62.7%).

The review by Guan Zunxin reported that Huang Heqing applied electrical stimulation to the auricular heart point of hypertensive patients.[27] Persons with stage I hypertension showed decreased blood pressure within two 30-minute sessions, whereas patients with stage II or stage III hypertension improved after 30 treatments; overall effectiveness rate reached 63.3%. Yu Peng examined the use of auricular plaster therapy for 72 cases of primary hypertension and 31 patients with hypotension. *Plaster therapy* refers to the procedure of taping a small ball or seed to a particular auricular point. The same auricular heart point that led to reduced blood pressure in hypertensive patients yielded increased blood pressure in hypotensive patients. In a controlled trial by Liu Wenyuan, 80 cardiac patients were divided to receive either auricular plaster therapy at the heart point or routine medications, such as nitroglycerin and isosorbide dinitrate. After 30 days, 33 patients (82.5%) in the auriculotherapy group, and only 10 patients (25%) in the medication group showed significant improvement. Sherkovina treated 61 hypertensive patients with needles bilaterally inserted into three to six auricular points and manipulated the sites for 20 to 25 minutes. The systolic pressure decreased by 25 mm Hg, and the diastolic pressure decreased by 5 mm Hg.

Williams et al conducted a randomized controlled trial of patients with borderline diastolic hypertension given electroacupuncture at either acupoints appropriate for treating hypertension or at nonacupuncture points.[32] An evaluator blinded to group assignment found a significantly greater reduction in those patients given true electroacupuncture than in those patients in the sham acupuncture group. In a crossover study, Ballegaard et al investigated the effect of acupuncture on hypertension as opposed to the effects of a placebo pill.[33] The 23 male subjects received 30 minutes of acupuncture or a placebo pill. Both the subjects and the observer monitoring the data were blinded to the treatment being applied. Blood pressure was significantly lower when patients received acupuncture rather than placebo.

Blood pressure changes in patients with systemic hypertension were examined by Haung and Liang.[34] A total of 30 patients received daily treatment by a needle inserted into one of two points on the external ear. The auricular heart acupoint was needled on some days, whereas the auricular stomach acupoint was treated on alternate days. Significant changes were found with the heart acupoint but not with the stomach acupoint. Yu et al studied the effect of auricular acupressure in 291 patients with essential hypertension.[35] Semen vaccarie seeds were attached to the ear acupoints with adhesive plaster and were pressed three times each day. A medication group received one tablet of *fufang jiangya*. Both the auricular acupressure and the medication group showed reductions in blood pressure, particularly for those with only stage I essential hypertension.

Zhou et al studied the efficacy of auricular acupressure in 41 hypertension patients categorized by their TCM symptoms of Type A versus Type B behavior patterns.[36] After three months of treatment, yang-deficient patients showed the greatest improvement in diastolic pressure. Blood pressure changes were found in yin-deficient patients who exhibited Type A behavior and yang deficient patients exhibiting Type B behavior. Chiu et al performed acupuncture in 50 patients with untreated essential hypertension.[37] After 30 minutes of acupuncture, systolic pressure decreased from 169 to 151 mm Hg, diastolic pressure decreased from 107 to 96 mm Hg, and heart rate decreased from 77 to 72 bpm. No significant changes were found in vasopressin or cortisol concentrations. Li et al[38] studied electroacupuncture at ST 36 in 13 dogs whose blood pressure was elevated by intravenous infusion of norepinephrine. Significant reductions in blood pressure by electroacupuncture were observed for all 13 dogs, and this hypotensive effect from electroacupuncture was reversed by the opiate antagonist naloxone.

CLINICAL PROCEDURES

A wide variety of clinical texts have provided specific guidelines for using auricular acupuncture points for the treatment of cardiovascular disorders.[1-3,9,19,20,39-41] Clinical application of the research findings in the field of auricular acupuncture are amazingly uncomplicated, once a practitioner is open to the rather unconventional concept that specific points on the auricle can affect the heart and the cardiovascular system. Sometimes, simple observation of the inferior concha region of the external ear can reveal an underlying disorder. In one of my earliest experiences with auricular diagnosis, I observed white, flaky skin covering the heart point in the inferior concha of a colleague. He also had a distinctive, diagonal, earlobe crease. Upon suggestion that he might consult his family physician for a medical evaluation, he made an appointment with his physician that next week. During that visit he was immediately referred for cardiac bypass surgery. The high degree of skin flakiness had suggested that his coronary condition was quite severe and conventional diagnostic tests confirmed that impression. At other times, both the Chinese heart point found in the inferior concha and the European heart point located on the antihelix chart can appear as a red spot or as rough skin protrusion.

More precise determination of a reactive heart point can be obtained by the use of an electrodermal point locator, as is shown in Figure 16-4. The surface of the external ear must first be cleaned with alcohol and allowed to dry. This procedure allows the removal of skin oils, ear wax, facial make-up, and hair sprays from the skin. Such substances will raise the electrodermal resistance of the auricle and interfere with the ability to correctly detect auricular reflex points that are electrically conductive because of pathology in the corresponding organ. Commercially available point locators are usually spring-loaded to maintain constant pressure on the skin. They can be either monopolar, with only one electrical lead touching the skin of the ear, or bipolar, with a central lead surrounded by a cylindrical tube. Bipolar leads provide more precise differential amplification of the reactive ear acupoint. A light or a sound indicates to the practitioner when an electrically conductive point has been found. Although detection of such ear points can lead to diagnosis of a previously unknown disorder, electrical point finders often are used to determine the most appropriate auricular loci to treat because of their reduced skin resistance.

The most common form of treating auricular acupuncture points has been the insertion of acupuncture needles. The appropriate ear points are first

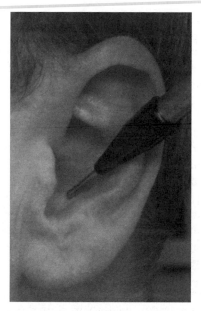

Fig 16-4. Photograph of a electrical point locator applied to the external ear.

determined with an electrical point finder and then the probe is pressed more firmly into the skin. This technique leaves a small indentation in the skin that lasts for approximately 1 minute. During this brief time, a needle can be inserted into the auricle and is usually left in place for 20 minutes. Short, half-inch needles are inserted to a shallow depth into the external ear as they are less likely to fall out than would longer needles. Needles can be inserted into both locations for the Chinese heart points on the auricle, at the European locations for the heart on the antihelix, and hypertension acupoints on the posterior sides of the auricle. Electroacupuncture is applied by first attaching microgator clips to needles inserted into at least two ear points. The electrode leads are then connected to a commercially available electrical stimulator. The frequency of stimulation is often set to a series of 2-Hz pulses alternated with a series of 100 Hz pulses. Intensity of stimulation is gradually increased until the patient can feel a slight tingliness in the ear, and then the amount of current is reduced to sub-threshold levels.

Noninvasive electrical stimulation of auricular acupuncture points is provided by transcutaneous electrical stimulation. After cleaning the auricle with alcohol and allowing it to dry, an electrical probe is slid over the skin of the external ear. When a point of low skin resistance is detected, the practitioner presses a button and immediately stimulates the reactive ear point for 10 to 30 seconds. The frequency is usually set at 5 Hz or 10 Hz and the intensity at 20 to 80 microamps. After one auricular point has been detected and stimulated, the practitioner continues to search for reactive points in other areas of the ear. The same ear points that are used for needle acupuncture or electroacupuncture are also used for transcutaneous electrical stimulation. These ear points include the

Chinese heart points in the inferior concha and on the superior tragus and the European heart points on the anterior and posterior antihelix body. The practitioner could also stimulate the hypertension points found in the superior triangular fossa and the inferior tragus. After treating ear points specifically related to the heart, auricular master points—such as shen men, point zero, sympathetic, and endocrine points—are then stimulated. In Oriental medicine, the small intestines meridian is the yang channel which corresponds to the heart meridian, thus the auricular small intestines point is also included in auriculotherapy treatments of coronary disorders. Other supplemental ear points for coronary disorders and hypertension include the adrenal gland, occiput, kidney, liver, and spleen.

For maintenance of auriculotherapy treatment actions in the time period between treatment sessions, and sometimes as the primary treatment, Chinese acupuncturists have developed the application of small balls or seeds taped onto the auricle. Called *auricular plaster therapy* or *otopoint acupressure*, reactive ear points are first determined with a point finder and then forceps are used to precisely place a small pellet over a specific auricular loci. These pellets are held in place by an adhesive tape that is pressed onto the auricle, as shown in Figure 16-5. Patients are often encouraged to press on these ear pellets several times a day to continue the stimulation. For more intense stimulation, press needles are inserted into reactive ear points rather than ear pellets. Application of acupuncture needles, electrical stimulation, and press pellets have all been shown to alleviate coronary artery disorders and hypertension.

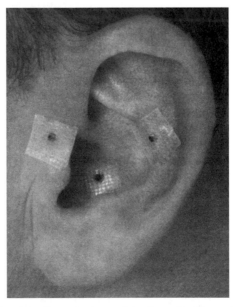

Fig 16-5. Ear seeds placed on the coronary points, hypertension points, master points, and supplemental points.

TRAINING AND CERTIFICATION

Auricular acupuncture is taught in the United States at most colleges of acupuncture and Oriental medicine as either a course on ear acupuncture or as part of a course on microsystems. Most of these courses only provide information on the location of Chinese ear acupuncture points, but there is usually extensive practical training on correct needle techniques and the use of ear pellets. The Council of Colleges of Acupuncture and Oriental Medicine (CCAOM) can be reached at its website www.accaom.org for a list of acupuncture colleges in different regions of the country. A UCLA extension course for physicians provides postgraduate training in medical acupuncture that includes teaching of both the Chinese and European systems of auricular acupuncture. Further information about this course can be obtained at the American Academy of Medical Acupuncture's (AAMA) internet site, www.medicalacupuncture.org. Training in both the Chinese and European auricular systems is provided by the Auriculotherapy Certification Institute (ACI), which also offers certificates in auriculotherapy and auricular acupuncture. The ACI website address is www.auriculotherapy.org. Each of these organizations can provide professional training to healthcare professionals who seek to expand their knowledge of auricular acupuncture.

CONCLUSION

Auriculotherapy is based upon the principle that specific treat areas of the external ear can be used to alleviate pathology in correspondent areas of the body. Clinical application of this procedure derives from both the principles of TCM and from the pioneering work of Dr. Paul Nogier. Specific changes in the morphology, tenderness, and electrical resistance of the skin over the external ear have revealed particular regions related to cardiovascular disorders. Insertion of needles, electrical stimulation, and taping of ear pellets have all been found to alleviate coronary disorders and hypertension, thus providing a simple yet effective treatment for relieving such conditions. Auriculotherapy can be easily integrated with other alternative medicine and conventional medical procedures for assisting patients suffering from cardiovascular disorders.

REFERENCES

1. Huang HL: Ear acupuncture, New York, 1974, Rodale Press.
2. Huang LC: Auriculotherapy: diagnosis and treatment, Bellaire, TX, 1996, Longevity Press.
3. Nogier P: Treatise of auriculotherapy, Moulins-les Metz, France, 1972, Maisonneuve.
4. Chen G, Lu P: History of auricular acupuncture in China, Presentation at International Consensus Conference on Acupuncture, Auriculotherapy, and Auricular Medicine, Las Vegas, August 14, 1999, 7-9.

5. Oleson T, Kroening R: A comparison of Chinese and Nogier auricular acupuncture points, Am J Acupunct 11:205-223, 1983.

6. World Health Organization: A standard international acupuncture nomenclature: memorandum from a WHO meeting, 68:165-169, 1990.

7. Akerele O: WHO and the development of acupuncture nomenclature: overcoming a tower of Babel, Am J Chin Med 1:89-94, 1991.

8. Oleson T: Origins of auriculotherapy in Asia and Europe, Presentation at International Consensus Conference on Acupuncture, Auriculotherapy, and Auricular Medicine, Las Vegas, August 14, 1999, 1-6.

9. Oleson T: Auriculotherapy manual: Chinese and Western systems of ear acupuncture, ed 3, London, 2003, Churchill Livingstone.

10. Dale R: The micro-acupuncture system, Am J Acupunct 4:7-24, 1976.

11. Oleson T: The role of auricular acupuncture in neurologic disorders. In Weintraub W, editor: Alternative and complementary treatment in neurologic illness, Philadelphia, 2001, Churchill Livingstone, 221-233.

12. Dale R: Acupuncture meridians and the homunculus principle, Am J Acupunct 19:73-75, 1991.

13. Shiraishi T, Onoe M, Kojima T, Sameshima Y, Kageyama T: Effects of auricular stimulation on feeding-related hypothalamic neuronal activity in normal and obese rats, Brain Res Bull 36:141-148, 1995.

14. Alimi D, Geissmann A, Gardeur D: Auricular acupuncture stimulation measured on functional magnetic resonance imaging, Med Acupunct 13:18-21, 2002.

15. Sjolund B, Terenius L, Eriksson M: Increased cerebrospinal fluid levels of endorphins after electroacupuncture, Act Physiol Scand 100:382-384, 1977.

16. Clement-Jones V, Mc Loughlin L, Lowery P et al: Acupuncture in heroin addicts: changes in met-enkephalin and beta-endorphin in blood and cerebrospinal fluid, Lancet 2:380-383, 1979.

17. Pert A, Dionne R, Ng L et al: Alterations in rat central nervous system endorphins following transauricular electroacupuncture, Brain Res 224:83-93, 1981.

18. Oleson T: Differential application of auricular acupuncture for myofascial, autonomic, and neuropathic pain, Med Acupunct 9:23-28, 1998.

19. Nogier P: From auriculotherapy to auriculomedicine, Moulins-les-Metz, France, 1983, Maisonneuve.

20. Wexu M: The ear gateway to balancing the body: a modern guide to ear acupuncture, New York, 1975, ASI Publishers.

21. Bergsmann O, Hart A: Differences in electrical skin conductivity between acupuncture points and adjacent skin areas, Am J Acupunct 1:27-32, 1973.

22. Romoli M, Vettoni F: Alterations in the skin of the auricle and correlation with chronic disease, Minerva Med 73:725-730, 1982.

23. Oleson T, Kroening R, Bresler D: An experimental evaluation of auricular diagnosis: the somatotopic mapping of musculoskeletal pain at ear acupuncture points, Pain 8:217-229, 1980.

24. Saku K, Mukaino Y, Ying H, Arakwa K: Characteristics of reactive electropermeable points on the auricles of coronary heart disease patients, Clin Cardiol 16:415-419, 1993.

25. Lichstein E, Chaddie K, Naik D, Gupta P: Diagonal earlobe crease: prevalence and implications as a coronary risk factor, New Engl J Med 290:615-616, 1974.

26. Mehta J, Homby R: Diagonal earlobe crease as a coronary risk factor, New Engl J Med 291:260, 1974.

27. Guan Z: Review on the experimental research on auricular points and their diagnostic and therapeutic mechanism. Intl J Clin Acupunct 12(3): 265-275, 2001.

28. Romoli M, Tordini G, Giommi A: Diagonal ear-lobe crease: possible significance as cardio-vascular factor and its relationship to ear-acupuncture. Acupunct Electother Res 14(2):149-154, 1989.

29. Huang L: Auricular Diagnosis. Bellaire, TX, Longevity Press, 1999.

30. Chen GS: On auricular acupuncture. Second International Symposium on Auricular Medicine. Beijing, China, October 21, 1995:37–48.

31. Kober A, Scheck T, Schubert B, et al: Auricular acupressure as a treatment for anxiety in prehospital transport settings. Anesthesiology 98(6):1328-1332, 2003.

32. Williams T, Mueller K, Cornwall MW: Effect of acupuncture-point stimulation on diastolic blood pressure in hypertensive subjects: a preliminary study. Physical Therapy 7(7):523-529, 1991.

33. Ballegaard S, Muteki T, Harada H, et al: Modulatory effect of acupuncture on the cardiovascular system: a cross-over study, Acupunct Electother Res 18:103-115, 1993.

34. Haung H, Liang S: Acupuncture at otopoint heart for treatment of vascular hypertension, J Tradit Chin Med 12(2):133-136, 1992.

35. Yu P, Li F, Wei X, Wu R, Fu C: Treatment of essential hypertension with auriculoacupressure, J Tradit Chin Med 11(1):17-21, 1991.

36. Zhou R, Zhang Y, Lu Y: Hypotensive effect of ototherapy in relation to sympathetic and dispositional types of patients, J Tradit Chin Med 12(2):124-128, 1992.

37. Chiu YJ, Chi A, Reid IA: Cardiovascular and endocrine effects of acupuncture in hypertensive patients, Clin and Exp Hypertension 19(7):1047-1063, 1992.

38. Li P, Sun F, Zhang A: The effect of acupuncture on blood pressure: the interrelation of sympathetic activity and endogenous opiods, Acupunct Electother Res 8:45-56, 1983.

39. Kropej H: The fundamentals of ear acupuncture, Heidelberg, 1984, Haug.

40. Rubach A: Principles of ear acupuncture: microsystem of the auricle, Stuttgart, 2001, Thieme.

41. Strittmatter B: Ear acupuncture, Stuttgart, 2003, Thieme.

CHAPTER 17

Chelation Therapy

William H. Frishman, MD
Andrew I. Wolff, MD

C helation therapy is a process of using specific molecules (chelating agents) to form complexes that inactivate heavy metals (metal ions), which can then be safely excreted in the urine. The most popular application of this therapy has been in heavy-metal toxicity, in which the binding of chelating agents to these metals forms soluble, inactive complexes that are eliminated via the urine.[1-3] This use of chelation therapy is a well established and accepted treatment approach.

However, a more intriguing and controversial aspect of chelation therapy lies in its use in the treatment of human diseases, especially atherosclerotic diseases.[4-7] The management of cardiovascular disease with this therapy involves the multiple administrations of intravenous ethylenediaminetetraacetic acid (EDTA) supplemented with some "nutrients" (vitamins C, B complex, B_6, heparin, and magnesium sulfate)[8-10] and was initiated in the early to middle 1950s, when a group from Michigan first reported on its use in the treatment of atherosclerotic cardiovascular diseases.[4,8] This initial report generated tremendous controversy regarding the benefits of chelation therapy that have continued to this day. The focus of the arguments for and against chelation therapy have related to efficacy, safety, and mechanisms of benefit of this treatment.[4,8,9,11-15] Despite the ongoing controversies, estimates suggest that more than 800,000 patient visits per year in the United States are dedicated to chelation therapy.[16]

In chelation a metal ion is bound by a complex organic molecule with affinity for that metal ion; the ion serves as the chelating agent, or ligand. Usually the chelating agent has a heterocyclic ring structure, in which the metal ion is bound by two or more ions within the complex molecule.[1,17]

The following summarizes some of the arguments for and against the use of chelation therapy with EDTA and deferoxamine (iron chelation) in the treatment of cardiovascular diseases and presents clinical experiences in which its use has been applied or advocated.

EDTA

EDTA is a known chelating agent that can bind divalent ions such as calcium. EDTA is not specific for this metal because it can also bind other divalent and trivalent cations as well as trace elements such as zinc, copper, lead, and iron, transporting them in a bound form out of the body via urine.[1,18,19] However, EDTA's ability to displace and immobilize calcium ions by chelation has prompted its use in atherosclerotic vascular diseases, as is discussed below. Proponents of chelation therapy for the treatment of cardiovascular diseases (especially atherosclerosis-mediated diseases) agree that vascular injury and smooth-muscle cell proliferation initiate the atherosclerotic cascade and that proteins, carbohydrates, and lipids (cholesterol esters) are major components of atherosclerotic plaques. However, they also believe that other critical factors exist in this pathogenesis, including mineral metabolism—specifically calcium deposition. Calcium is very highly integrated with cholesterol in atheromatous lesions.[4,8,18,20]

Evidence supporting the importance of calcium deposition in atherosclerotic disease served as the theoretical background for using chelation therapy (EDTA) to decalcify complex atherosclerotic plaque in blood vessels (Box 17-1). This same evidence would allow EDTA to serve as a therapeutic approach in patients with angina pectoris, intermittent claudication, and other atherosclerosis-mediated cardiovascular diseases.[4,8,19]

Another rationale for EDTA chelation therapy in cardiovascular diseases is that it can decrease platelet aggregability by either irreversibly altering the platelet calcium ratio or by altering a critical pathway in platelet aggregation that requires increased calcium (e.g., the platelet glycoprotein [GP] IIb/IIIa), and this inhibition of aggregation is obviously important in reducing complications from atherosclerotic disease.[21-23]

Free-radical reduction with EDTA is another proposed mechanism that is believed to be important for the treatment of cardiovascular diseases. EDTA

Box **17-1** **Theoretical Benefits of Using EDTA Chelation Therapy in Coronary Artery Disease**

1. Decalcification of complex atherosclerotic plaques
2. Decreased platelet aggregability
3. Reduction in oxygen-derived free radicals
4. Lowering of serum iron
5. Lowering of serum cholesterol

reduces iron and copper levels from cell membranes. These metals are important catalysts in the lipid peroxidation of long-chain unsaturated fatty acids and oxidation of LDL, which generate free radicals that disrupt membrane architecture and consequently promote cellular injury and atherosclerosis.[24,25] Furthermore, some investigators have reported that chelation therapy, by removing calcium, results in a demonstrable increase in vascular dilation, a decrease in peripheral resistance, and an increase in blood flow.[26] EDTA also stimulates parathormone release, which, in turn, might mobilize calcium from the plaques and retard progressive calcification.[27] EDTA may also have an indirect effect by lowering serum iron levels and serum cholesterol.[28,29]

Arguments made against these proposed beneficial actions of EDTA and its use in the management of heart disease include the contention by critics that although calcium is seen in atherosclerotic plaques, its role in stabilizing the plaque may not be significant enough to warrant it being the target of therapy for heart disease.[13-15] For instance, some contend that because most stabilized atherosclerotic lesions contain cholesterol and its esters, collagen, lipoproteins, proteoglycans, and elastic fibers as primary components, with calcification occurring only as the final step in chronic atherosclerosis, agents that mobilize serum calcium (like EDTA) may not be effective in altering the initiation or progression of atherosclerotic disease.

CLINICAL EXPERIENCES WITH EDTA

Peripheral Vascular Disease

Several studies have used intravenous EDTA infusions to treat patients with peripheral vascular disease (PVD) and intermittent claudication. Most of the reports have been either retrospective experiences or individual case studies that have described how EDTA infusions were able to relieve or improve the symptoms of PVD.[18,30-32] In one of these studies, Casdorph and Farr described how four patients with severe PVD and facing possible amputation of their lower extremities were successfully treated with intravenous and topical antibiotics, debridement, hyperbaric oxygen, and multiple EDTA infusions.[32] Only one patient ended up with amputation of three toes. The investigators believe that EDTA was the main therapeutic ingredient of the treatment regimen.

In a large retrospective study, Olszewer and Carter evaluated 2870 patients with symptomatic vascular disease who received EDTA and found that these subjects' clinical symptoms significantly improved.[7] The drawback of the study was the lack of controls and its retrospective design. However, this same group then set out to conduct a controlled, double-blind study of sodium/magnesium EDTA in PVD. They started with 10 male patients with known PVD from diabetes or atherosclerosis. All patients had intermittent claudication but no rest pain or gangrene. The parameters they used to follow the effects of EDTA included peripheral vascular signs (skin disturbances, temperature, hair changes, etc.), kidney function, blood pressure, and blood pressure index that compared the ankle systolic blood pressure to the arm systolic blood pressure, as well as time exercising on a treadmill and bicycle stress tests. The 10 patients were randomly and equally divided into two groups, receiving either ampules of 10 mL of EDTA or distilled water. Both treatment groups also received the usual administered nutritional additives to the intravenous solution, which included vitamin C, B complex, B_6, heparin, and magnesium sulfate. Disodium EDTA was used in a dose of 1.5 g for each infusion. After 10 treatments (chelation and placebo), the results indicated that some patients were improving significantly and that others were not. The investigators then broke the study code and realized that the experimental group (those receiving EDTA infusions) showed significant improvement, whereas the placebo group did not. The study was then switched to a single-blind, and all patients received EDTA treatment. After this switch, the placebo group improvement was comparable to the EDTA-treated group, as measured by the distance walked and the arm-ankle BP index. This study was significant in supporting earlier descriptive and less objective studies that showed basically the same results.

In contrast, a large, double-blind multicenter study of 153 patients with PVD, half of whom received placebo or EDTA, found no differences in symptomatic relief between control and treatment groups.[33] The same investigators also studied 30 patients on EDTA and followed their treatment with angiograms and transcutaneous oxygen-tension measurements and reported no positive benefits with chelation therapy.[34] In addition, the results of a single-center, double-blind, randomized, controlled trial[12] failed to show any benefit from chelation therapy in a group of patients with intermittent claudication. In this study, 32 patients were randomized into treatment and control groups. The investigators used subjective measurements of patient improvement combined with the objective measurements of walking distance and ankle/brachial pulse indices.

Coronary Artery Disease

The first clinical use of chelation therapy for cardiovascular disease was for treatment of angina pectoris secondary to coronary artery disease (CAD).[8] The rationale for the study was based on the observation that coronary artery atheromas (the pathologic basis for angina) are formed by calcium-cholesterol integration in a matrix that includes proteoglycans and lipoproteins.

EDTA was used because of its known ability to bind and remove calcium.[4,8,18] In this first study, a total of 20 patients with established angina pectoris were treated with a solution of 5 g disodium EDTA in 500 mL of 5% glucose or normal saline given intravenously.[8] Each treatment solution was infused for 2.5 to 4 hours in a regimen of 5 g/d times 5 days a week. Each patient received 35 infusions. Nineteen of the 20 patients treated with these infusions were relieved of their symptoms. Furthermore, the ECG abnormalities associated with old myocardial infarcts present in some patients before EDTA were normalized after treatment.

Kitchell et al treated 38 patients with severe angina for 1 to 2 months with repeated infusions of EDTA.[35] Patient progress was based on individual perception of improvement and measured exercise tolerance. The investigators reported significant symptomatic relief in approximately 75% of the patients, and 40% showed evidence of ECG improvement between 6 and 12 of beginning

EDTA therapy. However, by 18 months, 32% of the patients had died from their disease, and only approximately 40% still maintained their achieved benefit from EDTA treatment. These same investigators then attempted a placebo-controlled study of EDTA in nine relatively sick angina patients and found that only two of these patients showed consistent improvement from the chelation treatment. The investigators concluded that EDTA had no significant benefit in the treatment of CAD.[35]

In another group of 18 patients with angina pectoris associated with CAD, EDTA infusions improved clinical symptoms.[35] The patient response to treatment was assessed by documenting clinical symptoms and measuring left ventricular (LV) ejection fraction via cardiac nuclear scintigraphy with technetium-99m before and after EDTA treatment. Twenty infusions of EDTA in 3-gram doses led to complete clinical improvement and complete cessation of the anginal pain in all but two patients. There was also a significant (6%) improvement in LV ejection fraction.

In 1993, Hancke and Flytlie, in a retrospective study of 470 patients, reported on the dramatic benefit obtained with EDTA treatment on patients previously scheduled to undergo coronary artery bypass for their CAD.[36] Of 92 patients referred for surgical management of their diseases, only 10 required surgical intervention after EDTA chelation therapy. This report also described a series of CAD patients whose abnormal exercise ECG ST segments normalized after EDTA treatment. Furthermore, the authors went on to imply that EDTA chelation therapy was safe because after 6 years of follow-up, no serious side effects were observed. The findings of Van der Schaar showed that patients with various atherosclerotic vascular diseases receiving EDTA had better exercise tolerance than control patients, thus suggesting a benefit from chelation therapy.[37]

One case report described a patient with angina secondary to atherosclerosis of the right coronary artery in whom EDTA therapy provided both symptomatic relief and a normalized treadmill ECG stress test after 5 months of therapy. However, the patient's symptoms later worsened and required angioplasty. These investigators believed that EDTA was not effective in dissolving the blockade because angiography of the arteries before and after angioplasty showed significant occlusion. They concluded that EDTA chelation therapy is not beneficial.[14]

Other Cardiovascular Diseases

In 1961, Soffer and colleagues performed an uncontrolled study that looked at the effects of EDTA or chelation therapy in patients with arrhythmia.[38] In that study, the investigators administered EDTA infusions to 58 patients with different dysrhythmias for approximately 28 months. They found that chelation therapy abolished ventricular premature contractions in 12 of 18 patients, increased the ventricular rate in all patients with complete heart block, and improved arteriovenous (AV) conduction in 6 of 12 patients. Furthermore, they found that EDTA treatment slowed the ectopic atrial rate in patients with atrial tachycardia. In 9 of 11 patients with atrial fibrillation who were receiving digitalis, the addition of EDTA further slowed the ventricular rate. The therapeutic principle behind the effect of EDTA on digitalis toxicity was based on the effective binding of calcium in serum, because calcium is known to affect cell membrane permeability, especially in the presence of digitalis. The conclusion at that time was that EDTA could abolish ectopic ventricular beats, terminate ventricular tachycardia, and improve AV nodal conduction in patients with heart block.[38] However, additional studies and the advent of better and more effective medications for dysrhythmias and digitalis toxicity ultimately countered these findings.[14] Twenty-three years after his initial report, Soffer, one of the early chelation proponents, wrote an editorial that condemned the use of this treatment for cardiovascular disease for lack of scientific proof of its efficacy.[39]

CLINICAL RECOMMENDATIONS

The major questions concerning EDTA chelation revolve around its efficacy and safety. The perception is that no generally accepted scientific evidence from well conducted studies justifies its universal use, despite some studies that show its efficacy. A meta-analysis found that evidence supported the use of EDTA in the treatment of cardiovascular diseases.[40] However, most of the studies included in the analysis were not controlled. Not a single reputable cardiovascular society has endorsed chelation therapy for the treatment of cardiovascular disease, including the recent ACC/AHA guidelines update for the management of patients with stable angina pectoris.[41]

Nonetheless, how safe is chelation therapy? The concerns regarding the safety of EDTA treatment have been addressed by the proponents of this therapy with the publication of guidelines for its safe use.[10] However, it is well known that EDTA is not a benign drug when high doses are administered over a short period of time. Some of the adverse effects that have been reported with high doses of EDTA include nephrotoxicity; bone marrow depression; hypocalcemic tetany; allergic reactions; insulin shock; hypotension; thromboemboli; ECG changes, including cardiac arrhythmias; and prolongation of the prothrombin time.[14,17,42,43]

It seems that the general acceptance of EDTA chelation therapy in the treatment of cardiovascular diseases certainly requires more mainstream basic science studies and better-designed clinical research studies to establish its efficacy and safety. Recently, the results of the Canadian Program to Assess Alternative Treatment Strategies to Achieve Cardiac Health (PATCH) trial showed no benefit with chelation therapy in patients with CAD regarding exercise-tolerance, quality of life measurements, and indices of endothelial function.[44-46]

In addition, a large definitive, placebo-controlled, multicenter RCT trial has been initiated by the NIH to assess EDTA with regard to clinical symptoms, clinical outcomes, healthcare use, and plasma markers of oxidative stress and endothelial activation.[47] The study population will comprise 2372 patients aged 50 or older who have had a myocardial infarction more than 6 months before enrolling. Each participant will be randomized to receive either the standard chelation solution or a placebo. Both groups will additionally be randomized to receive high-dose or low-dose vitamin/mineral supplements. The study will consist of 40 infusions: 30 weekly infusions followed by 10 bimonthly infusions. Each participant will be followed throughout the 28-month course with the primary endpoint being a composite of all-cause mortality, myocardial infarction, stroke, hospitalization for angina, and hospitalization for congestive heart failure. The study will secondarily examine quality of life and cost effectiveness among other factors. The trial is currently in the recruitment phase.[48,49]

The use of ultrafast CT scan to evaluate the efficacy of EDTA on coronary artery calcification with clinical correlations has been suggested as a means to evaluate treatment efficacy in future chelation trials. As previously stated, no reputable cardiovascular society has endorsed EDTA chelation therapy for the treatment of cardiovascular disease, including the 2002 American College of Cardiology/American Heart Association guidelines update for the treatment of chronic stable angina.[41] Chelation therapy with EDTA should therefore remain a last resort choice for cardiovascular disease treatment and certainly should not replace accepted medical and surgical therapies.[50-52]

DEFEROXAMINE AND DEFERIPRONE

The role of iron in the pathogenesis of atherosclerosis, particularly CAD, has generated much interest. Several epidemiologic studies have found an association between markers of increased iron stores and increased risk of CAD and acute coronary events.[53-55] Salonen et al followed 1931 randomly selected men with no clinical evidence of CAD at the time of inclusion in a 5-year observational study.[53] They found that men with serum ferritin 200 μg/L had a 2.2-fold (95% CI, 1.2 to 4.0; p <.01) risk factor-adjusted risk for acute myocardial infarction in comparison to men with a lower serum ferritin. The dietary intake of iron also showed a significant and direct correlation with the incidence of acute coronary events. The adverse effects of iron seem to be independent of or potentiated by other risk factors such as hypercholesterolemia. Morrison et al also found an increased risk of fatal myocardial infarction in male as well as female patients with increased serum iron levels.[54]

Studies have also shown an increased risk of acute myocardial infarction in carriers of the hemochromatosis gene Cys 282 Tyr mutation.[56] These epidemiologic observations are not surprising, considering that iron is an important element in cellular metabolism and growth. Iron is found in many enzymes and proteins involved in electron shuttling and oxygen binding and transport. Besides its normal physiologic activity, iron has an important role in the generation of oxygen free radicals, specifically the highly reactive hydroxyl radical generated by the superoxide driven Haber-Weiss reaction.[57] Iron can also directly activate platelets.[58] Its activation is mediated by hydroxyl radical formation and involves pyruvate kinase activity. A recent clinical study demonstrated an association between increased iron stores and impaired endothelial function in patients with hereditary hemochromatosis.[59]

However, a theoretical link associating iron and atherosclerosis is still not clear. A Canadian study failed to show any relation between serum ferritin levels and angiographically confirmed CAD.[60] Another study from Iceland followed men and women for up to 8.5 years and found no association between risk of myocardial infarction and elevated serum ferritin levels.[61] However, a study from Iran did show an association of increased ferritin levels with premature coronary artery stenosis in men only.[55]

Deferoxamine is the most widely used iron chelator and has been used experimentally in non–iron overload conditions to interfere with free-radical production during myocardial reperfusion after an ischemic injury and in other cardiovascular conditions.[62] Besides its role as an iron chelator and antioxidant, some authors suggest that deferoxamine might have an effect on vascular smooth-muscle proliferation.[63]

CLINICAL USE

In animal studies and in small patient trials, deferoxamine preserved myocardial function and energy metabolism after postischemic reperfusion. From these studies, there is evidence of reduced oxygen free radical generation as a possible mechanism of benefit.[64-66] However, not all studies have shown benefit in protecting against myocardial ischemia-reperfusion injury.[67]

One reported case described a patient with severe iron overload cardiomyopathy who was treated successfully with chelation therapy.[68] In addition, chelation therapy with oral deferiprone can be used to improve heart function (LV ejection fraction) in patients with thalassemia major who are transfusion-dependent.[69]

Deferoxamine has also been tried as a treatment to prevent or limit cardiotoxicity associated with anthracycline chemotherapy. One mechanism proposed for anthracycline cardiomyopathy is the generation of oxygen free radicals by anthracycline-iron-complexes. Deferoxamine and other iron chelators appear to prevent anthracycline cardiotoxicity while preserving the tumoricidal effects of chemotherapy.[64,70]

CLINICAL RECOMMENDATION

As with EDTA, the experience with deferoxamine in prevention and treatment of cardiovascular disease needs to be established with more substantial clinical trials before it can be recommended. Deferoxamine is also associated with substantial toxicity involving multiple organ systems.[62]

CONCLUSION

Although a theoretical basis exists for the use of various chelation therapies for the prevention and treatment of cardiovascular disease, its therapeutic use still remains investigational until more definitive clinical studies demonstrate whether the treatment is efficacious and safe.

REFERENCES

1. Cranton EM, editor: A textbook on EDTA chelation therapy, J Adv Med 2:1-416, 1989.
2. Diagnostic and therapeutic technology assessment: chelation therapy, JAMA 250:672 1983.
3. Elihu N, Anandasabapathy S, Frishman WH: Chelation therapy in cardiovascular disease: ethylenediaminetetraacetic acid and deferoxamine, J Clin Pharmacol 38:101-105, 1998.
4. Clarke NE, Clarke CN, Mosher RF: The "in vivo" dissolution of metastatic calcium: an approach to atherosclerosis, Am J Med Sci 229:142, 1955.
5. Blumer W, Cranton EM: Ninety percent reduction in cancer mortality after chelation therapy with EDTA, J Adv Med 2:183-187, 1989.
6. Olszewer E, Carter JC: EDTA chelation therapy in chronic degenerative disease, Med Hypotheses 27:41-49, 1988.
7. Olszewer E, Carter JP: EDTA chelation therapy a retrospective study of 2870 patients, J Adv Med 2:197-211, 1989.
8. Clarke NE, Clarke C, Mosher R: Treatment of angina pectoris with disodium ethylene tetraacetic acid, Am J Med Sci 232:654-666, 1956.
9. Morgan K: Myocardial ischemia treated with nutrients and intravenous EDTA chelation: report of two cases, J Adv Med 4:47-56, 1991.
10. Cranton EM: Protocol of the American College of Advancement in Medicine for the Safe and Effective Administration of EDTA Chelation Therapy, Laguna Hills, CA, 1989, American College of Advancement in Medicine.
11. Godfrey ME: EDTA chelation as a treatment of arteriosclerosis, NZ Med J 103:162-163, 1990.
12. van-Rij AM, Solomon C, Parker SG, Hopkins WG: Chelation therapy for intermittent claudication: a double-blind, randomized, controlled trial, Circulation 90:1194-1199, 1994.
13. Soffer A: Chelation therapy for atherosclerosis, JAMA 233:1206-1207, 1975.
14. Wirebaugh SR, Geraets DR: Apparent failure of edetic acid chelation therapy for treatment of coronary atherosclerosis, DICP 24:22-25, 1990.
15. Rathmann KL, Golithly LK: Chelation therapy of atherosclerosis, Drug Intell Clin Pharm 8:1000-1003, 1984.
16. Eisenberg et al: Trends in alternative medicine use in the United States, 1990–1997: results of a follow-up national survey, JAMA 280: 1569-1575, 1998.
17. Magee P: Chelation treatment for atherosclerosis, Med J Aust 142: 514-515, 1985.
18. Boyle AJ, Clarke NE, Mosher RE, McCann DS: Chelation therapy in circulatory and sclerosing diseases, Fed Proc 29:243-251, 1961.
19. Olszewer E, Sabbag FC, Carter JA: A pilot double-blind study of sodium-magnesium EDTA in peripheral vascular disease, J Natl Med Assoc 82:173-177, 1990.

20. Ross R: The pathogenesis of atherosclerosis: an update, N Engl J Med 314:488-500, 1986.
21. Peerscke EL, Grant RA, Zucker MB: Decreased association of 45 calcium with platelets unable to aggregate due to thrombasthenia or prolonged calcium deprivation, Br J Haematol 46:247-256, 1980.
22. Kindness G, Frackelton JP: Effect of ethylene diamine tetraacetic acid (EDTA) on platelet aggregation in human blood, J Adv Med 2:519-530, 1989.
23. Fitzgerald LA, Phillips DR: Calcium regulation of the platelet membrane glycoprotein IIb/IIIa complex, J Biol Chem 260:11366-11374, 1985.
24. Cranton EM, Frackelton JP: Free radical pathology in age-associated diseases: treatment with EDTA chelation, nutrition and antioxidants, J Hol Med 6:6-37, 1984.
25. Deucher DP: EDTA chelation: an antioxidant strategy, J Adv Med 1:182-190, 1988.
26. Walker M, Gordon G: The chelation answer. How to prevent hardening of the arteries and rejuvenate your cardiovascular system, New York, 1982, M Evans.
27. Mallette LE, Hollis BW, Dunn K et al: Ten weeks of intermittent hypocalcemic stimulation does not produce functional parathyroid hyperplasia, Am J Med Sci 302(3):138-141, 1991.
28. Perry HM, Schroeder HA: Depression of cholesterol levels in human plasma following ethylenediamine tetraacetate and hydralazine, J Chron Dis 2:520-533, 1995.
29. Rudolph CJ, McDonagh EW, Barber RK: Effect of EDTA chelation on serum iron, J Adv Med 4:39-45, 1991.
30. Lamar CP: Chelation therapy of occlusive arteriosclerosis in diabetic patients, Angiology 15:379-395, 1964.
31. Lamar CP: Chelation endarterectomy for occlusive atherosclerosis, J Am Geriatr Soc 14:272-294, 1966.
32. Casdorph HR, Farr CH: EDTA chelation therapy, III: treatment of peripheral arterial occlusion, an alternative to amputation, J Hol Med 5:3, 1983.
33. Guldager B, Jelnes R, Jorgensen SJ et al: EDTA treatment of intermittent claudication: a double-blind, placebo-controlled study, J Intern Med 231:261-267, 1992.
34. Sloth-Nielsen J, Guldager B, Mouitzen C et al: Arteriographic findings in EDTA chelation therapy on peripheral arteriosclerosis, Am J Surg 162:122-125, 1991.
35. Kitchell JR, Palmon F Jr, Aytan N, Meltzer LE: The treatment of coronary artery disease with disodium EDTA: a reappraisal, Am J Cardiol 11:501, 1963.
36. Hancke C, Flytlie K: Benefits of chelation therapy in atherosclerosis: a retrospective study of 470 patients, J Adv Med 6:161, 1993.
37. Van der Schaar P: Exercise tolerance in chelation therapy, J Adv Med 2:563, 1989.

38. Soffer A, Toribara T, Sayman A: Myocardial responses to chelation, Br Heart J 23:690-694, 1961.

39. Soffer A: Chelation clinics: an abuse of the physician's freedom of choice, Arch Intern Med 144:1741-1742, 1984.

40. Chappell LT, Stahl JP: The correlation between EDTA chelation therapy and improvement in cardiovascular function: a meta-analysis, J Adv Med 6:139-160, 1993.

41. Gibbons RJ, Abrams J, Chatterjee K et al: ACC/AHA 2002 guideline update for the management of patients with chronic stable angina, a summary article: a report of the American College of Cardiology/American Heart Association Task Force on Practice Guidelines (Committee on the Management of Patients with Chronic Stable Angina), J Am Coll Cardiol 41:159-68, 2003.

42. Riordan HD, Cheraskin E, Dirks M, Schultz M, Brizendine P: Electrocardiographic changes associated with EDTA chelation therapy, J Adv Med 1:191-194, 1988.

43. Riordan HD, Cheraskin E, Dirks M et al: EDTA chelation/hypertension study: Clinical patterns as judged by the Cornell Medical Index questionnaire, J Ortho Med 4:91-95, 1989.

44. Knudtson ML, Wyse DG, Galbraith PD et al: Chelation therapy for ischemic heart disease: a randomized, controlled trial, JAMA 287:481-486, 2002.

45. Anderson TJ, Hubacek J, Wyse G, Knudtson ML: Effect of chelation therapy on endothelial function in patients with coronary artery disease: PATCH substudy, J Am Coll Cardiol 41:420-425, 2003.

46. Laslett L: Chelation theapy: new proof of lack of efficacy, Prev Cardiol Spring: 92-93, 2002.

47. Holden C: Alternative medicine: NIH trial to test chelation therapy, Science 297:1109, 2002.

48. NIH: NIH Launches large clinical trial on EDTA chelation therapy for coronary artery disease, *http://nccam.nih.gov/news/2002/chelation/pressrelease.htm.*

49. Clinical Trial: 4rial to assess chelation therapy. *www.clinicaltrials.gov/ct.*

50. Quan H, Ghali WA, Verhoef MJ et al: Use of chelation therapy after coronary angiography, Am J Med 111:686-691, 2001.

51. Frishman WH: Chelation therapy for coronary artery disease: panacea or quackery? (editorial), Am J Med 111:729-730, 2001.

52. Frishman WH, Retter A, Misailidis J et al: Innovative pharmacologic approaches to the treatment of myocardial ischemia. In Frishman WH, Sonnenblick EH, Sica DA, editors: Cardiovascular Pharmacotherapeutics, ed 2, New York, 2003, McGraw Hill, 655-690.

53. Salonen JT, Nyyssonen K, Korpela H et al: High stored iron levels are associated with excess risk of myocardial infarction in eastern Finnish men, Circulation 86:803-811, 1992.

54. Morrison HI, Semenciw RM, Mao Y, Wigle DT: Serum iron and risk of fatal acute myocardial infarction, Epidemiology 5:243-246, 1994.

55. Haidari M, Javadi E, Sanati A et al: Association of increased ferritin with premature coronary stenosis in men, Clin Chem 47: 1666-1672, 2001.

56. Tuomainen TP, Kontula K, Nyyssonen K et al: Increased risk of acute myocardial infarction in carriers of the hemochromatosis gene Cys282Tyr mutation: a prospective cohort study in men in eastern Finland, Circulation 100:1274-1279, 1999.
57. Maza SR, Frishman WH: Therapeutic options to minimize free radical damage and thrombogenicity in ischemic/reperfused myocardium, Med Clin North Am 72:227-242, 1988.
58. Pratico D, Pasin M, Barry OP et al: Iron-dependent human platelet activation and hydroxyl radical formation: involvement of protein kinase C, Circulation 99(24):3118-3124, 1999.
59. Gaenzer H, Marschang P, Sturm W et al: Association between increased iron stores and impaired endothelial function in patients with hereditary hemochromatosis, J Am Coll Cardiol 40:2189-2194, 2002.
60. Solymoss BC, Marcil M, Gilfix BM et al: The place of ferritin among risk factors associated with coronary artery disease, Coron Artery Dis 5(3):231-235, 1994.
61. Magnusson MK, Sigfusson N, Sigvaldason H et al: Low iron-binding capacity as a risk factor for myocardial infarction, Circulation 89:102-108, 1994.
62. Voest EE, Vreugdenhil G, Marx JJM: Iron-chelating agents in non-iron overload conditions, Ann Intern Med 120:490-499, 1994.
63. Porreca E, Ucchino S, Di Febbo C et al: Antiproliferative effect of desferrioxamine on vascular smooth muscle cells in vitro and in vivo, Arterioscler Thromb 14:299-304, 1994.
64. DeBoer D, Clark R: Iron chelation in myocardial preservation after ischemia-reperfusion injury: the importance of pretreatment and toxicity, Ann Thorac Surg 53:412-418, 1992.
65. Ambrosio G, Zweier J, Jacobus W et al: Improvement of postischemic myocardial function and metabolism induced by administration of deferoxamine at the time of reflow: the role of iron in the pathogenesis of reperfusion injury, Circulation 76:906-915, 1987.
66. Menasche P, Antebi H, Alcindor LG et al: Iron chelation by deferoxamine inhibits lipid peroxidation during cardiopulmonary bypass in humans. Circulation 82(Suppl IV):IV390-396, 1990.
67. Reddy BR, Wynne J, Kloner RA, Przyklenk K: Pretreatment with the iron chelator deferoxamine on transferrin receptors: the cell cycle and growth rates of human leukaemic cells, Cardiovasc Res 25:711, 1991.
68. Rudolph CJ, McDonagh EW, Barber RK: Effect of EDTA chelation on serum iron, J Adv Med 4:39-45, 1991.
69. Anderson LJ, Wonke B, Prescott E et al: Comparison of effects of oral deferiprone and subcutaneous desferrioxamine on myocardial iron concentrations and ventricular function in beta-thalassaemia, Lancet 360:516-520, 2002.
70. Frishman WH, Sonnenblick EH: Environmental factors in cardiac hypertrophy and failure. In Molecular Mechanisms of Cardiac Hypertrophy and Failure, edited by Walsh RA. Lancaster UK, Parthenon Publishing. In press.

CHAPTER 18

Aromatherapy In Cardiac Conditions

Alan R. Hirsch, MD

The lay aromatherapy literature is replete with pronouncements that different essential oils can be used for a panoply of cardiac conditions. Aromas said to improve the body's circulation include angelica, carrot seed, chamomile, garlic, lemon, neroli, black pepper, peppermint, rose, spikenard, black spruce, yarrow, ylang-ylang,[1] rosemary,[1,2] thyme, basil, marjoram, and clove.[2] Hypertension is said to be relieved with the aromas of clary, sage,[1,3] juniper,[1] lavender,[1,3] mandarin,[1] yarrow, ylang-ylang,[1,3] melissa,[2,3] neroli,[2] and marjoram,[2,3] *Cananga odorata*, citrus limon (per.), *lavandula angustifolia, lavandula-x-intermedia* 'super,' *ocimum basilicum* var. album, *origanum majorana*, and *melaleuca viridiflora*.[4]

Hypotension, on the other hand, is reported to respond to the smells of black pepper and rosemary.[1]

Paradoxically, the aromas of garlic[1,3] and ginger[1,2] are proclaimed to relieve both hypertension and hypotension. Although lemon aroma is recommended as a treatment of hypertension,[3] Schnaubelt lists hypertension as a contraindication to its use.[5]

Khella is claimed to dilate coronary blood vessels.[5] Ylang-ylang is promoted for its use in reducing palpitations.[5] Heart tonic effects are ascribed to the aroma of incilagraveoleus[3] and neroli.[6]

The specific claims of cardiovascular effects of aromatherapy are discussed in this chapter.

DEFINITION AND RATIONALE

Aromatherapy, as used here, is inhalation of an aroma, which, through stimulation of the olfactory or trigeminal nerves, causes a therapeutic effect.

300

This does not include concurrent therapies applied with the aromas, such as massage, talking, pressure points, and so on because the other approaches in and of themselves may have therapeutic effects. If these were used concurrently, it would be impossible to assess whether the benefit was due to the aromatherapy or to one of the nonaroma interventions.

Theoretically, why should odors affect the heart? An odorant's influence on the cardiovascular system may be primarily based on its effects on the limbic system—in particular, the lateral nucleus of the amygdala. To better understand aromatherapy's possible mode of action, the neuroanatomy and neurophysiology of olfaction are reviewed.[7-10]

Upon inhalation, an odorant passes the nasal turbinates and eventually reaches the olfactory epithelium at the top of the nose. Once an odorant passes through the olfactory epithelium, it stimulates the olfactory nerve, which consists of unmyelinated olfactory fila and has the slowest conduction rate of any nerves in the body. The olfactory fila pass through the cribiform plate of the ethmoid bone and enter the olfactory bulb.[10,11] Different odors localize in different areas of the olfactory bulb.

Inside the olfactory bulb is a conglomeration of approximately 2000 glomeruli. Four different cell types make up the glomeruli: processes of receptor cell axons, mitral cells, tufted cells, and second-order neurons that give off collaterals to the granule cells and to cells in the periglomerular and external plexiform layers. The mitral and tufted cells form the lateral olfactory tract and establish a reverberating circuit with the granule cells: the mitral cells stimulate firing of the granule cells, which in turn inhibit firing of the mitral cells.

A reciprocal inhibition exists between the mitral and the tufted cells. This results in a sharpening of olfactory acuity. The olfactory bulb receives several efferent projections, including the primary olfactory fibers, the contralateral olfactory bulb and the anterior nucleus, the prepiriform cortex (inhibitory), the diagonal band of Broca with neurotransmitters acetylcholine and gamma aminobutyric acid, the locus coeruleus, the dorsal raphe, and the tuberomamillary nucleus of the hypothalamus.

The olfactory bulb's efferent fibers project into the olfactory tract, which divides at the olfactory trigona into the medial and lateral olfactory stria. These project to the anterior olfactory nucleus, the olfactory tubercle, the amygdaloid nucleus (which in turn projects to the ventral medial nucleus of the hypothalamus, a feeding center), the cortex of the piriform lobe, the septal nuclei, and the hypothalamus—in particular the anterolateral regions of the hypothalamus—which are involved in reproduction. The neurotransmitters by which the olfactory bulb conducts its information include glutamate, aspartate, N-acetyl-aspartyl-glutamate, cholecystokinin, and gamma aminobutyric acid.

The anterior olfactory nucleus receives afferent fibers from the olfactory tract and projects efferent fibers, which decussate in the anterior commissure and synapse in the contralateral olfactory bulb. Some of the efferent projections from the anterior olfactory nucleus remain ipsilateral and synapse on internal granular cells of the ipsilateral olfactory bulb.

The olfactory tubercle receives afferent fibers from the olfactory bulb and the anterior olfactory nucleus. Efferent fibers from the olfactory tubercle project to the nucleus accumbens and to the striatum. Neurotransmitters of the olfactory tubercle include acetylcholine and dopamine.

The primary olfactory cortex, which is the area on the cortex where olfaction is localized, includes the prepiriform area, the periamygdaloid area, and the entorhinal area. Afferent projections to the primary olfactory cortex include the mitral cells, which enter the lateral olfactory tract and synapse in the prepiriform cortex (lateral olfactory gyrus) as well as in the corticomedial part of the amygdala. Efferent projections from the primary olfactory cortex extend to the entorhinal cortex (area 28), the basal and lateral amygdaloid nuclei, the lateral preoptic area of the hypothalamus, the nucleus of the diagonal band of Broca, the medial forebrain bundle, the dorsal medial nucleus and submedial nucleus of the thalamus, and the nucleus accumbens.[9]

It should be noted that the entorhinal cortex is both a primary and a secondary olfactory cortical area. Efferent fibers from the cortex project via the uncinate fasciculus to the hippocampus, the anterior insular cortex (next to the gustatory cortical area), and the frontal cortex. This connection is demonstrated pathophysiologically in temporal lobe epileptic patients, who have uncinate or insular fits. These are manifested by the phantageusia of a metallic taste or a burning rubber phantosmia.[12]

The left insular cortex is the center of cardiac autonomic control, and left insular stroke patients demonstrate increased heart rate variability (R-R) and increased vanillylmandelic acid production. This suggests a shift away from parasympathetic and toward sympathetic predominance.[13] Theoretically, odorants acting on the same insular nucleus may activate the parasympathetic center, thus reducing sympathetic discharge, heart rate variability, and vanillylmandelic acid levels.

Some of the efferent projections of the mitral and tufted cells decussate in the anterior commissure and form the medial olfactory tract. They then synapse in the contralateral paraolfactory area and contralateral subcallosal gyrus. The exact function of the medial olfactory stria and tract is unclear. The accessory olfactory bulb receives afferent fibers from the bed nucleus of the accessory olfactory tract and the medial and posterior corticoamygdaloid nuclei. Efferent fibers from the accessory olfactory bulb project through the accessory olfactory tract to the same afferent areas (e.g., the bed nucleus of the accessory olfactory tract and medial and posterior corticoamygdaloid nuclei). It is of note that the medial and posterior corticoamygdaloid nuclei project secondary fibers to the anterior and medial hypothalamus, which are areas associated with reproduction. Therefore the accessory olfactory bulb in humans may be the mediator for human pheromones.[14]

Some unique aspects of the anatomy of the olfactory system are worthy of mention. Smell is the only sensation that reaches the cortex before reaching the thalamus. The only sensory system that is primarily ipsilateral in its projection, olfaction does not depend upon the cortex, as has been demonstrated in decorticate cats.

Neurotransmitters of the olfactory cortex are multiple and include glutamate, asparatate, cholecystokinin, luteinizing hormone–releasing hormone, and somatastatin. Virtually all known neurotransmitters are present in the olfactory bulb. Perception of odors modulates olfactory neurotransmitters within the olfactory bulb and the limbic system. Thus odorant modulation of neurotransmitter levels in the olfactory bulb, tract, and the limbic system intended for transmission of sensory information may have unintended secondary effects on a variety of different behaviors and disease states that are regulated by the same neurotransmitters. For instance, odorant modulation of dopamine in the olfactory bulb/limbic system may potentially affect manifestations of Parkinson's disease. Nonolfactory mesolimbic override to many of the components of Parkinson's disease have been well documented (e.g., motoric activation associated with emotional distress and fear of injury in a fire).

The olfactory bulb projects directly to the amygdala, without first being transmitted to the neocortex.[15,16] The central amygdala projects through the bed nucleus of the stria terminalis to the paraventricular hypothalamus.[7] The paraventricular hypothalamus in turn releases corticotropin-releasing factor, which transmits to the infundibulum, thus causing the anterior pituitary to release adrenocorticotropic hormone (ACTH).[17] In turn, ACTH induces the adrenal cortex to produce corticosteroids, the chronic production of which may be a mediator of the stress response.

Alternately, the olfactory amygdaloid connections may act to change the baseline setting of the amygdala, so it is less responsive to visceral sensory input from the nucleus tractus solitarius, thus inhibiting parasympathetic outflow from the baroreceptor reflex and causing chronically elevated blood pressure.[18]

More directly, the amygdala may be involved in the maintenance of hypertension by increasing sympathetic discharge, thus causing vasoconstriction as well as sympathetic projections to the adrenal medulla, which causes epinephrine release and induces vasoconstriction.[19]

Odorants may act indirectly on the amygdala to stimulate sympathetic discharge as well. Odorants, like ammonia or smelling salts, act on the ascending reticular formation, thus discharging norepinephrine neurons from the locus ceruleus, serotonin-containing neurons in the dorsal raphe nucleus, and cholinergic neurons in the lateral dorsal tegumentum and parabranchial area.[20] These project diffusely to the forebrain and limbic system as well as the amygdala.

Moreover, aromatherapy may influence cardiovascular function through its mood-altering effects and associated impact on the limbic symptoms and its connection. The insular cortex, the central nucleus of the amygdala, and the lateral hypothalamus integrate emotional tone and olfactory sensation and function to coordinate descending efferent projections involved in regulation of the heart and blood vessels.[21]

AROMATHERAPY'S EFFECTS ON THE AUTONOMIC NERVOUS SYSTEM

Central nervous system control of cardiovascular activity traditionally has been centered on the autonomic nervous system, with subcortical nuclei projections to the parasympathetic and sympathetic preganglionic cells. However, aromatherapy-induced cardiovascular changes may involve a multitude of other descending neural cardiovascular pathways that arise anywhere from the cortex through the brainstem.[22-26] These include the frontal lobes[27,28] (medial agranular region),[29] sigmoid cortex,[30] subcallosal gyrus,[31] septal area,[32] cingulate gyrus,[33-35] and temporal lobes.[33] The insula of the temporal lobe, the area classically delineated as the primary focus of gustatory hallucinations in temporal lobe epilepsy, mediates emotional stress-induced change in heart rate and cardiac rhythm.[36-39] Afferent projections to the amygdala come from the insular and orbitofrontal cortices, the parabrachial nucleus, and the nucleus tractus solitarius (the brainstem taste center).[40-42] The amygdala integrates these,[43] and efferent projections from the amygdala and tegmentum regulate the autonomic nervous system.[44,45]

The medial hypothalamic nuclei which receive afferent olfactory imput, project descending fibers into the midbrain, periaqueductal gray, reticular formation, and intermediolateral nuclei of the spinal cord. These areas then act to modulate arrhythmogenesis.[46] Efferent fibers from the infralimbic cortex project to the lateral hypothalamus.[47] The lateral hypothalamus in turn processes the autonomic component of emotion with descending efferent projection to the periaqueductal gray matter, the parabrachial region, parvicellular formation, dorsal vagal nucleus, and spinal cord.[48,49]

Thus a variety of anatomic means allow odorants to influence cardiac and vascular function: through their effect on neural pathways—not, as many lay aromatherapy books state, by the odorant directly entering the blood stream and relaxing the blood vessels or by directly acting on the heart itself.

CARDIOVASCULAR EFFECTS OF AROMATHERAPY

Given the preceding information, what is the evidence that odorants actually do affect cardiovascular function? Scientific studies that specifically demonstrate the efficacy of aromatherapy in cardiovascular disease are sorely lacking. Four parameters of cardiovascular function have been evaluated: blood pressure, R-R variability, heart rate, and coagulability.

EFFECTS ON BLOOD PRESSURE

Over 100 years ago, Vaschide noted an increase in blood pressure in response to exposure to unpleasant odors with trigeminal components.[50]

Unpleasant, trigeminally stimulating odors induce a variety of effects consistent with the induction of pain. Pain, through its activation of the reticular activating system and amygdala, then induces elevations in blood pressure, blood cortisol levels, and epinephrine discharge as described previously. By inducing a generalized sympathetic discharge, pain can cause transient elevations in blood pressure and cardiac irritability, thus potentially having adverse effects on cardiac status.

Irritating odors have been demonstrated to cause an elevation in blood pressure.[51,52] An aromatherapy approach would be to eliminate irritating odors from the environment of those with unstable, elevated blood pressure and cardiac arrhythmias. Therefore the hospital custodian may be the real true aromatherapist!

On the other hand, over 2 decades ago, Eccles[53] noted that unpleasant, irritating odorants stimulated the apneic reflex with closure of the larynx and a generalized parasympathetic response, with a decrease in both heart rate and blood pressure. Thus while trigeminal stimuli can decrease heart rate, lay aromatherapists have not endorsed the use of such aromatic agents as ammonia or galbanum (vomitus) for this purpose.

Tomonobu et al measured the effects of a malodor, the rotting odor of Welsh onion, and an unnamed pleasant essential oil combination.[54] Outcome measures included heart rate, heart rate variability, systolic blood pressure, and diastolic blood pressure. Of the 10 female subjects aged 20 to 27 years exposed to the odors for 6 minutes, the rotting Welsh onion odor increased heart rate variability, systolic blood pressure, and diastolic blood pressure. The effect of the malodor may have been mediated by the induction of stress, thus activating the autonomic nervous system. This is consistent with what is seen in response to pain and suggests a trigeminally induced response. At six minutes, the pleasant aroma had no effect on these parameters.

Stress may be the key to understanding an aroma's effect on blood pressure. Baba et al reported an elevation in systolic and diastolic blood pressures in 28 untreated hypertensive men on working days.[55] This was attributed to job-related stress. This would imply that a possible mechanism of aromatherapy to reduce blood pressure would be through stress reduction (or relaxation). A mild reduction in systolic blood pressure is an indicator of anxiolysis.[56] However, studies have addressed the anxiolytic effects of aromatherapy in the clinical setting, with ambiguous results. In a case-controlled study of 36 men with public-speaking anxiety, jasmine and apple spice were no more effective than the odorless control condition in reducing speech anxiety.[57]

Likewise, no clear efficacy has been demonstrated for aromatherapy for anxiety reduction in patients confined to the hospital. Aromas of marjoram, lavender, rose, eucalyptus, geranium, chamomile and neroli were used in combination with massage and music therapy to treat 69 terminally ill patients.[58] An 80% rate of success, defined as "deriving benefit in some way," was found, but this must be viewed cautiously because (1) statistical significance was not determined; (2) treatments ancillary to the aromatherapy, including talking, massage or music, may have provided the benefit; (3) concomitant medical treatment (e.g., to decrease pain) may have caused the beneficial effects ascribed to aromatherapy; (4) different odors were used for each subject, and (5) no consideration was given to hedonics, olfactory ability, a control group, expectation bias, or examiner bias.

Likewise, Dunn et al assessed systolic and diastolic blood pressure, heart rate, and rhythm in 122 ICU patients in response to massage with or without 1% essential oil of lavender (*lavendula vera*) or rest.[59] No statistically significant effect was observed.

Similarly, a randomized, double-blind trial of aromatherapy compared two different species of lavender and massage in 24 postoperative ICU cardiac patients. No statistically significant self-perceived anxiolytic effect of either species of lavender was found.[60]

In a randomized controlled trial, Stevenson assessed the effects of foot massage over 20 minutes with or without the essential oil of neroli.[61] No effect on mean blood pressure, systolic blood pressure, diastolic blood pressure, and heart rate was found in the 25 postcardiac surgery patients who received neroli in comparison to those receiving the nonodorized oil, although the neroli group experienced reduced anxiety. These results may not be generalizable to other paradigms in the use of aromatherapy because these subjects all wore oxygen facemasks during the period of intervention, thus inhibiting the inhalation of the neroli aroma.

Twelve ICU/CCU patients were assessed for changes in systolic blood pressure and heart rate in response to a 20-minute massage with lavender oil in comparison to an equal number of nonaromatherapy massage control patients.[62] Measurements were obtained immediately upon completion and at 20 and 30 minutes after treatment. A decrease in systolic blood pressure between 11 and 15 mm Hg was seen in six of the aromatherapy group and in five of the massage only group—clearly not a significant difference. A reduction in heart rate of between 11 and 15 beats per minute occurred in 11 of the aromatherapy patients, whereas only seven of the massage group experienced this reduction. However, the results of this study should be viewed with skepticism because no statistical significance was reported; no blinding occurred; olfactory ability was not assessed; and most importantly, because 42% of the aromatherapy group were on ventilators, the aroma presented would not have even reached the olfactory epithelium for these patients to smell it.

No change in heart rate or blood pressure in 24 postcardiac surgery patients was noted after a 20-minute exposure to a combination of lavender (*lavandula angustifolia* and *lavandula burnatti*).[60]

Given Stahl's findings, favorable effects from aroma in postcardiac surgery patients are not expected.[63] Significant orthonasal olfactory loss is observed immediately after surgery and 2 weeks after discharge amongst patients admitted for coronary artery bypass graft, valve replacement/repair, and thoracic aneurysm repair. Thus because these patients suffer from significant olfactory impairment, how aromatherapy could be therapeutic in these individuals is hard to understand.

Those odorants said to mitigate stress-induced elevation in systolic blood pressure include nutmeg oil, mace extract, neroli oil, valerian oil, myristicin, elemicin, and isoelemicin.[64] These beneficial claims cannot be critically evaluated because published versions of these studies are not available in the scientific literature.

Hirsch and Colavincenzo attempted to demonstrate an impact of aromas on mean arterial pressure as a surrogate of anxiety level in 27 normotensive white men.[65] Blood-pressure measurements were obtained at rest and under the stress of taking a test involving mental mathematical calculations, a paradigm of anxiety induction.[66] Subjects took the test twice and wore a surgical mask each time. Masks were impregnated with a hedonically pleasant odor, no odor, or a hedonically negative odor. The order of presentation of masks was randomized in a single-blinded fashion. The odorants tested included green apple, lavender, mesquite chips, roasting meat, pink grapefruit, cucumber, gardenia, peppermint, meat blend in olive oil, tobacco leaf, and peach. Despite expectations, no significant effect on mean arterial pressure was found with any odor in comparison to the blank.

Nonaromatic therapeutic modalities, which are provided concurrently with the aroma by lay aromatherapists, may be the primary mediators of the anecdotal efficacy of aromatherapy for the treatment of hypertension. Lay aromatherapists talk with the patient and provide massage and companionship, which tends to make the patient comfortable, independent of any odor effect. Talking, independent of aroma, has been shown to influence blood pressure in both normotensive and hypertensive individuals.[67] Also, degree of happiness has been demonstrated to be inversely proportional to systolic blood pressure, with a greater effect in those with labile blood pressure.[68] Thus by just making clients happier, aromatherapists can reduce blood pressure, independent of any specific effect of odor.

Confirming the principle of the general affective theory of aromatherapy, Vernet-Maury et al reported that pleasant odorants induced happiness and surprise, whereas unpleasant odorants evoked anger, fear, and disgust, with the associated autonomic nervous system responses.[69] However, this report should be viewed skeptically because the exact autonomic nervous system responses were not described.

A single-blind study measured changes in systolic blood pressure in four normosmics in response to a variety of odorants.[51] Whereas a change of 2 mm Hg was defined as significant, no effect was seen in response to the inhalation of orange, lavender, bergamot, cloves, and peppermint. No consistent effect was seen with wintergreen, menthol, eucalyptus, camphor, ether, chloroform, xylol, asafetida, butyric acid, pyridine, and ammonia. An elevation in systolic blood pressure was observed with inhalation of the trigeminal irritants formalin, Ar.Sp. ammonia, acetic acid, and oil of mustard. These effects from inducers of blood pressure elevation are not surprising because trigeminal nerve stimulation produces pain, and discharge of any nerve-mediating pain is known to induce an autonomic sympathetic response, including an increase in blood pressure.

To establish the effects of lavender as an aromatherapeutic agent for cardiac function, Romine et al[70] studied its effects on 10 undergraduate men after exercise. Cardiac parameters measured included diastolic blood pressure, systolic blood pressure, mean arterial pressure, pulse pressure, and heart rate. No statistically significant effect was found on any of the variables in comparison to the no odor control, thus casting doubt on lavender's efficacy as a therapeutic agent for cardiovascular conditions.

On the other hand, nutmeg odor, combined with an unnamed other fragrance, reduced stress (mental arithmetic) induced blood pressure elevation in comparison to the same unnamed fragrance without nutmeg.[71] However, in the resting, nonstress state, the nutmeg-unnamed fragrance combination had no effect. The validity of these findings cannot be confirmed because the odorants assessed are unknown.

Finally, an inhaled odorant's effect on blood pressure was assessed in a double-blind, controlled, randomized study of normosmic and anosmic, awake and anesthetized adults.[51] No significant effect was noted with inhalation of hedonically positive odors, but inhalation of an irritant (ammonia) caused an increase in blood pressure.

Based on this review of the literature, a measurable reduction in blood pressure as a manifestation of odorant-induced anxiolysis has not been demonstrated.

EFFECTS ON R-R VARIABILITY

Yagyu measured the coefficient variation of ECG R-R intervals, a cardiac indicator of autonomic nervous system function.[72] Baseline odor-free measurements were compared to lavender and jasmine odors in five men and five women. No significant effect was seen in response to lavender or jasmine. However, the seven subjects who liked the fragrance experienced increase of the ECG R-R interval. This was possibly due to the relaxation effect of the aromas, thus inducing a parasympathetic predominance with an associated increase of the R-R interval. These findings are in concordance with the "general affective theory of aromatherapy", which suggests that the specific odor is unimportant and rather that the relevant factor is the affective valence of the odor.[73,74]

Inoue et al[75] assessed the effects of jasmine tea aroma in lower and higher concentrations in 10 healthy volunteers. The subjects were subdivided based on jasmine tea odor hedonics. The investigation demonstrated a decreased heart rate and increased parasympathetic activity (based on R-R variability) in both hedonic groups upon exposure to the low-level odorant. With higher odorant level exposure, similar findings were also seen in the positive hedonic group. In the negative hedonic group, increased sympathetic activity was observed. Although these results should be viewed cautiously because of the lack of olfactory assessment or any discussion of statistical significance, the hedonic segregation would tend to confirm the general affective theory of aromatherapy.

Nagai et al[76] similarly assessed the impact of sweet fennel oil on ECG R-R interval, heart rate, and systolic and diastolic blood pressure in 12 subjects, while the subjects performed arithmetic problems. Although the findings regarding heart rate, systolic blood pressure, and diastolic blood pressure were not revealed, a decrease in R-R interval ($p < 0.05$) was reported. No mention of hedonic rating was described. Thus whether these findings represent effects of sweet fennel oil or rather a further confirmation of Yagyu's previously mentioned study and findings as a manifestation of the "general affective theory of aromatherapy" is unknown.[72,74]

Bensafi et al assessed heart rate variation in relation to hedonics, familiarity, arousal, and intensity with a variety of odorants. In a single-blinded study, six odorants (isovaleric acid, thiophenol, pyridine, l-menthol, isoamyl acetate, and 1-8 cineole) were randomly presented to six healthy right-handed men and women.[77]Odorant pleasantness was found to correlate with heart rate variation (p <0.05). No significant effect of arousal, familiarity, or intensity on heart rate variation was seen. Heart rate variation correlating with hedonics has been reported with other sensory modalities and again confirms the lack of importance of the specific aroma but rather supports the general affective theory of aromatherapy.[74] This study may come under criticism because no olfactory tests had been performed. A lack of subject knowledge regarding poor olfactory ability appears to be the rule rather than the exception;[78] therefore, self-reports cannot be reliable alternatives to olfactory screening. Five of the 12 subjects in this study were current smokers; because smoking can also markedly reduce olfactory ability, it must be controlled for.[79]

In another study, 16 subjects with unknown olfactory status were presented "pleasant odors."[80] Those odors that activated the central nervous system, as defined by concurrent measurements of contingent negative variation, increased heart rate variations (as measured by the ECG R-R interval). Sedating odors did the opposite. This implies that some odorants may act to promote cardiac stability in those subjects with presumably normal cardiac function. Because the specific odorants tested were not revealed and neither the olfactory ability nor the hedonic perception of the subjects was assessed, the implications of this study remain speculative.

In a randomized crossover controlled open-label study, 10 healthy women, aged 19-21 years, of unknown olfactory status, soaked their feet for 10 minutes with and without the essential oil of lavender.[81] Cardiac function assessed included heart rate and ECG R-R variability. No statistically significant effect was seen with this treatment.

EFFECT ON HEART RATE

A change in heart rate occurs with any sudden change in sensory experience; therefore, it is not surprising that odors could cause transient changes in heart rate.[82]

In demonstrating the importance of hedonic considerations and thus the "general affective theory of aromatherapy", Alaoui-Ismalli et al assessed the effects on heart rate of hedonically pleasant or unpleasant aromas on 15 volunteers.[83] The odors that were rated pleasant were lavender, camphor, and ethyl acetoacetate; the unpleasant aromas were acetic acid and butyric acid. The effects on heart rate correlated with hedonic evaluation, such that the exposure to pleasant odorants induced brachycardia in comparison to unpleasant odorants, which were associated with tachycardia. A postulated mechanism for these findings is such that the aroma induced a mood state concordant with the odorant hedonic valence and emotional valence has been demonstrated to be inversely related to heart rate.[84,85]

On the other hand, Brauchli et al[86] found no significant effect on heart rate amongst five men exposed to either the hedonically pleasant aroma of phenylethyl alcohol or the unpleasant aroma of valeric acid. Warrenberg and Schwartz[87] measured heart rate in 28 college students when exposed to apple, neroli, galbanum, and non-odor conditions. Regardless of hedonics, no effect on heart rate was observed for any of the odorants tested. Torii et al[88] found that amongst four male perfumers studied, no effect was observed in heart rate from exposure to jasmine, chamomile, or lavender.

Inhalation of (R)-(negative) linalool, a major odor component in jasmine tea, was reported to cause a reduction in heart rate in seven healthy volunteers, whereas inhalation of its enantiomer (S)–(+)–linalool elicited an increase in heart rate.[89] However, neither the extent of the hedonic ratings, change of heart rate, or statistical significance were reported.

In a test of aromas of carrot seed, petit grain, sage, and grapefruit, time required for return to baseline heart rate after exercise was not related to odor tested but rather correlated with odor hedonics: the quickest recovery rate was seen with use of the best liked aroma.[90] These results further substantiate the "general affective theory of aromatherapy". However, the number of subjects tested, the duration change in comparison to the lack of odor, and the mention of any statistically significant findings were not reported.

Transient heart rate reduction is a physiological concomitant of the mental process of attention. Therefore odorants that purportedly enhance attention should reduce heart rate, and those that sedate should increase heart rate. Kikuchi et al tested this hypothesis.[91] They found that the odor of lemon, a traditional stimulant, reduced heart rate in a concentration-dependent manner, whereas the aroma of rose, a putative sedating odor, increased heart rate, independent of strength. These results should be viewed cautiously because the number of subjects, the amount of change in heart rate, and statistical significance were not reported on.

Louis and Kowalski[92] found no statistically significant effect of lavender oil (*lavandula angustifolia*) on heart rate or blood pressure in 17 conscious, orientated hospice patients.

In a double-blinded study, Simpson et al evaluated the effects of lavender and peppermint on four normosmic male and female college students.[93] During 15 minutes of exercise, heart rate was assessed every 3 minutes. No statistically significant effect was found for either odor.

Exposure to the sight and aromas of a variety of breakfast foods by sham feeding was performed on seven healthy, nonobese subjects.[94] No change in heart rate or blood pressure was seen. However, a significant drop in cardiac output occurred. This cardiac output reduction may have been due to pooling of blood in the splanchnic area with an associated decrease in cardiac venous return. However, because both sight and odor were provided simultaneously in this sham feeding, whether all the observed effects were visually rather than olfactorily mediated is unknown.

Independent of its cardiac effect, aromatherapy may have efficacy for cardiac patients hospitalized in cardiac ICUs. In a study that was not randomized, not double-blinded, and not age-controlled, Woolfson and Hewitt gave aromatherapy and massage in 20-minute sessions twice a week to 12 patients; another 12 patients received massage only.[62] The aromatherapy patients were massaged with lavender oil in an odorless almond oil base, and the massage only patients were massaged with almond oil only. Observations were recorded at the beginning and end of each 20-minute session and 30 minutes after treatment. All sessions were conducted in midafternoon. Approximately 50% of the patients were in the CCU, and the others were in the ICU; 50% were artificially ventilated. The authors stated that half of the aromatherapy patients and 41% of massage-only patients reported a decrease in pain—not a statistically significant difference, thus indicating that aromatherapy was no better than massage alone. Given their selection of patients, however, one would not anticipate that aromatherapy would be effective, because the pathway for olfactory input is compromised by artificial ventilation.

An explanation for the lack of sound experimental data supporting the efficacy of aromas as a treatment for hypertension and tachycardia may relate to the basic pathophysiology of these conditions. Isometric stress stimulates both the adrenergic and noradrenergic systems, thus resulting in a substantial increase in blood pressure by increasing cardiac output, with an increase in both heart rate and total peripheral vascular resistance. On the other hand, mental stress stimulates only the adrenergic system, with an increase in cardiac output and heart rate without a change in peripheral vascular resistance.[95] Because aromatherapy is thought to act by reducing mental stress, the secondary cardiac effects will be related to a reduction in adrenergic activity, without noradrenergic effects. Therefore any decrease in blood pressure that is observed will be milder and more difficult to demonstrate.

In a broad perspective, aromatherapy may not benefit cardiac health directly, through direct actions on heart rate, blood pressure, or cardiac contractility but rather, indirectly by inducing a positive affect—that is, making people happier. This happier mood state would act to reduce depressive feelings.[96] Because mental depression is associated with a threefold to fourfold relative risk of coronary heart disease (similar to hypertension and dyslipidemia), aromatherapy may act to alleviate depression and in this way indirectly reduce heart disease.[97]

EFFECTS ON COAGULABILITY

Aromatherapy may improve cardiovascular function through hemostatic effects. Among normosmic sympathotonic subjects (as defined by ECG R–R interval, a measure of autonomic nervous system activity), subthreshold olfactory stimulation by oxytocin shortened the blood-clotting time.[98] This suggests that in susceptible individuals, a subthreshold level of odorants (and presumably, a suprathreshold level of odorants) may actually promote hemostasis and thus enhance the likelihood of an ischemic stroke or myocardial infarction.

Although it has not been described, hypothetically, other odorants could also act in the opposite direction, inhibiting hemostasis and acting like low-dose aspirin, thus reducing the likelihood of an ischemic cardiovascular event.

POTENTIAL RISKS OF AROMATHERAPY

Before using aromatherapy in cardiac conditions, one must consider the potential risks of treatment. Adverse reactions can occur among patients with diseases that predispose to the development of side effects; this can also occur in the population as a whole.

Certain diseases make patients particularly susceptible to the adverse effects of aromatherapy. Approximately 40% of migraine sufferers report osmophobia, whereby an odorant induces a migraine headache.[99] A wide range of odorants can act as migraine triggers and depend upon the individual; they include perfume, cigarette smoke, and food odors.[100]

Asthmatic patients who are exposed to common odors can suffer a worsening of their respiratory status, independent of their olfactory ability. In a survey of 60 asthmatic patients, 57 (95%) described respiratory symptoms upon exposure to common odors, including insecticides (85%), household cleaning agents (78%), perfume and cologne (72%), cigarette smoke (75%), fresh paint (73%), automobile exhaust or gas fumes (60%), and cooking aromas (37%).[101] Room deodorant and mint candy can also induce respiratory distress. Four subjects who underwent an odor challenge with four squirts of a popular cologne were shown to have an immediate decline in 1-second forced expiratory volume (18% to 58% reduction).[101]

Among persons who suffer complaints consistent with multiple chemical sensitivities, 24% of the men and 39% of the women reported that odors precipitated their complaints.[102] However, double-blind studies have failed to demonstrate odorant-induced multiple chemical sensitivity symptoms.[103]

Inhalation of some odorants can produce measurable levels of the odorants in the blood.[104] Because many common fragrances contain naphthalene-related compounds (including menthol and camphor), individuals with G6PD deficiency may be at risk from aromatherapeutic exposures.[105]

A variety of essential oils have been reported to precipitate seizures in epileptic patients. Whether these effects can occur by inhalation alone, as opposed to ingestion or percutaneous absorption, is unclear. Proconvulsant odorants include rosemary, fennel, hyssop, sage, and wormwood.[7]

Because aromatherapeutic inhalation of essential oils can produce detectable levels in the blood, these compounds, like any pharmacologic agents, may induce adverse drug-drug interactions in persons receiving other medications. Such interactions could enhance the metabolism of anticonvulsants, pain medications, or antihypertensive agents, for example, thus predisposing an epileptic patient to seizure, a chronic pain patient to withdraw from medication, or a previously stable patient to uncontrolled hypertension. Jori et al[106] demonstrated that the inhalation of eucalyptol by rats increased the activity of hepatic microsomal enzyme systems, thus decreasing the effect of pentobarbital.

Odorants can produce harmful side effects not only in persons predisposed to disease but also in the healthy population. Airborne-induced allergic contact dermatitis is a recognized result of aromatherapeutic inhalation of tea tree oil (melaleuca oil).[107] Examples of common melaleuca oil allergens include: d-limonene, aromadendrene, alpha-terpinene, 1,8-cineole (eucalyptol), terpinen-4-ol, p-cymene, and alpha-phellandrene. Because of the highly volatile nature of essential oils, their common constituents and cross-sensitization, DeGroot postulated that the same airborne-induced contact dermatitis could occur with several other essential oils, including lavender and a mixture of eucalyptus, pine, and peppermint.[107] Bridges suggested that if odorants can sensitize the respiratory system as they do the skin, they could not merely exacerbate but actually precipitate asthma.[108]

CONCLUSION

Just as with any therapy, aromatherapy practitioners must weigh the relative risk-to-benefit ratio for the aromatherapeutic treatment of cardiovascular conditions. This author does not believe that the available scientific literature supports—nor does the risk-to-benefit ratio justify—traditional aromatherapy for managing cardiovascular disease. However, evidence-based medicine does suggest possible efficacy of aromatherapy for the following: (1) the elimination of malodors and trigeminal stimulations in the ambient environment; and (2) the use of hedonically positive aromas to induce happiness, decrease depression and by these mechanisms to affect favorably perhaps the risk of cardiovascular disease.

REFERENCES

1. Damian P, Damian K: Aromatherapy scent and psyche. using essential oils for psychological and physical well-being, Rochester, VT, 1995, Healing Arts Press, 225, 228.
2. Keville K, Green M: Aromatherapy: a complete guide to the healing art, Freedom, CA, 1995, The Crossing Press, 135, 31.
3. Feller, RM: Practical aromatherapy. understanding and using essential oils to heal the mind and body, New York, 1997, Berkley Books, 163.
4. Price S, Price L: Aromatherapy for health professionals, New York, 1995, Churchill Livingstone, 165-166.
5. Schnaubelt K: Advanced aromatherapy: the science of essential oil therapy, Rochester, VT, 1995, Healing Arts Press, 49, 74, 95.
6. Tisserand R: The Art of aromatherapy, New York, 1988, CW Daniel Co., Ltd.
7. Brodal A: Neurological anatomy in relation to clinical medicine, ed 3, vol 10, New York, 1969, Oxford University Press, 640-697.
8. Scott JW, Harrison TA: The olfactory bulb: anatomy and physiology. In Finger TE, Silver WL, editors: Neurologiology of taste and smell, New York, 1987, John Wiley & Sons, 151-178.
9. Price JL: The central olfactory and accessory olfactory systems. In: Finger TE, Silver WL editors: Neurologiology of taste and smell, New York, 1987, John Wiley & Sons, Inc., 179-203.
10. Adams RD, Victor M, Ropper AH: Principles of Neurology, ed 6, New York, 1997, McGraw Hill, 227-236.
11. Hirsch AR, Wyse JP: Posttraumatic dysosmia: central vs peripheral, J Neurol Orthop Med Surg 14:152-155, 1993.
12. Acharya V, Acharya J, Luders H: Olfactory epileptic auras (abst), Neurol 46:A446, 1996.

13. Laowattana S, Lima, J, Zeger S, Goodman S, Oppenheimer S: Left insular stroke increases risk of adverse cardiac outcome though impairment of cardiac parasympathetic tone, Neurology 60:1:A520, 2003.

14. Hirsch AR: Scentsational sex, Boston, 1998, Element Books.

15. LeDoux JE: Emotion circuits in the brain, Annu Rev Neurosci 23: 155-184, 2000.

16. LeDoux JE: Emotional memory systems in the brain, Behav Brain Res 58:1-2:69-79, 1993.

17. Brodal A: Neurological anatomy in relation to clinical medicine, ed 3, vol 10, New York, 1969, Oxford University Press, 698-787.

18. Cechetto D, Gelb AW: The amygdala and cardiovascular control, J Neurosurg Anesthesiol 13:4:285-287, 2001.

19. Reis DJ, LeDoux JE: Some central neural mechanisms governing resting and behaviorally coupled control of blood pressure, Circulation 76: I-2-9, 1987.

20. Hobson JA: Current concepts, sleep: biochemical aspects, New Engl J Med 281:1468-1470, 1969.

21. Salamon E, Kim M, Beaulleu J, Stefano GB: Sound therapy induced relaxation: down regulating stress processes and pathologies, Med Sci Monit 9:RA116-RA121, 2003.

22. Holstege G: Some anatomical observations on the projections from the hypothalamus to brainstem and spinal cord: an HRP and autoradiographic tracing study in the cat, J Comp Neurol 260:98-126, 1987.

23. Holstege G, Meiners L, Tan K: Projections of the bed nucleus of the stria terminalis to the mesencephalon, pont, and medulla oblongata in the cat, Exp Brain Res 58:370-391, 1985.

24. Hopkins DA, Holstege G: Amygdaloid projections to the mesencephalon, ports and medulla oblongata in the cat, Exp Brain Res 32:529-547, 1978.

25. Kuypers HGJM, Maisky VA: Retrograde axonal transport of horseradish peroxidase from spinal cord to brainstem cell groups in the cat, Neurosci Lett 1:9-14, 1975.

26. Swanson LW, Kuypers HG: The paraventricular nucleus of the hypothalamus: cytoarchitectonic subdivisions and organization of projections to the pituitary, dorsal vagal complex, and spinal cord as demonstrated by retrograde fluorescence double-labeling methods, J Comp Neurol 194:555-570, 1980.

27. Crouch RL, Thompson JK: Autonomic functions of the cerebral cortex, J Nerv Ment Dis 89:328-334, 1939.

28. Hsu S, Hwang K, Chu H: A Study of the cardiovascular changes induced by stimulation of the motor cortex in dogs, Am J Physiol 137:468-472, 1942.

29. Buchanan SL, Valentine J, Powell DA: Autonomic responses are elicited by electrical stimulation of the medial but not lateral frontal cortex in rabbits, Behav Brain Res 18:51-62, 1985.

30. Schiff M: *Untersutchungen ueber die motorischen Functionen des Grosshirns*, Arch Exp Pathol Pharmakol Naunyn Schmiedeberg 3:171-179, 1875.

31. Hoff EC: The role of the cerebral cortex in the central nervous regulation of cardiovascular function, Confin Neurol 9:166-176, 1949.

32. de la Torre JC, Stefano GB: Evidence that Alzheimer's disease is a microvascular disorder: the role of constituitive nitric oxide, Brain Ret Rev II:1581-1585, 2000.

33. Maclean PD: Discussion, Physiol Rev 40:113-114, 1960.

34. Smith WK. The functional significance of the rostral cingular cortex as revealed by its responses to electrical excitation, J Neurophysiol 8: 241-254, 1945.

35. Ueda H: Arrhythmias produced by cerebral stimulation, Jpn Circ J 26:225-230, 1962.

36. Fimiani C, Liberty T, Aquirre AJ et al: Opiate, rannabinoid, and eicosanoid signaling converges on common intracellular pathways: nitric oxide coupling, Prostaglandins 57:23-34, 1999.

37. Russchen FT: Amygdalopetal projections in the cat, I, cortical afferent connections: a study with retrograde and anterograde tracing techniques, J Comp Neurol 206:159-179, 1982.

38. Calaresu FR, Ciriello J: Projections to the hypothalamus from buffer nerves and nucleus tractus solitarius in the cat, Am J Physiol 230:130-136, 1980.

39. Melville KI, Blunt G, Shister HE, Silver MD: Cardiac ischemic changes and arrhythmias induced by hypothalamic stimulation, Am J Cardiol 12:781-791, 1963.

40. Yasui Y, Itoh K, Kaneko T: Topographical projections from the cerebral cortex to the nucleus of the solitary tract in the cat, Exp Brain Res 85:75-84, 1991.

41. Friedman R, Zuttermeister F, Benson H: Letter to the editor, New Engl J Med 329:1201, 1993.

42. Bonvallet M, Bobo EG: Changes in phrenic activity and heart rate elicited by localized stimulation of amygdala and adjacent structures, Clin Neurophysiol 32:1-16, 1972.

43. Davis M: The role of the amygdala in fear and anxiety, Annu Rev Neurosci 15:553-575, 1992.

44. Allen GV, Saper GB, Hurley KM. Cechetto DF: Organization of visceral and limbic connections in the insular cortex of the rat, J Complement Neurol 311:1-16, 1901.

45. Kapp ES, Schwaber JS, Driscoll PA. Frontal cortex projections to the amygdaloid central nucleus in the rabbit, Neuroscience 15:327-346, 1985.

46. Beattie J, Brow GR, Long CNH: Physiological and anatomical evidence for the existence of nerve tracts connecting the hypothalamus with spinal sympathetic centers, Proc R Soc Lond B, 106:253-275, 1930.

47. Hurley KM, Herbert H, Moga MM, Saper GB: Efferent projections of the infralimbic cortex of the rat, J Complement Neurol 308:249-276, 1991.

48. Hosoya Y, Matsushita M: Brainstem projections from the lateral hypothalamic area in the rat, as studied with autoradiography, Neurosci Lett 24:111-116, 1981.
49. ter Horst GJ, Luiten PG, Kuipers F. Descending pathways from hypothalamus to dorsal motor vagus and ambiguus nuclei in the rat, J Autonomic Nerv Syst 11:59-75, 1984.
50. Vaschide N: *L'Expérience de webor et l'olfaction en milieu liquide.* Cited in Douek E: The sense of smell and its abnormalities, Edinburgh, 1974, Churchill Livingstone, 93.
51. Allen WF: Effect of various inhaled vapors on respiration and blood pressure in anesthetized, unanesthetized, sleeping and anosmic subjects, Am J Physiol 1988:620-632, 1929.
52. Yammoto C, Iwama K: Arousal reaction of the olfactory bulb, Jpn J Physiol 11:335, 1961.
53. Eccles R. Neurological and pharmacological considerations. In Proctor DF, Andersen L editors: The nose: upper airway physiology and the atmospheric environment, Amsterdam, 1982, Elsevier, 191-214.
54. Tomonobu N, Hagino I, Watanuki S, Yokoyama N, Funada Y: Effect of odor preference on the autonomic nervous system, Chem Senses 26:296, 2001.
55. Baba S, Ozawa J, Nakamoto Y, Ueshima H, Omae T: Enhanced blood pressure response to regular daily stress in urban hypertensive men, J Hypertens 8:647-655, 1990.
56. Langewitz W, Ruddel H, Von Eiff AW: Influence of perceived level of stress upon ambulatory blood pressure, heart rate, and respiratory frequency, J Clinl Hypertens 3:743-748, 1987.
57. Spector IP, Carey MP, Jorgensen RS et al: Cue-controlled relaxation and "aromatherapy" in the treatment of speech anxiety, Behav Cog Psychotherap 21:239-253, 1993.
58. Evans B: An audit into the effects of aromatherapy massage and the cancer patient in palliative and terminal care, Complement Therap Med 3:239-241, 1995.
59. Dunn C, Sleep J, Collett D: Sensing an improvement: an experimental study to evaluate the use of aromatherapy, massage and periods of rest in an intensive care unit, J Advanced Nurs 21:1:34-40, 1995.
60. Buckle J: Does it matter which lavender essential oil is used? Nursing Times 89(20):32-35, 1993.
61. Stevenson CJ: The psychophysiological effects of aromatherapy massage following cardiac surgery, Complement Therap Med 2(1):27-35, 1994.
62. Wolfson A: Intensive aromacare, Intl J Aromatherapy 4(2):12-13, 1992.
63. Stahl B, Bartoshuk LM, Funk M: Taste/smell dysfunction in cardiac surgical patients. AChemS 25th Annual Meeting Abstract Book No. 432, p. 108, 2003.
64. European Patent 0183 436 B 2 (published March 7, 1991). Cited in Jellinek JS. Aroma-chology: a status review, Cosmetics & Toiletries Magazine 109:83-101, 1994.

65. Hirsch AR, Colavincenzo ML: An investigation into the effects of certain odors upon anxiety, J Neurol Orthop Med Surg 22:47-53, 2002.
66. Eliot RS, From stress to strength. New York, 1994, Bantam, 66-92.
67. Lynch JJ, Long JM, Thomas SA, Malinow KL, Katcher AH: The effects of talking on the blood pressure of hypertensive and normotensive individuals, Psychosom Med 43(1):25-33, 1981.
68. James GD, Yee LS, Harshfield GA, Blank SG, Pickering TG: The influence of happiness, anger, and anxiety on the blood pressure of borderline hypertensives, Psychosom Med 48(7):502-508, 1986.
69. Vernet-Maury E, Alaoui-Ismaili O, Rousmans S et al: Olfaction/emotion connexion: comparison between autonomic and verbal responses (abst), ECRO XIII(108):121, 1998.
70. Romine IJ, Bush AM, Geist CR: Lavender aromatherapy in recovery from exercise, Perceptual and Motor Skills 88:756-758, 1999.
71. Warren D, Warrenburg S: Mood benefits of fragrance, Perfumer & Flavorist 18:9-16, 1993.
72. Yagyu T: Neurophysiological findings on the effects of fragrance: lavender and jasmine. Integrative Psychiatry, New York, 1994, Elsevier, 62-67.
73. Buchbauer G: Biological effects of fragrances and essential oils. Perfumer & Flavorist 18:19-24, 1993.
74. Hirsch AR. Aromatherapy: art, science, or myth? In Weintraub MI, Micozzi MS, editors: Alternative and complementary treatment in neurologic illness, New York, 2001, Churchill Livingstone, 128-150.
75. Inoue N, Kuroda K, Sugimoto A, Kakuda T, Fushiki T. Autonomic nervous responses according to preference for the odor of jasmine tea, Biosci Biotechnol Biochem 67(6):1206-1214, 2003.
76. Nagai H, Nakagawa M, Nakamura M et al: Effects of odors on humans (II): reducing effects of mental stress and fatigue, Chem Senses 16:198, 1992.
77. Bensafi M, Rouby C, Farget V, Bertrand B, Vigouroux M, Holley A: Autonomic nervous system responses to odours: the role of pleasantness and arousal, Chem Senses 27:703-709, 2002.
78. Nordin S, Monsch AU, Murphy C: Unawareness of smell loss in normal aging and alzheimer's disease: discrepance between self-reporting and diagnosed smell sensitivity, J Gerentol 50:187-192, 1995.
79. Frye RE, Schartz B, Doty RL: Dose-related effects of cigarette smoking on olfactory function, JAMA 263:1233-1236, 1990.
80. Oguri M, Iwaki T, Ogata S, Okazaki Y, Torii S: Coincidental variations between heart rate and contingency negative wave during odor condition, Chem Senses 16:197-198, 1992.
81. Saeki Y: The effect of foot-bath with or without the essential oil of lavender on the autonomic nervous system: a randomized trial, Complement Therap Med 8(1):2-7, 2000.
82. Douek E: The sense of smell and its abnormalities, Edinburgh, 1974, Churchill Livingstone.

83.   Alaoui-Ismalli O, Vernet-Maury E, Dittmar A, Delhomme G: Odor hedonics: connection with emotional response, Chem Senses 22(3):237-248, 1997.

84.   Stemmier G: The autonomic differentiation of emotions revisited: convergent and discriminant validation, Physiology 26:617-632, 1989.

85.   Hubert W, DeJohn-Meyer R: Autonomic neuroendocrine and subjective responses to emotion-inducing film stimuli, Intl J Pyschophysiol 11:131-140, 1991.

86.   Brauchli P, Ruegg PB, Etzweller F, Zeier H: Electrocortical and autonomic alteration by administration of a pleasant and an unpleasant odor, Chem Senses 20:505-515, 1995.

87.   Warrenburg S, Schwartz GE: A psychophysiological study of three odorants, Chem Senses 13:744, 1990.

88.   Torii S, Fukuda H, Kanemoto H et al: Contingent negative variation (CNV) and the psychological effects of odor. In Van Toller S, Dodd GH, editors: Perfumery: the psychology and biology of fragrance, New York, 1988, Chapman Hall.

89.   Kuroda K, Inoue N, Ito Y et al: Effects of the major odor component (R)-(−)-linalool, in jasmine tea on autonomic nervous system (abst), Chem Senses 28:J10, 2003.

90.   Yamaguchi M, Kawaki H, Kishi Y, Ikeda N, Tonoike M: The effect of the perfume of essential oil of the natural plant in the exercise test (abst), Chem Senses 28:J26, 2003.

91.   Kikuchi A, Tanida M, Uenoyama S, Abe T, Yamaguchi H: Effect of odors on cardiac response patterns and subjective states in a reaction time task, Psychologica 51:74-82, 1992.

92.   Louis M, Kowalski SD: Use of aromatherapy with hospice patients to decrease pain, anxiety, and depression and to promote an increased sense of well-being, Am J Hospice Palliative Care 19(6):381-386, 2002.

93.   Simpson WF, Coady RC, Osowski EE, Bode DS: The effect of aromatherapy on exercise performance, Kinesiology On-Line.09.22, 2001.

94.   Andersen HB, Jensen W, Madsbad S et al: Sham-feeding decreases cardiac output in normal subjects, Clin Physiol 12:439-442, 1992.

95.   Grossman E, Oren S, Garavaglia GE, Schmieder R, Messerli FH. Disparate hemodynamic and sympathoadrenergic responses to isometric and mental stress in essential hypertension, Am J Cardiol 64:42-44, 1989.

96.   Bunker SJ, Colquhoun DM, Esler MD et al: Stress and coronary heart disease: psychosocial risk factors, Med J Aust 178:272-276, 2003.

97.   Khawaja IS, Feinstein RE: Cardiovascular effects of selective serotonin reuptake inhibitors and other novel antidepressants, Heart Dis 5: 153-160, 2003.

98.   Sudakov KV, Uryvaev YV, Petrov GA: Odogenic change of blood coagulation in humans, Integrat Physiologic Behav Sci 33:3:150-154, 1999.

99.   Blau JN, Solomon F: Smell and other sensory disturbances in migraine, J Neurol 232:275-276, 1985.

100. Hirsch AR, Kang C: The effect of inhaling green apple fragrance to reduce the severity of migraine: a pilot study, Headache Quarterly 9:159-163, 1998.

101. Shim C, Williams, Jr. MH: Effect of odors in asthma, Am J Med 80: 18-22, 1986.

102. Miller CS. Chemical sensitivity: symptom, syndrome or mechanism for disease? Toxicology 111:69-86, 1996.

103. Ross PM, Whysner J, Covello VT et al: Olfaction and symptoms in the multiple chemical sensitivities syndrome, Prevent Med 28:467-480, 1999.

104. Stimpfl T, Nasel B, Nasel C et al: Concentration of 1,8-cineol in human blood during prolonged inhalation, Chem Senses 20(3):349-350, 1995.

105. Olowe SA, Ransome-Kuti O: The risk of jaundice in glucose-6-phosphate dehydrogenase deficient babies exposed to menthol, Acta Paediatr Scand 69:341-345, 1980.

106. Jori A, Bianchetti A, Prestini PE: Effect of essential oils on drug metabolism, Biochem Pharmacol 18(9):2081-2085, 1969.

107. DeGroot AC: Airborne allergic contact dermatitis from tea tree oil, Contact Dermatitis 35:304-305, 1996.

108. Bridges B: Fragrances and health (letter), Environ Health Perspect 107:A340, 1999.

CHAPTER 19

The Effects of Music Therapy in Cardiac Healthcare

Suzanne B. Hanser, EdD

Susan E. Mandel, MEd

"I just went to bed and I listened to that tape. And I let it work. Breathing into your heart is difficult because all the memories flood back and there are many of them. And when you go from the heart to the soul, that, I think, touched me in a spot... I don't know if I'd ever been to that place before, that deeply, that comfortably, that quietly. And when it was over I was relaxed... I took the whole feeling into a beautiful sleep. I have never felt so rested in my entire life. And I've been warm and fuzzy inside ever since. Nothing ever got through to me like this."

This quotation is from 72-year-old Eve, 5 months after undergoing triple coronary artery bypass surgery. During her initial music therapy session, Eve described the anxiety she felt during her hospitalization. She went home and implemented a strategy of utmost simplicity, listening to music prescribed by the music therapist. The therapist instructed Eve to breathe into her heart and to imagine beautiful places while she listened to the music. This resulted in a surprising outcome, 12 hours of a restful night's sleep and continuing "warm and fuzzy" effects for some time to come. At the end of her fourth and last music therapy session, while listening to music, Eve imagined walking across a footbridge to a huge bush of fragrant lilacs, and stated, "spring smell . . . new beginning . . . new life." At the conclusion of this session, she commented, "My journey is just beginning. I'm on my way." Several months after her music therapy sessions, she reported that she had never had such low blood-pressure readings before her "epiphany," as she calls her first experience, breathing with the music and letting it take her to a wondrous place. She stated that she no longer feels "roiling anxiety in my ribcage" and notes that "everything will go the way it's going to go."

This chapter is about music therapy, an established profession with national organizations around the world and a growing body of research literature to support its applications. It presents an overview of the discipline of music therapy and describes techniques that music therapists use with patients who have various forms of cardiac disease. It focuses on music-facilitated mind-body techniques indicated for ameliorating symptoms caused by stress or disequilibrium. It also discusses how nurses, physicians, other health practitioners and family caregivers may use music to help patients relax, distract themselves from pain, anxiety, or depression and enhance the quality of their lives.

INTRODUCTION TO MUSIC THERAPY

Music therapy has been defined as "a systematic process of intervention wherein the therapist helps the client to promote health, using music experiences and the relationships that develop through them as dynamic forces of change."[1] Some would cite biblical David's soothing Saul with the lyre as an ancient form of music therapy. Shamans and healers of many cultures have used music in their rituals and healing practices from ancient times.[2] In today's medical and health maintenance institutions, music therapists function as part of a team that assists patients with symptoms and coping mechanisms while developing the creative and competent parts of the person. Music therapy is included in many departments of integrative medicine and offers mind-body techniques designed to introduce positive thoughts, familiar images, pleasant associations, cheerful memories, peaceful mood, and enjoyable feelings. Listening to music may alone bring about an automatic change in mood. A pleasant memory or association may come to mind immediately and flood the listener with wonderful thoughts. Breathtaking images of places far and wide may also be elicited in the imagination of the listener. The effects may be profound relaxation, a peak experience of joy, or a depth of understanding or insight. It is up to the music therapist with knowledge of and input from the individual patient to select the most appropriate music and guide the individual to the most successful outcome.

Engaging in a more active music therapy experience gives many a sense of competence, control, comfort, and general well-being. Mastering beautiful music is a goal that people often see as unobtainable. Music therapists involve people in an aesthetically pleasing music activity through success-oriented techniques, whereby they contribute to the musical performance or composition by adding their note or sound, phrase or melody, drum beat or more sophisticated accompaniment. They participate at whatever level they are capable and gain a sense of positive self-efficacy or esteem. Music therapists are adept at presenting opportunities for participants to improvise, perform, sing, move to, or talk about music, which is especially meaningful or appropriate for their unique needs. They may work individually, in dyads, or in groups. Patients may experience music with family members of all ages when it is important to promote a sense of unity or support, or they may prefer to make or hear music all alone to engender a more solitary mood of peace and comfort.

A qualified music therapist must be board-certified in the United States and must have completed a degree from an approved program, performed a clinical internship, passed the National Board Certification Examination, and participated in continuing education. The American Music Therapy Association provides standards of practice, a code of ethics, competency-based models of practice, and guidelines for the approval of educational training programs and clinical internships.[3] The World Federation of Music Therapy supports music therapists across the globe with information and resources on professional associations, clinical practice, and publications.[4]

Music therapists assess the needs of their clients, determine their musical background and preferences, set goals and objectives consistent with the treatment plan, implement the indicated research-based protocols, and evaluate the impact of music therapy. They use all styles and genres of music, as appropriate, and may introduce any musical selection, instrument, song, improvisation, or experience. They apply techniques of composition or songwriting for people who want to express themselves in new and creative ways. They use music instruction to rehabilitate or compensate, as with the person who learns to play the recorder to enhance breath control or physically weak patients who state that they always wanted to learn to play an instrument. Music therapists are able to identify and adapt suitable instruments, such as a guitar tuned to open chords, which allows free strumming without any need to position the fingers on the fingerboard. They also use specialized protocols, such as guided imagery through music,[5] music-facilitated stress reduction,[6] and music-assisted relaxation and imagery.[7]

MUSIC RESEARCH IN CARDIAC CARE

After experiencing his third myocardial infarction (MI), Jim enrolled in a research experiment designed to determine whether music therapy in addition to cardiac rehabilitation could reduce stress more effectively than cardiac rehabilitation alone. Jim is a 65-year-old patient with diabetes who had undergone coronary artery bypass surgery 8 years earlier. He acknowledged that he was "really bummed out" after his last attack because he has actively maintained healthy lifestyle changes during this period, including full participation in unmonitored cardiac rehabilitation. Jim stated that he tried to put his concern "in a closet and shut the door." During music therapy sessions, Jim learned how to use music-assisted relaxation and imagery (MARI) to reduce every day stress at home. He continued listening to the prescribed music regularly and frequently. He said he wanted to "saturate myself with calming music for 2 weeks." He reported feeling much better, committed to continuing his music listening regimen to maintain good health. He practices replaying his preferred music in his head when actual recordings are not available.

Research has shown that, for a large number of cardiac patients like Jim, listening to music improves psychosocial, physiological, emotional, and overall health status. In fact, nurses, physicians, and surgeons have observed that the act of listening to music by itself is extremely helpful to many of their patients. They have contributed considerable experimental research to the body of literature.

ACUTE MYOCARDIAL INFARCTION

Patients recovering from acute myocardial infarction (AMI) have experienced reduced heart and respiratory rates as well as state anxiety accompanied by greater myocardial oxygen demand after listening to 20 minutes of music. These effects were significantly different than a control group. In addition, 1 hour after listening to music, patients maintained their reduced anxiety and heart and respiratory rates.[8] These results replicated similar findings of an earlier investigation.[9] In another study, patients who presented with AMI listened to 22 minutes of three classic compositions by Bach, Beethoven, and Debussy daily over 3 days of hospitalization. In comparison to a control group, those who listened to this music significantly reduced their reported anxiety.[10] Another experimental investigation compared music listening with a control group and also a relaxation practice for AMI patients. The music condition consisted of a relaxation exercise followed by listening to 20 minutes of one of three cassette tapes developed by the experimenter. The relaxation condition involved the same induction, a quiet environment, a comfortable body posture, repeating a word or sound, and a passive approach to intruding thoughts. These groups were comparable in reducing stress, anxiety, heart rate, and cardiac complications while raising peripheral temperature. These changes were significantly better than those observed in the control group.[11]

All of these significant effects notably occurred after patients listened to one or a few short selections of music that were not of their choice. Thus it is interesting that a study of the influence of an advice and relaxation audiotape that used a music tape of the patient's choice as a comparison condition found that both types of tapes were equally effective to improve anxiety and quality of life for AMI patients.[12]

Joan is a 72-year-old patient who attended her first music therapy for stress management session 2 months after experiencing an AMI. Joan underwent angioplasty and stent placement 5 weeks before her first music therapy session, and a second stent placement 1 month after her first music therapy session. She described herself as "highstrung" but did not think that "anything bad was going to happen to me." Joan reported enjoying violin music and following her first music therapy session, began listening to recorded music (Kobialka, "Timeless Motion") for 1 hour daily in the afternoon. At the conclusion of her third and final music therapy session, Joan described experiencing a white light, smelling flowers, and being accompanied by a figure in a white robe in "God's meadow," remarking that "music soothes the soul." Although she noted that she needs constant activity ("I only sit in a chair that moves,") Joan stated that she now plans to sit quietly and listen to her music daily in the afternoon.

One year after her music therapy treatment, Joan wrote a note to the music therapist; stating: "I'm listening to Mr. Kobialka's tape as I write. His music soothes my soul. If only everyone could understand what a wonderful part music can play in one's life. I can't read notes or play a musical instrument, yet I love music. My body just seems to unwind as I listen. You were a great help to me, teaching how music therapy can keep you calm and accept what life brings."

CORONARY ARTERY BYPASS GRAFT AND OTHER PROCEDURES

The music interventions studied in patients who have undergone coronary artery bypass graft (CABG) surgery have been more involved (see Chapter 27). Postsurgical patients listened to their choice of five musical tapes, or watched a 30-minute videocassette of peaceful scenes accompanied by music, or experienced 30 minutes of undisturbed rest. The music listening group reported significantly less pain than the resting group, and the video group reported significantly improved sleep as compared with the control group.[13] A related study found significant changes in mood for the patients who listened to music, although a generalized relaxation response was evident for patients in all three conditions.[14]

In response to the ill effects of noise annoyance for CABG patients, an investigation was undertaken to evaluate a compact disc blending ocean wave sounds with pieces of Mozart, Beethoven and Donizetti. Noise annoyance was, indeed, lower during the 15 minutes of music listening. During the first postoperative day, both heart rate and systolic blood pressure were also reduced. In this quasi-experimental repeated-measures design, all patients enjoyed listening to the music.[15] It is interesting that, in another study, ocean sounds alone enhanced sleep depth, awakening, returning to sleep, sleep quality, and a total evaluation of sleep in CABG patients.[16]

Another group of investigators researched the effects of guided imagery along with music. Randomly assigned patients undergoing a variety of cardiac surgical procedures listened to a music and imagery tape twice before surgery and twice after surgery. They heard music only during the induction of anesthesia and in the recovery room. Patient reports of anxiety and pain on visual analogue scales and their length of hospital stay were significantly lower for those in the imagery with music group as opposed to the control group.[17]

One study of taped suggestions versus music versus a blank tape via headphones involved CABG patients listening to one of these intraoperatively and postoperatively. The music was "Dreamflight II" by Herb Ernst, and it was also the background music for the suggestion tapes. Researchers found no differences between the conditions on hospital stay, narcotic use, or nurse ratings of progress or anxiety, depression, activities of daily living, and cardiac symptomatology. Unfortunately, the investigators did not evaluate whether the patients preferred listening to this music.[18]

While patients awaited cardiac catheterization, their anxieties were significantly reduced through listening to music. Heart rate and systolic blood pressure were significantly lower in those who heard music while these measures increased in control subjects.[19] In a different study, an increased sense of control and relaxation were accompanied by decreased anxiety.[20]

In fact, none of the experiments involving cardiac surgery patients reviewed here took patients' preferences into account in designing a music program. Given this limitation, it is surprising to find the many significant differences that appear in the literature as a function of music listening. It seems reasonable to conclude that if investigator-selected music has an impact, then music selected by the patient and administered by a music therapist who is trained to assess, observe and provide live music experiences should expect even greater effects.

Yet, music listening also has its limits. In a study of pain during chest tube removal after cardiac surgery, listening to self-selected music did not affect the patients' pain in comparison to listening to white noise or to nothing at all. Most patients did, however, report that they enjoyed hearing the music.[21] Although only a single study, this finding is somewhat consistent with a metaanalysis of music in medical and dental settings which reports that music listening is generally more effective with chronic pain than with acute and severe pain.[22]

Elton is a 77-year-old patient who began attending music therapy for stress management sessions 5 months after his second double coronary artery bypass graft surgery, aortic valve repair, and subsequent hospitalization for an aneurysm. Elton stated, "I can't get myself together" and complained of panic attacks, depression, and sleep apnea. Elton discussed his anxiety about how he would die: "I'm afraid to fall asleep and never wake up." Elton described the relaxation music and imagery tape that he received during his heart surgery as "mournful."

During Elton's first session, the music therapist incorporated recorded light jazz music by Kenny G. Elton reported a diminished stress level from 10 to 1.5 (on a scale of 0 to 10) from start to conclusion of the session. He stated that he experienced dancing images. While strumming the Omnichord to a waltz rhythm, Elton described ballroom dancing movements.

Elton listened to a specially-designed music and imagery tape twice daily. He stated that music therapy is "the best therapy you can get." Elton reported sleeping regularly through the night since listening to the music. At the end of four sessions, Elton also reported that his panic attacks were "cooling down." He noted that he listens to music in conjunction with using an inhaler to ease his breathing difficulty. He also uses music and imagery to reduce leg pain.

CORONARY CARE UNITS

Symphonic music paired with nature sounds was effective in reducing blood pressure, respiratory rate, and psychologic distress in cardiac patients who required bed rest.[23] But other research in coronary care units yield inconsistent results for music listening. One investigation by a music therapist used music previously found in preliminary studies and years of clinical experience to evoke positive moods in patients with little energy. Patients had some choices in musical styles, and this meticulous selection may have contributed to findings that heart rate, anxiety, and depression were significantly reduced while toleration of pain was also improved.[5] Other researchers confirm decreased heart rates[24] and reductions in diastolic and systolic blood pressure for these patients.[25,26] However, light classic investigator-selected music was not effective in aiding patients' anxieties.[27] A choice of music by Halpern, classic-instrumental, or country western music was equally effective as white noise or uninterrupted rest in reducing anxiety in coronary care patients.[28] Clearly, proper care in selecting music must be a part of every research experiment designed to determine the efficacy of music listening.

Bea was far more anxious than her husband who was being treated for coronary artery disease on the coronary care unit. She became extremely agitated when she learned that her husband, Carl, would require bypass surgery. She was concerned that she would not be able to care for herself without him at home, and this compounded her worries about his health and longevity. Now, with the prospect of surgery, she was despondent and cried uncontrollably.

The music therapist entered Carl's hospital room to find him arguing vociferously with his wife. She asked them about the problem and the couple agreed that something had to be done about the anxious state that both patient and wife were experiencing. She asked them about their musical taste and learned that they enjoyed hearing the dance music that was popular when they were dating.

On her next visit, Bea brought in some of their favorite music. Bea and Carl agreed to listen to these recordings before interacting about anything else. After hearing a Benny Goodman song, they laughed and reminisced about dancing until early morning. They embraced and cried in each other's arms. They promised each other to think about the music that was so symbolic of their love whenever stress or anxiety intervened and to begin every conversation with the smile that accompanied that memory.

Carl's surgery went well and Bea reminded herself of their relationship and their music whenever she felt panicky.

Pediatric Cardiac Care

Music therapists have an important role in the pediatric cardiac care setting. In the intensive care unit, music therapy offers distraction, quality of life, and a sense of normalcy to children and families. Singing is a way to motivate children to enhance deep breathing and breath control. For transplant patients, music provides meaningful, successful activities. Music experiences focus on abilities, not disabilities, and offer a creative way to communicate and express feelings. Even the dying child benefits from passive music activities that provide peace and comfort.[29]

Katie was a 13-year-old and had been interested in music before her heart transplant. After her transplant, in isolation, she relished every opportunity to acquire new musical abilities and display them whenever she could. She learned to play the recorder and the keyboard and improvised on the xylophone. Katie pursued her interest in learning music many months later upon her return to school. Two years after her transplant she wrote: "Music therapy really helped me after my transplant. Even though I played the piano and the recorder beforehand, the music helped me become more relaxed. For a couple of days after going to the cardiac ward I would only walk to the bathroom in the isolation room and back. But after I started playing these musical instruments and others, I felt stronger and started to move around outside my room to other places like the playroom."[29]

CARDIAC REHABILITATION

Cardiac rehabilitation programs provide progressive cardiac services from prevention to rehabilitation in inpatient and outpatient settings. Cardiac rehabilitation incorporates structured, monitored exercise and education to help patients develop habits to enjoy a healthy life. In one setting, preferred music had a tendency to decrease perceived exertion, improve mood, and lessen the perceived passage of time in four patients with cardiovascular disease who undertook a cardiac rehabilitation exercise program.[30]

In another setting, the music therapy for stress management program in cardiac rehabilitation exists in the outpatient clinics at two different hospital sites. The program is funded jointly by the hospital's administration and grant support for research. The program's music therapy services are provided contractually. The second author, Susan E. Mandel, describes the music therapy program currently under investigation at Lake Hospital System in Ohio.

A review of patient records from two outpatient clinics revealed that 63% of the patients enrolled in monitored exercise (Phase II) cardiac rehabilitation were identified with stress as a risk factor during their initial evaluations. Additional patients recognized the impact of stress on their well-being during their participation in rehabilitation sessions. With this high incidence of stress as a risk factor for cardiovascular disease in mind, clinical trials of the music therapy for stress management program were developed.

In the small group or individual music therapy sessions, live and taped music are used in combination with verbal discussion to encourage expression of feelings and to reduce anxiety. Patients describe a variety of stressful issues in their lives. These issues may be related to chronic health problems or other situations. Music may be suggested by the music therapist or requested by the patient or family member. Music therapy techniques for verbal self-expression included song lyric writing, interpretation of song lyrics, and identification of song lyrics or titles, which suggest stressors and coping techniques. Patients also express themselves nonverbally through improvisation on the Q-chord (Suzuki), which is an instrument used for accompaniment, and/or hand drums. Sessions conclude with a MARI session. MARI is the music therapist's systematic application of music, cued relaxation techniques, and verbally guided imagery to facilitate the patient's relaxation response. A variety of music, relaxation techniques, and imagery are combined, based on the patient's expressed or observed needs and preferences. The live MARI experience is individually taped for the patient's personal use.

Sue previously attended music therapy for stress management sessions along with cardiac rehabilitation after bypass surgery 2 years earlier. At that time, Sue stated that she experienced angina and increased fibromyalgia pain with stress. Sue listed the angina, pain, stress at work, and lack of rest at home as her main stressors in rank order. During a music therapy session, Sue stated that although she had a will to live, she was "no good to anyone" at that time and felt "on the edge all the time." Sue did not return for music therapy until 2 years later.

Sue, at age 50, began cardiac rehabilitation once again, to treat unstable angina. During her music therapy assessment, Sue revealed her lifetime history of stress-related problems. She also acknowledged her anxiety related to angina, which recurs two to three times weekly. Sue expressed a desire to resume playing "worshipful" piano music. Sue remarked that her leisure time activities are limited by her pain and fatigue. She stated that her life ended at the time of her bypass surgery and that she simplified her life to the point of having "no life."

During the third music therapy session, Sue stated that she listens to her MARI tape on most nights and places a walkman and headset beside her bed as "the key" to her regular listening. Sue noted that listening to the MARI tape helps her to cope with insomnia and "gives [her] strength" to deal with fibromyalgia pain.

Sue stated that she had begun to play hymns on her home keyboard for a few minutes at a time, and she recognized that the absence of music in her life had been difficult for her. The music therapist sang "Amazing Grace" and observed that Sue seemed to withhold her emotional response to the music. Sue expressed that the music was "too much," explaining that she has felt emotionally blocked for 11 years since her father's death. Sue stated that in that past she had written prayers beginning with a Psalm and then recited a Psalm. When asked to continue verbally composing a prayer, she requested a pen and paper. As the music therapist played a recorded version of "Amazing Grace," she wrote: "Thank you Lord that when you seem distant I can know that it is I who have moved away and not you."

During a subsequent music therapy session, the music therapist recorded relaxation suggestions that begin with the feet and move upward through the body. Sue later reported that listening to this MARI tape is highly effective in helping her cope with recent pain associated with foot neuropathy resulting from diabetes. During her final music therapy session, Sue stated that "energy and how to spend it is a big thing... Stress takes a lot of energy. Relaxation is a slowing down." The patient noted that she previously thought that she was "going to go until I dropped" and that she is making changes "while it's still a choice." Sue stated that she is journaling, listening to her own spiritual music, and feeling "more peace."

CONCLUSION

This chapter has presented research, clinical cases, and techniques to demonstrate how music therapy may be integrated successfully into cardiac healthcare. It is a privilege to work with the creative power within every person to make music and respond to music. As Ralph Waldo Emerson stated, "no man ever forgot the visitations of that power to his heart and brain, which created all things anew, which was the dawn in him of music."[31]

REFERENCES

1. Bruscia KE: Defining music therapy, Gilsum, PA, 1998, Barcelona, 20.
2. Davis WB, Gfeller KE, Thaut MH: An introduction to music therapy, ed 2, Boston, 1999, McGraw-Hill.
3. AMTA Member Sourcebook, Silver Spring, Md., 2002, American Music Therapy Association.
4. *http://www.musictherapyworld.de*
5. Bonny HL, West M: Music listening for intensive coronary care units, Music Ther 3:4, 1983.
6. Hanser SB: Music therapy to reduce anxiety, agitation, and depression, Nurs Home Med 10:286, 1996.
7. Mandel SE: Music for wellness: music therapy for stress management in a rehabilitation program, Music Ther Persp 14:38, 1996.
8. White JM: Effects of relaxing music on cardiac autonomic balance and anxiety after acute myocardial infarction, Am J Crit Care 8:220, 1999.
9. White JM: Music therapy: an intervention to reduce anxiety in the myocardial infarction patient, Clin Nurs Spec 6:58, 1992.
10. Bolwerk CL: Effects of relaxing music on state anxiety in myocardial infarction patients, Crit Care Nurs Q 13:63, 1990.
11. Guzzetta CE: Effects of relaxation and music therapy on patients in a coronary care unit with presumptive acute myocardial infarction, Heart Lung 18:609, 1989.
12. Lewin RJ, Thompson DR, Elton RA: Trial of the effects of an advice and relaxation tape given within the first 24 hours of admission to hospital with acute myocardial infarction, Int J Cardiol 82:107, 2002.
13. Zimmerman L, Neiveen J, Barnason S, Schmaderer M: The effects of music interventions on postoperative pain and sleep in coronary artery bypass graft (CABG) patients, Schoolarly Inq Nurs Prac 10:153, 1996.
14. Barnason S, Neiveen J, Zimmerman L: The effects of music interventions on anxiety in the patient after coronary artery bypass grafting, Heart Lung 24:124, 1995.
15. Byers JF, Smyth KA: Effect of a music intervention on noise annoyance, heart rate, and blood pressure in cardiac surgery patients, Am J Crit Care 6:183, 1997.
16. Williamson JW: The effects of ocean sounds on sleep after coronary artery bypass graft surgery, Am J Crit Care 1:91, 1992.
17. Tusek DL, Cwynar R, Cosgrove DM: Effect of guided imager on length of stay, pain and anxiety in cardiac surgery patients, J Cardiovasc Mgmt 20:22, 1999.
18. Blankfield RP, Zyzanski SJ, Flocke SA et al: Taped therapeutic suggestions and taped music as adjuncts in the care of coronary-artery-bypass patients, Am J Clin Hypertens 37:32, 1995.
19. Hamel WJ: The effects of music intervention on anxiety in the patient waiting for cardiac catheterization, Intensive Crit Care Nurs 17:279, 2001.

20. Robichaud-Ekstrand S: The influence of music in coronary heart disease (CHD) patients' relaxation levels, J Cardiopulm Rehab 19:304, 1999.
21. Broscious SK: Music: an intervention for pain during chest tube removal after open heart surgery, Am J Crit Care 8:410, 1999.
22. Standley JM: Music research in medical/dental treatment: an update of a prior meta-analysis. In Furman CE, editor: Effectiveness of music therapy procedures: documentation of research and clinical practice, Silver Spring, Md., 1996, National Association for Music Therapy.
23. Cadigan ME, Caruso NA, Haldeman SM et al: The effects of music on cardiac patients on bed rest, Prog Cardiovasc Nurs 16:5, 2001.
24. Davis-Rollan C, Cunningham SG: Physiologic responses of coronary care patients to selected music, Heart Lung 16:370, 1987.
25. Webster C: Relaxation, music and cardiology: the physiological and psychological consequences of their interrelation, Aust and Occup Ther J 20:9, 1973.
26. Stone SK, Rusk F, Chambers A: The effects of music therapy on critically ill patients in the intensive care setting, Heart Lung 18:291, 1989.
27. Eliot D: The effects of music and muscle relaxation on patient anxiety in a coronary care unit, Heart Lung 23:27, 1994.
28. Zimmerman LM, Pierson MA, Marker J: Effects of music on patient anxiety in coronary care units, Heart & Lung 17:560, 1988.
29. Dun B: A different beat: music therapy in children's cardiac care, Mus Ther Persp 13:35, 1995.
30. Macnay SK: The influence of preferred music on the perceived exertion, mood, and time estimation scores of patients participating in a cardiac rehabilitation exercise program, Mus Ther Persp 13:91, 1995.
31. Emerson RW: Essay V: love. In Ralph Waldo Emerson essays, Boston, 1980, Houghton Mifflin, 175.

CHAPTER 20

Reflexology

Donald A. Bisson, RRPr

R eflexology is a focused pressure technique, usually directed at the feet or hands. It is based on the premise that zones and reflexes on different parts of the body correspond to and are relative to all parts, organs, and glands of the entire body. Stimulation of these reflex areas in disease assists the body to correct, strengthen, and reinforce itself by returning to a state of homeostasis. In Asian cultures, reflexologists sometimes use electrical or mechanical devices. However, these are discouraged in North America.

The oldest documentation of the use of reflexology is found in Egypt in an ancient Egyptian papyrus depicting medical practitioners treating the hands and feet of their patients. Dr. William Fitzgerald (1872-1942) is credited with being the father of modern reflexology. His studies brought about the development and practice of reflexology in the United States.

Dr. Fitzgerald's studies found that pressure in the nose, mouth, throat, tongue, hands, feet, joints, and so on deadened definite areas of sensation and relieved pain. This led to the discovery of *zone therapy*. In the early years, Dr. Fitzgerald worked mainly on the hands. Later, the feet became very popular as a site for treatment, and over the years, hand reflexology was not used as much. In his book on zone therapy in 1917, Dr. Fitzgerald spoke about working on the palmar surface of the hand for any pains in the back of the body, and working on the dorsal of the fingers for any problems on the anterior part of the body. The distal joints were squeezed, then the medial, and then the proximal joints by clasping the hands. Another remarkable hand reflex that Dr. Fitzgerald found was for helping morning sickness in pregnancy or an upset stomach. This was by working the first and second zones on the backs of the hands with deep pressure and also the palmar surface of the wrist and forearm. He spoke further of finger squeezing for eye and ear troubles. Thyroid problems were also helped, he said, by pressing upon the joints of the thumb, first and second fingers.

Dr. Joe Shelby Riley learned zone therapy from Dr. Fitzgerald. Dr. Riley carried the techniques out to finer points and made the first detailed diagrams and drawings of the reflex points and zones located on the feet and hands.

In this chapter, reflexology as an alternative medicine is described, and the experiences with this technique to treat cardiovascular disease are reviewed.

THEORY OF REFLEXOLOGY

Manipulating specific reflexes removes stress and activates a parasympathetic response in the body to enable the blockages to be released by a physiological change in the body. With stress removed and circulation enhanced, the body is allowed to return to a state of homeostasis.

CONVENTIONAL ZONE THEORY

Conventional zone theory (CZT) is the foundation of hand and foot reflexology. An understanding of the CZT and its relationship to the body is essential to understanding reflexology and its applications (Figure 20-1).

Zones are a system for organizing relationships between various parts, glands, and organs of the body and of the reflexes. Ten equal longitudinal or vertical zones run the length of the body from the tips of the toes and the tips of the fingers to the top of the head. From the dividing centerline of the body, five zones exist on the right side of the body and five zones on the left side. These zones are numbered one to five from the medial side (inside) to the lateral side (outside). Each finger and toe falls into one of the five zones (e.g., the left thumb is in the same zone as the left big toe, zone 1).

The reflexes are considered to pass all the way through the body within the same zones. The same reflex, for example, can be found on the front and also on the back of the body, and on the top and on the bottom of the hand or foot. This is the three-dimensional aspect of the zones.

Reflexology zones are not to be confused with acupuncture and acupressure meridians.

Pressure applied to any part of a zone will affect the entire zone. Every part, gland, or organ of the body represented in a particular zone can be stimulated by working any reflex in that same zone. This is the foundation of zone theory and foot reflexology.

In addition to the longitudinal zones of CZT, reflexology also uses the transverse zones (horizontal zones) on the body and feet or hands. The purpose is to help fix the image of the body by mapping it onto the hands or feet in a proper perspective and location. The following four transverse zone lines are commonly used: transverse pelvic line, transverse waistline, transverse diaphragm line, and transverse neck line.

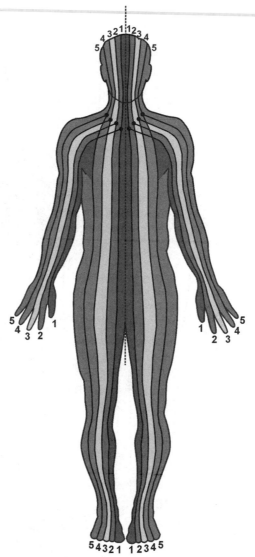

Fig 20-1. Longitudinal zones of the body.

INTERNAL ORGANS AND THE 3D ASPECT OF THE BODY

It is important to remember that internal organs lay on top, over, behind, between, and against each other in every possible configuration. The reflexes on the hands and feet that correspond to the parts, organs and glands, overlap as well. For example, the kidney reflexes on the foot chart (Figure 20-2) or hand chart (Figure 20-3) overlap with many other reflexes, just as the kidneys overlap other organs and parts of the body when viewed from the back or the front.

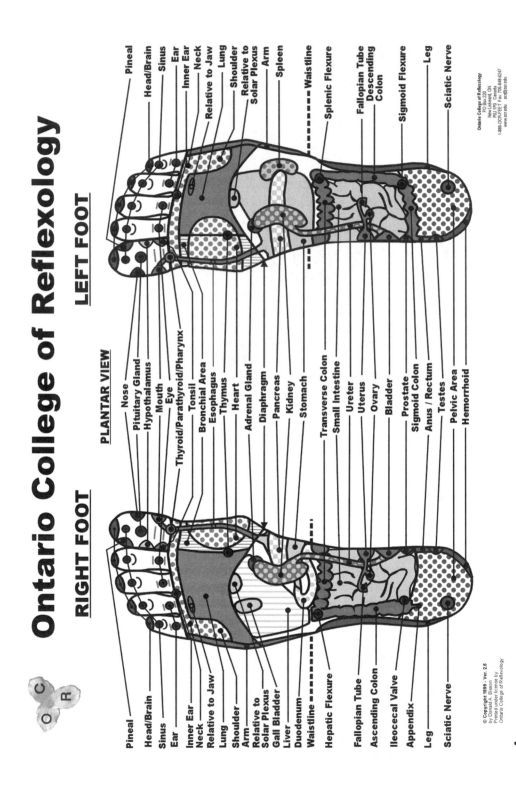

Fig 20-2. Foot reflexology chart.

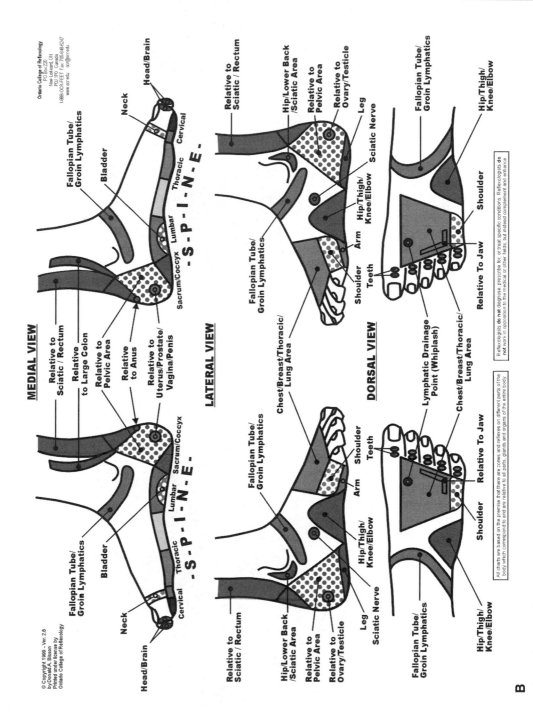

MEDIAL VIEW

LATERAL VIEW

DORSAL VIEW

© Copyright 1999 - Ver. 2.5
by Donald A. Bisson
Printed under license by
Ontario College of Reflexology

Ontario College of Reflexology
P.O. Box 220
New Liskeard, ON
P0J 1P0 Canada
1-888-OCR-FEET Fax: 705-648-6247
www.ocr.edu ocr@ocr.edu

Reflexologists **do not** diagnose, prescribe for, or treat specific conditions. Reflexologists do not work in opposition to the medical or other fields, but instead complement and enhance

All charts are based on the premise that there are zones and reflexes on different parts of the body which correspond to and are relative to all parts, glands and organs of the entire body.

B

Fig 20-2. Foot reflexology chart.

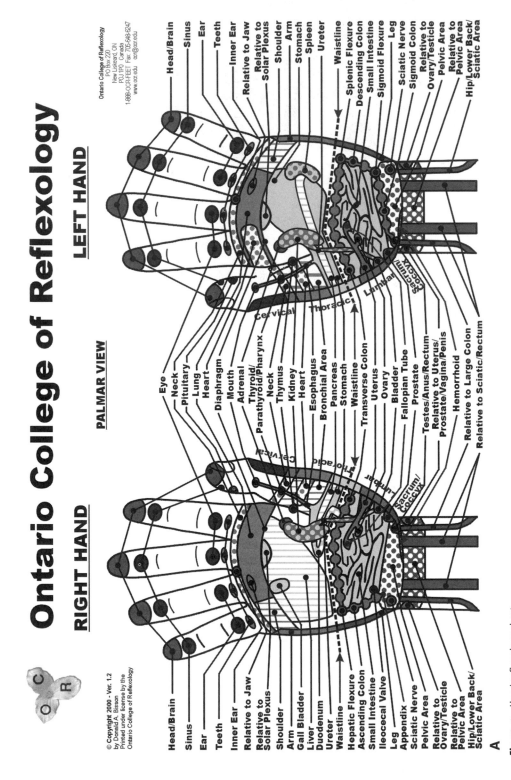

Fig 20-3. Hand reflexology chart.

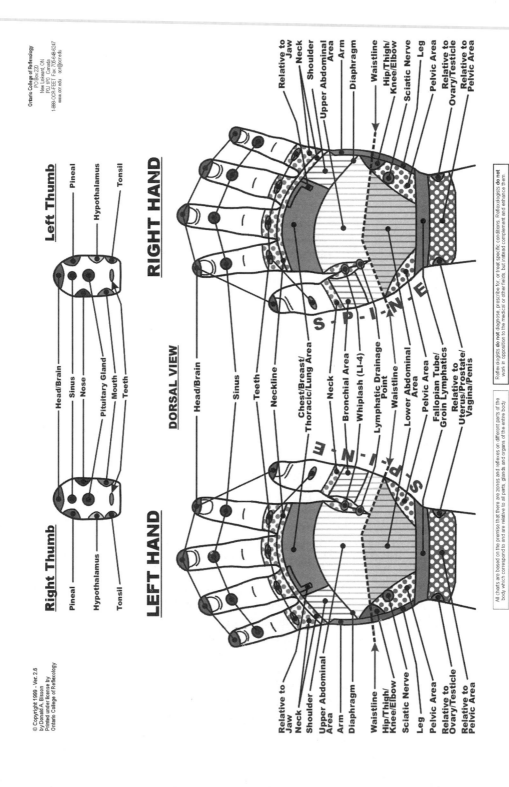

Left Thumb

Pineal — Pineal

Hypothalamus — Hypothalamus

Tonsil — Tonsil

Ontario College of Reflexology
PO Box 220
New Liskeard, ON
P0J 1P0 Canada
1-888-OCR-FEET Fax: 705-648-6247
www.ocr.edu   ocr@ocr.edu

RIGHT HAND

Relative to Jaw
Neck
Shoulder
Upper Abdominal Area
Arm
Diaphragm
Waistline
Hip/Thigh/Knee/Elbow
Sciatic Nerve
Leg
Pelvic Area
Relative to Ovary/Testicle
Relative to Pelvic Area

S - P - I - N - E

Right Thumb

Head/Brain
Sinus
Nose
Pituitary Gland
Mouth
Teeth

Pineal
Hypothalamus
Tonsil

DORSAL VIEW

LEFT HAND

Head/Brain
Sinus
Teeth
Neckline
Chest/Breast/Thoracic/Lung Area
Neck
Bronchial Area
Whiplash (LI-4)
Lymphatic Drainage Point
Waistline
Lower Abdominal Area
Pelvic Area
Fallopian Tube/Groin Lymphatics
Relative to Uterus/Prostate/Vagina/Penis

S - P - I - N - E

Relative to Jaw
Neck
Shoulder
Upper Abdominal Area
Arm
Diaphragm
Waistline
Hip/Thigh/Knee/Elbow
Sciatic Nerve
Leg
Pelvic Area
Relative to Ovary/Testicle
Relative to Pelvic Area

All charts are based on the premise that there are zones and reflexes on different parts of the body which correspond to and are relative to all parts, glands and organs of the entire body

Reflexologists **do not** diagnose, prescribe for, or treat specific conditions. Reflexologists **do not** work in opposition to the medical or other fields, but instead complement and enhance them

B

Fig 20-3. Hand reflexology chart.

Exception to The Zone Theory

The basic concept of the CZT is that the right foot or hand represents the right side of the body and that the left foot or hand corresponds to the left side. However, with the central nervous system, the right half of the brain controls the left side of the body and vice versa. In any disorders or problems that affect the brain or the central nervous system, a reflexologist will emphasize the reflexes or areas of the disorder on the opposite hand or foot. For example, the brain reflexes will be worked on the left foot or hand for strokes that caused paralysis on the right side of the body.

Zone-Related Referral Areas

Many people assume that the hands and feet are the only areas to which reflexology can be applied. However, reflexes exist throughout the 10 zones of the body, and they may present unlikely relationships within these zones. For example, a zonal relationship exists between the eyes and the kidneys. Because both lie in the same zone, working the kidney reflexes can affect the eyes.

Areas around a foot injury should be avoided and not be worked. An alternate part of the body in the same zone should be worked instead. For example, the arm is a reflection of the leg, the hand to the foot, the wrist to the ankle, and so forth. If any part of the arm is injured, the corresponding part of the leg can be worked and vice versa. Common problems such as varicose veins and phlebitis in the legs can be helped by working the same general areas on the arms.

This approach can be used to find other referral areas. Identify which zone(s) an injury has occurred in and trace it to the referral area. Tenderness in the referral area will usually help the reflexologist to find it.

Referral areas can give insights into the problem areas by showing the relationships to the areas in the same zone(s) that may be at the root of the problem. For example, a shoulder problem may be caused by a hip problem because the shoulder lies in the same zone as the hip.

Negative Feedback Loop

A reflexology session always begins on the right foot or hand and finishes on the left foot or hand. In addition, the reflexes on both feet or hands are worked from the bottom of the foot or hand at the heel, up to the top of the foot or hand and the toes or fingers.

To aid the body's self-regulation, a highly complex and integrated communication control system or network is required. This type of network is called a *feedback control loop*. Different networks in the body control diverse functions such as blood carbon dioxide levels, temperature, and heart and respiratory rates. Homeostatic control mechanisms are categorized as *negative* or *positive feedback loops*. The most important and numerous of the homeostatic control mechanisms involve negative feedback loops.

Negative feedback loops are *stabilizing mechanisms* (i.e., maintaining homeostasis of blood carbon dioxide [CO_2] concentration). As blood carbon dioxide increases, the respiratory rate increases to permit carbon dioxide to exit the body in increased amounts through expired air. Without this homeostatic mechanism, body carbon-dioxide levels rapidly rise to toxic levels, and death results.

The blood circulation loop is from the left side of the body to the right side. Fresh oxygenated blood enters the aorta from the left side of the body, into the body cells. Venous blood with carbon dioxide enters the vena cava on the right side of the body. By beginning a reflexology session on the right foot, we are helping to boost the loop by pushing venous or deoxygenated blood into the heart/lungs so that fresh oxygenated blood will be available to the body cells. The same reason applies for the direction that we work on the foot—*from the bottom of the foot upward* to bolster the homeostatic loop.

BENEFITS OF REFLEXOLOGY

Reflexology demonstrates the following four main benefits: (1) relaxation with the removal of stress; (2) enhances circulation; (3) assists the body to normalize metabolism; (4) complements all other healing modalities.

When the reflexes are stimulated, the body's natural electrical energy works along the nervous system to clear any blockages in the corresponding zones.

A reflexology session seems to break up deposits (felt as a sandy or gritty area under the skin), which may interfere with the flow of the body's electrical energy in the nervous system.

Reflexologists do not diagnose medical conditions unless qualified to do so. The only diagnosis made is a tender reflex. Nor are any blockages in any area of the body diagnosed other than in the reflexes. A reflexologist will refer to other qualified health care practitioners when services required are outside the reflexologist's scope of practice.

Similarly, reflexologists do not prescribe medications unless qualified to do so. The therapeutic intervention is limited to working the reflexes.

CARDIOVASCULAR INDICATIONS

A reflexologist will refer to other qualified healthcare practitioners when services are required outside the reflexologist's scope of practice. However, reflexology can assist in patient healing for some cardiovascular conditions.

Pressure on the corresponding reflexes should generally be decreased for heart problems, blood problems, and hypertension. A reflexology session may cause unnecessary strain in the cardiovascular system because of increased circulation. It may adversely affect patients with pacemakers and artificial heart valves.

Reflexology has been used as an adjunct therapy to relieve the symptoms of angina pectoris, to reduce the size of an aortic aneurysm, to normalize irregular heartbeats, and to treat hypertension and hypotension.

Reflexologists should refrain from working on the reflexes related to a thrombus or embolism. A reflexologist can work on reflexes to a stroke-affected area or after a myocardial infarction if the blood clot has been stabilized.

Much of the benefits from reflexology come from the relief of tension and stress. In hypertension and hypotension, reflexology may also have effects related to favorable action on hemodynamics and blood volume.

ADVERSE EFFECTS

The adverse effects of reflexology are minor and include fatigue (increase in parasympathetic activity), headache, nausea, increased perspiration, and diarrhea.

CREDENTIALING AND TRAINING

No legal or formal credentialing exists for reflexology. Certification is provided by certain educational institutions specializing in this training. A patient should look for a therapist who is certified and/or registered as a qualified reflexologist by a reputable organization. Also select a reflexologist who presents a professional attitude.

Many schools of reflexology exist to provide adequate training; their requirements range from 100 to 1000 hours of instruction. Look for a school that is established and, if possible, is recognized by the local governing body.

CONCLUSION

Reflexology is a form of manipulative therapy that has been used to treat various cardiovascular and noncardiovascular disorders. As with many alternative medical approaches, good scientific studies to confirm its benefit are lacking. It does appear to relieve stress, which in turn could reduce or minimize physical symptoms. At best, reflexology should only be used as an adjunct to proven therapies in the treatment of disease. The profession of reflexology also needs to be regulated.

SUGGESTED READINGS

Byers DC: Better health with foot reflexology, St. Petersburg, Florida, 1983, Ingham.

Carter M: Healing yourself with foot reflexology, New York, 1983, Prentice Hall.

Carter M: Helping yourself with foot reflexology, West Nyack, NY, 1969, Parker.

Fitzgerald WH, Bowers EF: Zone therapy, Columbus, Ohio, 1917, IW Long.

Issel C: Reflexology: art, science, and history, Sacramento, Calif., 1990, New
    Frontier.
Kunz K, Kunz B: Hand and foot reflexology: a self-help guide, New York,
    1984, Prentice Hall.
Marquardt H: Reflexotherapy of the feet, Stuttgart, 2000, Thieme.

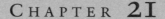

CHAPTER **21**

Sauna as a Therapeutic Option for Cardiovascular Disease

Yen Nguyen, MD

Nauman Naseer, MD

William H. Frishman, MD

T he basic sauna is a wood-paneled room with wooden platforms and a rock-filled electric heater. Humidity is created in the sauna by throwing water onto the heated rocks. The recommended humidity is between 40 to 70 grams of water vapor per kilogram of air.[1,2] The temperature should be between 80° C and 100° C at the level of the bather's head and 30° C at floor level.[2] A sauna should have adequate ventilation, with the air changed three to eight times per hour.[2] The size of the sauna should also be at least 3 m² to allow proper balance of heat, humidity and adequate ventilation. Bathing time is usually between 5 to 20 minutes, depending on an individual's tolerance of high temperature and humidity, separated by cooling-off periods and the oral intake of fluids.[3,4]

Although the sauna has been used for thousands of years, only recently have there been studies of this bathing method as a therapeutic modality for cardiovascular diseases. There have been reviews of the physiologic effects (Table 21-1) and benefits and risks (Table 21-2) of sauna bathing,[4-10] but this chapter will focus mainly on the available literature regarding sauna bathing as a therapeutic option for cardiovascular diseases.

HEMODYNAMIC EFFECTS OF SAUNA

The physiologic responses of the cardiovascular system have been extensively described and reviewed previously.[3-7,11,12] The increase in skin temperature in the sauna causes an increase in skin blood flow from 5% to 10% to 50% to 70% of cardiac output (CO).[12] CO is increased from 5 to 6 L/minute

Table **21-1**   PHYSIOLOGIC EFFECTS OF SAUNA BATHING

Physiologic Effect	Changes	References
Skin temperature	Increased up to 40° C	6
Sweating	Increased rate of secretion from 0.6 to 1.0 kg/hr at 80° to 90° C.	1,6
Blood flow to skin	Increased from 5% to 10% of cardiac output to 50% to 70% of cardiac output (from 0.5 to 7 L/minute)	12
Blood flow to internal organs	Renal blood flow is decreased by 0.4 L/minute	12
	Splanchnic blood flow is decreased by 0.6 L/minute	12
Blood flow to muscles	Blood flow to muscles is decreased by 0.2 L/minute	12
Heart rate	Increased up to 100 beat/minute during moderate sauna bathing in accustomed subjects	6, 13-16, 21
	Increased up to 150 beats/minute during intense sauna bathing or in unaccustomed subjects	16
Cardiac output	Increased from 5-6 L/minute to 9 to 10 L/minute	7, 12
Cardiac stroke volume	Unchanged	7
Systolic blood pressure	Unchanged	8, 15, 16, 21
	Or decreased by 8 to 31 mm Hg	9, 13, 14
	Or increased by 9 to 21 mm Hg	16
Diastolic blood pressure	Unchanged	13
	Or decreased by 6 to 39 mm Hg	8, 9, 14-16

Modified from Hannuksela M, Ellahham S: Benefits and risks of sauna bathing, Am J Med 110:118-126, 2001.

Table **21-2**   BENEFITS AND RISKS OF SAUNA BATHING

Benefits	Risks
• Sauna bathing lowers mean blood pressure in hypertensive patients[14,19,20] • Improves vascular endothelial function in patients with coronary risk factors[17] • Improves hemodynamics in patients with chronic congestive heart failure[15,18] • Improves lung function in patients with obstructive pulmonary diseases[30,31] • Alleviate pain in patients with rheumatic disease[32,33]	• Alcohol consumption while sauna bathing increases risk of hypotension, fainting, and arrhythmias[34] • Patients with severe aortic stenosis, unstable angina pectoris, recent myocardial infarction, decompensated heart failure, and cardiac arrhythmias are at increased risk of hypotension, fainting, reinfarction, arrhythmias, and sudden death[4,10,24] • Hypotension in patients on beta-blocker and short-acting nitroglycerin while sauna bathing[27,28,29]

to 9 to 10 L/minute.[7,12] Stroke volume remains the same and heart rate is increased to between 100 to 150 bpm, depending on level of tolerance to thermal exposure.[6,11] Renal blood flow is reduced by 0.4 L/minute, and blood flow to muscles is reduced by 0.2 L/minute.[12] The reported changes in diastolic and systolic blood pressure have been variable. Diastolic blood pressure has been reported to be unchanged[13] as well as being reduced by 6 to 39 mm Hg.[8,9,14-16] Systolic blood pressure has been reported as unchanged[8,15,16] as well as being reduced by 8 to 31 mm Hg[9,13,14] or being increased by 9 to 21 mm Hg.[16] For a more complete review, see Hannuksela et al.[5]

SAUNA AND ENDOTHELIAL DYSFUNCTION

Imamura et al reported improvement in vascular endothelial function in patients with coronary risk factors.[17] To assess endothelial function, researchers using high-resolution ultrasound measured brachial artery diameter at rest, during reactive hyperemia (flow-mediated endothelium-dependent dilation [FMD]), again at rest, and after sublingual nitroglycerin administration (endothelium-independent vasodilation [NTG]). Twenty-five men with at least one coronary risk factor (age group 38 ± 7 years) and 10 healthy men (control group 35 ± 8 years) were given sauna therapy once a day for 2 weeks. The sauna used was an infrared-ray dry sauna bath. The FMD measurement was significantly impaired in the risk group in comparison to the control group (4.0 ± 1.7% vs. 8.2 ± 2.7%, $p < 0.0001$), whereas the NTG measurement was similar (18.7 ± 4.2% vs. 20.4 ± 5.1%). Two weeks of sauna therapy significantly improved the FMD measurement in the risk group (4.0 ± 1.7% to 5.8 ± 1.3%, $p < 0.001$). In contrast, the NTG measurement did not change after 2 weeks of sauna therapy (18.7 ± 4.2% to 18.1 ± 4.1%).

In a study by Kihara et al, 20 patients (aged 62 ± 15 years) with New York Heart Association (NYHA) functional class II or III congestive heart failure (CHF) were treated in a dry sauna at 60°C for 15 minutes and then were kept on bed rest with a blanket for 30 minutes, daily for 2 weeks.[18] Ten control patients with CHF, matched for age, gender, and NYHA functional class, were placed on a bed in a temperature-controlled (24°C) room for 45 minutes. The FMD after 2 weeks of sauna treatment significantly increased from the baseline value, whereas NTG-induced dilation did not. This was associated with an improvement in clinical symptoms in 17 of the 20 actively-treated patients.

ROLE OF SAUNA IN CARDIOVASCULAR DISEASES

HYPERTENSION

Various studies by Winterfeld et al reported the positive effects of regular sauna bathing in hypertensive patients.[14,19,20] The mean blood pressure was lowered from 162/110 to 139/92 mm Hg in 180 hypertensive patients with other heart conditions.[14] In one study, a group of 47 individuals with hypertension were observed during a 3-month period of biweekly sauna bathing.[20] Mean blood pressure was lowered from 166/110 to 143/92 mm Hg. Winterfeld et al also did a long-term comparison (1- and 3-year follow-up) between sauna therapy and kinesiotherapy (running and swimming).[19] This study found that regular sauna therapy had a positive effect on the regulation of blood pressure and hemodynamics in patients with hypertension only, and was similar to that of kinesiotherapy in hypertensive patients with coronary heart disease.

CORONARY HEART DISEASE

Various investigators have studied the safety of sauna for coronary heart disease and have found that sauna bathing is well tolerated by patients with stable disease.[10,13,21]

In a recent study, Giannetti et al looked at whether sauna use caused myocardial ischemia in patients with coronary artery disease because of prior case reports of adverse cardiac events linked to sauna.[13] They reported that sauna bathing caused no clinical symptoms in 16 patients with coronary heart disease, although heart rate was increased by an average of $32 \pm 20\%$ ($p < 0.001$) and systolic blood pressure increased by an average of $13 \pm 6\%$ ($p < 0.001$). Reversible ischemia, as demonstrated by scintigraphy, occurred in 14 of 15 patients who completed the study, compared to baseline. Sauna-induced perfusion defects were highly correlated with exercise-induced scores ($p < 0.001$). No incidents of arrhythmia, electrocardiographic changes, or any other symptoms were observed. The study concluded that in patients with stable coronary artery disease, sauna use is clinically well tolerated but is associated with scintigraphically demonstrated myocardial ischemia.

As mentioned earlier, Winterfeld et al also reported positive effects on the regulation of blood pressure and hemodynamics in patients with coronary heart disease.[14,19]

CONGESTIVE HEART FAILURE

Significant studies from Kagoshima University in Japan have demonstrated that sauna can be a legitimate therapy for patients with CHF.

Tei et al first demonstrated that hemodynamics improve after sauna bathing in patients with chronic CHF.[15] In this study, 34 patients (mean age 54 ± 14 years; two in NYHA class II, 19 in NYHA class III, and 13 in NYHA class IV) were monitored before, during, and after a 15-minute sauna bath at 60° C. During the sauna bath, oxygen consumption increased almost 20% ($p < 0.01$); the heart rate increased almost 25% from 77 to 97 beats per minute (bpm, $p < 0.01$); the average systolic pressure was not significantly changed; the average diastolic blood pressure decreased from 78 to 70 mm ($p < 0.05$); and systemic vascular resistance decreased significantly ($p < 0.01$). However, 30 minutes after the sauna bath, the increase in oxygen consumption from control was not statistically significant, and the heart rate only increased an average of 5 bpm ($p < 0.01$), whereas diastolic blood pressure and systemic vascular resistance remained reduced to even lower values than those seen during sauna in comparison to the controls. The mean pulmonary artery, mean pulmonary capillary wedge, and mean right atrial pressures also decreased significantly during (p <0.05) and after (p <0.01) a sauna bath. The investigators concluded that hemodynamics improve after a sauna bath in patients with chronic CHF because of the reduction of both cardiac preload and afterload.[15]

In a study of hamsters, Ikeda et al hypothesized that the improvement observed with sauna therapy was mediated through modulation of arterial endothelial nitric oxide synthase.[22] In their study, hamsters were given sauna therapy at 39° C for 15 minutes followed by therapy at 30° C for 20 minutes once daily for 4 weeks. The control group hamsters were placed in the sauna system switched off at 24° C for 35 minutes. At the end of the study, hamsters in both the experimental and the control groups were sacrificed, and the endothelial nitric oxide synthase expression was quantified using immuno-histochemistry, a Western blot analysis, and reverse transcription polymerase chain reaction assay. The study proved that repeated sauna therapy up-regulates endothelial nitric oxide synthase expression.[22] In a subsequent study, Ikeda et al demonstrated that sauna therapy improves survival in cardiomyopathic hamsters with CHF.[23] Sixty cardiomyopathic hamsters were divided into two groups, one that received sauna therapy and the other a control group. The hamsters in the sauna group underwent therapy in an infrared ray dry sauna system at 39° C, followed by 30° C for 20 minutes, once a day, five times per week. The hamsters in the control group were placed in the same sauna system switched off for 35 minutes at room temperature (24° C) also once a day, five times a week. The results showed that the survival rate in the sauna group was significantly higher than that in the control group (p <0.01).[23]

As discussed earlier, Kihara et al performed a study on human subjects with chronic CHF and found that sauna treatment improved vascular endothelial function, thus resulting in improvement in cardiac function and clinical symptoms.[18] In the study, clinical symptoms improved in 17 of 20 patients, as indicated by a survey after two weeks of therapy. Vascular endothelial function, assessed by high-resolution ultrasound to measure the diameter of the brachial artery, also improved significantly from baseline value. The concentration of plasma brain natriuretic peptide was decreased after 2 weeks of therapy, thus suggesting an improvement in cardiac function. In addition, a significant correlation between the change in FMD measurement and the percent improvement in brain natriuretic peptide concentrations was found in the sauna-treated group. In contrast, none of the variables changed at the 2-week interval in the nontreated group.[18]

RISK OF SAUNA BATHING

Because of the heat load that one receives in a sauna, it is generally not recommended for patients with unstable angina, recent myocardial infarction, decompensated heart failure, cardiac arrhythmia, uncontrolled hypertension, and severe aortic stenosis.[4,10,24]

Although no adverse effect from sauna exists for healthy people receiving beta-blockers,[25,26] reports have described a hypotensive reaction caused by sauna use in hypertensive patients receiving beta-blockade[27,28] or short-acting nitroglycerin[29] because of the hypotensive effects of these medications. However, hypertensive patients receiving calcium channel blockers,[28] digitalis,[10] or diuretics[10] tolerate sauna well. Alcohol consumption during sauna bathing increases the risk of hypotension, arrhythmia, and sudden death.

CONCLUSION

Sauna bathing has the potential to be an effective therapeutic option for patients with hypertension or CHF, as well as for patients with known coronary heart disease risk factors. The common mechanism of action is improvement in vascular endothelial function, which results in a reduced cardiac preload and afterload. Although some studies suggest that the cardiovascular improvement happens at the level of genetic expression, whether this improvement is permanent or short-lived once sauna therapy is discontinued is unknown. It would also be interesting to know—provided that the improvement is permanent—if some of the damage on the cardiovascular system can be reversed by sauna therapy. Sauna bathing can be risky in patients who receive alcohol, beta-blockade, and nitrates.

Although one cannot dispute the demonstrated positive results of sauna therapy in patients with heart disease, ignoring possible confounding variables is difficult because a double-blinded placebo-controlled study in humans would be impossible to carry out with this type of therapy.

REFERENCES

1. Leppaluoto J: Human thermoregulation in sauna. Ann Clin Res 20: 240-243, 1988.
2. Helamaa E, Aikas E: The secret of good "loyly." Ann Clin Res 20: 224-229, 1988.
3. Kauppinen K: Facts and fables about the sauna. Ann NY Acad Sci 813:654-662, 1997.
4. Keast M, Adamo K: The Finnish sauna bath and its use in patients with cardiovascular disease. J Cardiopulmonary Rehabil 20:225-230, 2000.
5. Hannuksela M, Ellahham S. Benefits and risks of sauna bathing. Am J Med 110:118-126, 2001.
6. Hasan J, Karvonen MJ, Piironen P: Special review, part I: physiological effects of extreme heat as studied in the Finnish "sauna" bath. Am J Phys Med 45:296-314, 1966.
7. Hasan J, Karvonen MJ, Piironen P. Special Review. part II: physiological effects of extreme heat as studied in the Finnish "sauna" bath. Am J Phys Med 46:1226-1246, 1967.
8. Leppaluoto J, Tuominen M, Vaananen A et al: Some cardiovascular and metabolic effects of repeated sauna bathing. Acta Physiol Scand 128: 77-81, 1986.

9. Davies H: Cardiovascular effects of the sauna. Am J Phys Med 54: 178-185, 1975.

10. Eisalo A, Luurila OJ: The Finnish sauna bath and cardiovascular diseases. Ann Clin Res 20:267-270, 1988.

11. Kauppinen K, Vuori I: Man in the sauna. Ann Clin Res 18:173-185, 1986.

12. Vuori I: Sauna bather's circulation. Ann Clin Res 20:249-256, 1988.

13. Giannetti N, Juneau M, Arsenault A et al: Sauna-induced myocardial ischemia in patients with coronary artery disease. Am J Med 107: 228-233, 1999.

14. Winterfeld HJ, Siewert J, Strangfeld D et al: Effects of sauna therapy on patients with coronary heart disease with hypertension after bypass operation, after heart aneurysm operation and essential hypertension. Z Gesamte Inn Med 48:247-250, 1993.

15. Tei C, Horikiri Y, Park JC et al: Acute hemodynamic improvement by thermal vasodilation in congestive heart failure. Circulation 91: 2582-2590, 1995.

16. Kukkonen-Harjula K, Oja P, Laustiola K et al: Haemodynamic and hormonal responses to heat exposure in a Finnish sauna bath. Eur J Appl Physiol 58:543-550, 1989.

17. Imamura M, Biro S, Yoshifuku S et al: Repeated thermal therapy improves impaired vascular endothelial function in patients with coronary risk factors. J Am Coll Cardiol 38:1083-1088, 2001.

18. Kihara T, Biro S, Imamura M et al: Repeated sauna treatment improves vascular endothelial and cardiac function in patients with chronic heart failure. J Am Coll Cardiol 39:754-759, 2002.

19. Winterfeld HJ, Siewert H, Strangfeld D et al: Application of sauna for long-term treatment of hypertension in cardiovascular disorders: a comparison with kinesiotherapy. Schweiz Rundsch Med Prax 81: 1016-1020, 1992.

20. Siewert C, Siewert H, Winterfeld HJ et al: Changes of central and peripheral hemodynamics during isometric and dynamic exercise in hypertensive patients before and after regular sauna therapy. Z Kardiol 83:652-657, 1994.

21. Luurila OJ: Arrhythmias and other cardiovascular responses during Finnish sauna and exercise testing in healthy men and post-myocardial infarction patients. Acta Medica Scandinavica 64:1-60, 1980.

22. Ikeda Y, Biro S, Kamogawa Y et al: Repeated thermal therapy upregulates arterial endothelial nitric oxide synthase expression in Syrian golden hamsters. Jpn Circ J 65:434-438, 2001.

23. Ikeda Y, Biro S, Kamogawa Y et al: Effect of repeated sauna therapy on survival in TO-2 cardiomyopathic hamsters with heart failure. Am J Cardiol 90:343-345, 2002.

24. Luurila OJ: The sauna and the heart. J Intern Med 231:319-320, 1992.

25. Kukkonen-Harjula K, Oja P, Vuori I et al: Effects of atenolol, scopolamine and their combination on healthy men in Finnish sauna baths. Eur J Appl Physiol 69:10-15, 1994.

26. Vanakoski J, Seppala T: Effects of a Finnish sauna on the pharmacokinetics and hemodynamic actions of propranolol and captopril in healthy volunteers. Eur J Clin Pharmacol 48:133-137, 1995.

27. Iisalo E, Kanto J, Pihlajamaki K: Effects of propranolol and guanethidine of circulatory adaptation in the Finnish sauna. Ann Clin Res 1:251-255, 1969.

28. Luurila OJ, Kohvakka A, Sundberg S: Comparison of blood pressure response to heat stress in sauna in young hypertensive patients treated with atenolol and diltiazem. Am J Cardiol 64:97-99, 1989.

29. Barkve TF, Langseth-Manrique K, Bredensen J et al: Increased uptake of transdermal glyceryl trinitrate during physical exercise and during high ambient temperature. Am Heart J 112:537-541, 1986.

30. Laitinen LA, Lindqvist A, Heino M: Lungs and ventilation in sauna. Ann Clin Res 20:244-248, 1988.

31. Cox NJM, Oostendorp GM, Folgering HTM, van Heerwaarden CLA: Sauna to transiently improve pulmonary function in patients with obstructive lung disease. Arch Phys Med Rehabil 70:911-913, 1989.

32. Nurmikko T, Hietaharju A: Effect of exposure to sauna heat on neuropathic and rheumatic pain. Pain 49:43-51, 1992.

33. Isomaki H: The sauna and rheumatic diseases. Ann Clin Res 20: 271-275, 1988.

34. Roine R, Luurila OJ, Suokas A et al: Alcohol and sauna bathing: effects on cardiac rhythm, blood pressure, serum electrolyte and cortisol concentrations. J Intern Med 231:333-338, 1992.

CHAPTER 22

Prayer and Cardiovascular Disease

Jonathan E. E. Yager, MD

Jeffery A. Dusek, PhD

Suzanne W. Crater, RN, ANP-C

Mitchell W. Krucoff, MD

S tudies have shown that over 90% of people believe in God or a higher being.[1,2] Forty percent of Americans weekly attend mosques, synagogues, or churches.[3] When individuals become sick, many turn to prayer for comfort and solace. When caring for the sick, many include prayer.

Prayer has been a part of the human experience since early in history. Although people offer prayers for a myriad of reasons, one of the most consistent across the world's religions is the use of prayer and spiritually based healing practices during times of illness. Not surprisingly, early physicians found their base in religion, where the power of God or deities was considered the true source of healing effects. From Shamanic traditions to Chinese medicine, many healing traditions see tangible remedies such as herbal preparations not as a mechanistic tool for curing disease but as a tool through which the spirit or vital energy qi is released, enhanced, or otherwise made to flow. Even with the development of scientifically based allopathic medicine, prayer continues to be an integral part of the illness and healing experience for many individuals. Early hospitals were run by religious orders, the nursing profession was founded by nuns, and even today, most modern secular hospitals have chapels, chaplains, and services to attend to the spiritual needs of patients and families. Most religious congregations today conduct daily or weekly prayers on behalf of members who are ill, often naming them specifically, regardless of whether the subject is physically amongst the congregation during the prayer or away in a hospital.

Although the supportive nature of prayer is well understood, the direct therapeutic effects are not. Because the vast majority of concept and information about prayer is metaphoric rather than mechanistic, studying prayer as a therapy is a complex endeavor. Testing prayer as a therapy requires rigorous clinical trials. Although the literature in this area is growing, the field is still quite young. Trial designs are maturing; studies are being conducted on multiple diseases; and further investigations are being planned. To date, the quality of prayer trials varies considerably. Many of the earlier studies of prayer and healing have faulty methodology, which allows for justified criticism in interpreting their results, whereas others are quite provocative in their conclusions and challenge established healing paradigms. No prayer study in human subjects has shown a significant and reproducible treatment effect, although epidemiologic data are quite consistent in the indication that spirituality in an individual and in a community is associated with health-related benefits. Perhaps most importantly, no established mechanistic explanations for how prayer might heal exist to date. The very nature of prayer may even transcend modern scientific understanding, and because of this, explanatory models and scientific methodology such as testing the null hypothesis may not be appropriate in prayer trials.[4] However, as a practice that has been ubiquitous to civilization worldwide over the course of human history, the systematic exploration of prayer used for healing purposes and the relevance of these practices to modern health care cannot simply be overlooked.

This chapter introduces studies of prayer and cardiovascular disease. After defining terms and concepts which are paramount to the scientific investigation of prayer, the chapter will describe the major studies that have been conducted or are ongoing with regard to prayer and cardiac disease. We will also address larger systems-related issues with regard to studying prayer, including those related to informed consent and safety.

DEFINITION OF PRAYER

Certain terms and concepts must be defined to discuss studies of prayer. Prayer, in and of itself, can be many things. For some, it is the recitation of specific written passages, the performance of established rituals, or direct contact with another individual who has a connection to a higher power, energy, or intention. For others, it is a spontaneous expression of faith or spirituality without predetermined form. To study "prayer" as a standardized intervention for the purposes of health care, as many qualitative and quantitative aspects as possible must be rigorously defined.[4]

Furthermore, one must recognize that any clinical study cannot attempt or claim to study the effects of prayer *per se*. Families, friends, communities, and medical staff often pray for individuals who are ill, as might the individual by him or herself. Ultimately, given current knowledge, documenting or eliminating prayer for the sick from the hospital or healthcare environment is impossible. Ethically, any attempt to regulate or curtail these spontaneous prayers for recovery simply because an individual is participating in a study is equally problematic. Thus clinical investigations of the therapeutic benefits of prayer can, at best, examine the effects of "supplementary" prayer as a systematic addition to the care environment as a feature of study design.

Studies of prayer as therapy generally have examined a form of prayer called *intercessory prayer*, which has been defined as prayer that calls specifically "for aid to others."[5] Intercessory prayer can have many forms. *Distant healing* prayer, in which the individual or congregation performing the prayers is physically separated from the patient, potentially by thousands of miles, has been studied. Other studies have used direct, hands-on prayer, in which the spiritual healer actually touches the intended beneficiary. A third format includes multiple tiers of prayer, in which one tier prays specifically for a patient while another tier prays for the prayers of the persons praying for the patient. To date, no available data suggest either mechanistic or outcomes insights into differences across these methods, thus again emphasizing the importance of methodologic definition to support the comparability or utility of pooling data across studies.

Other standards that characterize the investigation of all new treatment strategies may also be relevant to the concept of prayer as therapy. Not all individuals who pray may do so with the same conviction, intention, experience, or fervor; thus the efficacy of an individual intercessor may vary. In most traditions, characteristics of prayer offered by an individual may differ from the prayers offered by a congregation. Although doing so may seem odd, one must consider classical issues related to dose response. The frequency and duration of prayers, the actual content of sacred or mystical passages, and whether or not the prayer is said in proximity to the patient or with the patient's awareness, all must be accounted for.

When studies of prayer as therapy are conducted as experiments on human research subjects, many consider the ethical requirements of informed consent and safety absolutely imperative.[5] The equipoise of how or whether simple awareness of prayer studies affects the patients who participate and the ramifications of these considerations on trial design will be considered in greater detail later in this chapter. In fact, most prayer studies conducted to date appear to assume that prayer therapy is safe and carries no untoward side effects. Conceptually, however, in the absence of mechanistic knowledge, it must at least be considered that even a loving healing prayer in some patients, in some illnesses, may cause unintended harm. In fact in many traditions, prayer's highest level of healing achievement is the freeing of the spirit from the body, which in a clinical trial would be identified as death. In some settings, such as incurable cancer trials, this may be a positive endpoint and recognized as such. If such a process is inadvertently engaged in patients struggling to survive a heart attack, however, harm could result. At the current state of early investigation and fundamental mechanistic ignorance, obligations to protect human subjects with safety monitoring and informed consent in study designs bear strong consideration.

PRAYER AS AN INTERVENTION

The design and conduct of any clinical trial is challenging, but few are as challenging as a trial designed to evaluate the efficacy of prayer. Without an accepted scientific basis for the potential effect of prayer on illness, identifying a "biologically plausible" endpoint to study in the trial is difficult. If the selected endpoint is not even relevant to the effects of prayer, study interpretation, especially of negative results, will be difficult. Second, the optimal timing, amount, and duration of prayer as well as optimal prayer methods are unknown, again in large part because of the lack of biologic knowledge on the basis of healing effects of prayer. Thus one might examine irrelevant clinical endpoints or administer an inadequate "dose" of prayer. This is particularly important because studies of prayer can at best look only at incremental benefit over and above whatever healing prayer and intention is ubiquitous in the environment, outside of the study design. Third, documentation of or specific instructions for how and when prayer is administered that supports a consistent study design produces changes in the prayer group's usual practice. This may affect the measurable therapeutic benefit and/or limit the generalizability of the trial results.

All of these considerations may be regarded essentially as key uncontrolled variables. An ideal study design would address each. The goal of the study—to elucidate mechanistic observations or to examine outcomes effects—must be clearly discerned. Although mechanistic knowledge may optimize outcomes studies, they do not depend on mechanistic knowledge *per se*. This notion is evidenced by the use of beta-blockers to reduce death rates after myocardial infarction, which is well proven in outcomes models even though to date the mechanism of this benefit remains elusive. Certain features, such as prayer in the culture at large, may be addressed by randomization. In other cases, relatively arbitrary decisions may need to be made largely from cultural practice or metaphoric beliefs. With due regard for all these issues, one must recognize that only through structured data collection and clinical studies can sufficient knowledge be gained to affect systematically health care practice and the curricula of health care training programs.

CURRENT STATUS OF RANDOMIZED CONTROLLED TRIALS OF PRAYER

Scientific studies of prayer reported in the peer review literature have been conducted over the past 30 years. The vast majority of these trials suffer from a range of design deficiencies, including heterogeneous nomenclature, endpoints of unclear clinical significance, and small sample sizes with inadequate statistical power, thus resulting in mixed and contradictory findings. The heterogeneity of these studies results in an inability to perform useful pooling or to conduct an overall meta-analysis of the published literature. The consistent impression that a measurable treatment benefit associated with prayer may in fact exist may result from a reporting and/or publication bias. Nonetheless, independent reviews and recommendation papers have concluded on a consensus basis that better-designed scientific investigations of prayer were needed and were of scientific and clinical import.[6,7]

Knowing this background, we turn to the first major study of intercessory prayer in cardiac patients, which was conducted by Byrd in 1982 in the

Coronary Care Unit (CCU) at San Francisco General Hospital.[8] Four hundred fifty consecutive patients were approached to participate in this study of intercessory prayer; 393 agreed. The patients were randomized to receive standard CCU care or standard CCU care plus distant intercessory prayer. The prayer intervention consisted of daily prayer for the individual by three to seven born-again Christian intercessors, who only knew the patient's first name and diagnosis. Intercessors were given updates about the patient's general condition and progress, and the prayer intervention lasted for the entire duration of each patient's stay in the CCU. The primary outcome measured was a nonstandardized, nonvalidated global assessment of the CCU stay that considered major complications, procedures, medications, and other interventions. Outcomes were rated as "good," "bad," or "intermediate" and were assessed by an individual who was blinded to the treatment group of the individual. More patients in the prayer group had "good" outcomes than in the standard care group (85% in comparison to 73%), and fewer had a "bad" outcome (14% in comparison to 22%). These differences were statistically significant.

Although numerous critics of this study appropriately note significant limitations of this trial (e.g., the unvalidated composite clinical score makes the clinical importance of the "significant" findings impossible to interpret), Byrd broke through several barriers in conducting a clinical investigation of prayer as a therapeutic intervention. Byrd combined scientific methodology with a blinded, prospective randomized clinical trial design and acknowledged that because prayer from patients, families, and others was not controlled for, he was, in essence, measuring "supplemental" therapeutic prayer, or incremental benefit, not prayer *per se*. This study was an important step in defining the limitations of prayer studies and in properly framing the context for future investigations. Importantly, Byrd also studied prayer not as a replacement to the high technology of standard care, but as an adjunct in addition to standard care. Finally, by publishing these findings in a peer-reviewed journal, Byrd set the stage for serious Western clinicians and scientists in the study of spiritual intervention in patients with heart disease.

The second major trial of intercessory prayer in patients with heart disease was published over 10 years after Byrd's groundbreaking study. In 1999 Harris and colleagues[9] studied more than 1000 patients in the CCU and deliberately borrowed many features from the Byrd study. Patients were randomized to receive standard CCU care with or without an offsite intercessory prayer intervention, and intercessors were given the first name of the patient for whom to pray. In contrast with the earlier study, however, intercessors were not informed of the diagnosis or of the patient's condition, and the prayer intervention that was prescribed by the study was for "a speedy recovery with no complications" and "for anything else that seemed appropriate to them" for a total of 28 days. Two outcome measures were employed. One was the "good" and "bad" outcome scale developed by Byrd. The other was an illness-scoring system called the MAHI (Mid-America Heart Institute) scale, which, although it is more detailed than the Byrd score, was equally unvalidated for clinical relevance.

Study results showed no difference in the Byrd score (i.e., investigators were unable to reproduce the earlier findings). In comparing the unweighted MAHI CCU score, which totaled the number of medications prescribed, procedures performed, and clinical events, the intervention group had 10% fewer "elements" than the control group had. Similarly, in analyzing a weighted score, the prayer group had an 11% improvement in comparison to the standard therapy arm. Both of these values achieved statistical significance, although, as with the Byrd study, the clinical meaning of these results is unclear.

In addition to studying a larger cohort of patients and the attempt to build upon the findings of an earlier study, the landmark feature of the Harris study was that informed consent was not obtained from patients and the CCU staff were not informed that a study was in progress. As explicitly discussed in the report of this trial, the investigators were concerned that knowledge about the study would affect the "spiritual terrain" of the CCU, and/or that patients might feel extra anxiety by worrying that they might *not* be receiving intercessory prayer. The study was reviewed and approved by the institutional review board at the MAHI, which allowed these theoretical concerns to override the use of the traditional informed consent process in the context of the assumption that patients who were either receiving or not receiving the prayer therapy could not have been harmed. This issue remains highly controversial. Furthermore, data from this study provide no insight into the concern that mere awareness of a prayer study might change the outcome of the study.

The third published CCU study involved 800 patients from the Mayo Clinic but tested a somewhat different research hypothesis, specifically asking if 26 weeks of remote prayer therapy initiated at the time of hospital discharge might affect long-term outcome.[10] In this trial, traditional clinical endpoints of death, coronary revascularization, rehospitalization, or an emergency department visit for a cardiac problem were analyzed. Follow-up extended for 6 months after discharge. Patients all gave informed consent to participate in the trial. In comparison to the earlier CCU studies, the specifics of the prayer intervention were not as strictly prescribed. Intercessors were not specifically directed how to pray but were asked to do so at least once per week. The content of the prayer was not predetermined, and in fact the authors acknowledge that a possible limitation in this study was that the "dose" of prayer was not standardized. Although it was conducted as a prospective, randomized study, the Mayo design uniquely stratified randomized treatment relative to risk categories.

Although several trends favored the prayer-treated group, no significant difference was seen between the prayer group and the control group with regard to the predefined clinical endpoints or in a quality of life score. Importantly, however, the trial studied hard endpoints of clear clinical relevance in a thoughtful study design. Two features of the data are notable as potential confounding variables. First, the event rate in the control population was lower than predicted for sample size calculation, meaning that the trends seen could represent a treatment effect underpowered for the cohort enrolled. In addition, patients were enrolled while still in the CCU, while the prayer therapy was not initiated until discharge from the CCU. With the assumption that time is linear in the effect of prayer on healing, this particular intervention may simply have been too late to reduce events in the CCU nor did it minimize post-CCU events.

The fourth published study of prayer in cardiovascular patients was the Monitoring and Actualization of Noetic Trainings (MANTRA) pilot study.[11] In this study offsite prayer was studied in parallel with other intangible ("noetic") modalities, including healing touch, stress relaxation, and imagery. This was conducted at the Veterans Affairs Medical Center in Durham, North Carolina and enrolled 150 male patients with acute coronary syndromes who were scheduled for urgent percutaneous coronary intervention (PCI) for clinical indications. The MANTRA pilot was a prospective, five-way randomized trial comparing the four noetic therapies with a standard care group. In three arms (healing touch, stress relaxation, and imagery) a trained practitioner administered therapy at the bedside before the PCI procedure. The other two-fifths of the patients remained double-blinded, with half receiving offsite prayer intervention and half receiving standard care. Although the MANTRA pilot was designed as a feasibility and safety study, the primary endpoints, like the Mayo Clinic protocol, consisted of standard clinical outcomes during the index hospitalization and mortality out to 6 months. No statistical differences between the groups were found; however, the study was not powered to show efficacy. A 27% absolute reduction of in-hospital complications was observed in the noetic groups overall compared to the standard care group, with the lowest absolute complication rate in-hospital observed in the off-site prayer group. At 6 months, mortality was lowest in the standard care and prayer groups, with a trend toward higher mortality in the three other noetic therapies.

Several features of the MANTRA pilot design were unique in comparison to previous published investigations of distant prayer in patients with heart disease. The male patient cohort was a pure coronary disease population who were being treated in the acute setting and enrolled just before an invasive procedure rather than CCU patients of mixed gender with mixed cardiac pathologies (arrhythmias, heart failure, valvular disease) as in previous trials. Unique descriptors in the study included documentation of patient awareness of nonstudy related prayer on his or her behalf as well as documentation of the pre-PCI presence of family, community members, or hospital chaplains. In the MANTRA pilot nearly 40% of all enrolled patients were aware of someone praying for their recovery outside of the study protocol, and more than two-thirds of patients were visited by family, community, or chaplains before the PCI, thus reinforcing the awareness that clinical trials in this area can examine only incremental benefit over and above what is already a part of the fabric of cultural healing systems in the United States. Finally, the MANTRA pilot prayer intervention arm was unique in its structure compared to previous trials. A total of nine prayer congregations covering a variety of ethnic belief systems (Catholic, Baptist, Fundamentalist, Moravian, Unitarian Christian; Jewish; Buddhist) dwelling across an array of time zones (Nepal, Jerusalem, France, east coast United States, midwest United States) were all provided with the patient's name, age, and illness for each patient assigned to prayer therapy. All prayer groups conducted their prayers wholly in accordance with their ethnic traditions—there were no prescribed instructions from the protocol.

In addition to prayer trials involving cardiac disease, other illnesses have also been studied in prospective randomized trials. Although many of these trials are significantly flawed, we will examine two of the better studies in detail, one trial that studied patients with infertility[12] and one that studied patients with the human immunodeficiency virus (HIV).[13] Both of these highlighted studies are provocative in their approach to trial design, and both provide clinically interpretable results.

The infertility study was conducted under the auspices of Columbia University. Study subjects included 219 women participating in an in-vitro fertilization (IVF) and embryo transfer program in Korea. Women were randomized to receive standard IVF therapy or standard IVF therapy plus a prayer intervention. The intervention method used a two-tiered or "prayer amplification" structure, with one group of intercessors praying directly for the women to have a successful pregnancy, while a second group of intercessors prayed specifically that the prayers of the first group would be answered. The intercessors who prayed directly for the patients received digital photos of the patients for whom they were praying. The primary study endpoint was the presence of a healthy term baby.

Like the staff of the MAHI study mentioned previously, the clinic staff caring for the patients were unaware of the study, and patients did not give informed consent to participate in a clinical trial. As mentioned previously, failure to obtain informed consent remains highly controversial and perhaps borderline unethical.

Interestingly, the results of this study constitute the most striking report of effects of prayer on somatic health. Twice as many women in the prayer group had successful pregnancies (50% as opposed to 26% in the control, which was also the typical success rate for that clinic), which was both highly statistically significant as well as obviously clinically relevant. This study is remarkable for the unique population studied; the unique structure of the prayer intervention; and the dramatic, clinically and statistically significant outcome findings, although to date these findings have not been confirmed.

A second study worthy of mention investigated the role of distant healing for patients with HIV disease. As opposed to most clinical prayer trials in which patients are "assigned" a certain intercessor or groups of intercessors, this trial allowed for a rotation between the patients and those praying for them. The authors designed this specifically to account for any differences in efficacy between intercessors. They chose not to view prayer as a necessarily binary intervention (that a patient would either receive or not receive prayer) but possibly one with varying degrees of intensity. Also, prayers in this trial came from intercessors of multiple different ethnic backgrounds (Christian, Jewish, Buddhist, Shamanic traditions, Native American) as well as other trainings that might or might not be characterized as prayer, such as graduates of bioenergetic and meditative healing schools.

In this trial, informed consent was obtained, but patients and physicians were blinded as to whether the individual was receiving prayer therapy. Intercessors were directed to pray for 1 hour per day for 6 consecutive days, specifically with "an intention for health and well-being." The intervention group spent fewer days in the hospital, had fewer total hospitalizations, had a less severe illness score, and had better mood. They also had fewer AIDS-defining illnesses and fewer outpatient doctor visits. There was no difference in CD4 lymphocyte counts between the two groups. However, concern that the investigators' decision to not correct for multiple comparisons likely improved the chances of finding a positive result remains. As was the case with the infertility trial described previously, these findings have not been replicated.

What makes this trial different from the others is the attention paid to rotating intercessors as well as the intermixture of "prayer" with "energy" or "intentionality" healing modalities in the treatment cohort. Although other trials may have used multiple intercessors or groups of intercessors for any given patient, this was the first to openly acknowledge that not all prayer may have the same "strength." Essentially, through the rotation this model provides a degree of quality control.

The previously mentioned studies illustrate a wide array of approaches as well as a central core of common design elements. All studies used prospectively defined therapies and outcomes, and all used randomized treatment assignments. On the other hand, the patient cohorts selected, the choice of endpoints, the characteristics of prayer intervention, and the overall study quality varied greatly across trials.

The studies also illustrate the important difference between statistical significance and clinical relevance. In spite of the negative results, the Mayo study[10] and MANTRA Pilot[11] used hard, easily reproducible endpoints of death, myocardial infarction, hospitalization, and revascularization. The infertility study[12] followed successful embryo implantations producing healthy term pregnancies, and the HIV study[13] documented healthcare use such as hospitalization and outpatient visits as well as the number of AIDS-defining illnesses and mood scales. Therefore interpreting the clinical relevance of the results is somewhat easier, although all the mechanistic questions remain unanswered by these data. The other CCU studies, on the other hand, report statistically significant differences in composite clinical scores, but because these scores have not been validated, what clinical conclusions can be drawn from the results remains unclear.

FUTURE TRIAL DESIGN AND INFORMED CONSENT

A recently published consensus paper describes recommendations for designing high quality studies of prayer.[5] The authors explore the different components and controversies of prayer research and base their suggestions on the standards of the Consolidated Standards of Reporting Trials (CONSORT) group.[14] It essentially recommends that high-quality prayer research endeavor to systematically define methodology and terminology with endpoints and statistical analyses defined *a priori*. As with other clinical trials, patient selection, randomization, data collection, and blinding are suggested as clinical trial tools that may help cope with an area full of uncontrolled variables and assumptions in the complete absence of mechanistic knowledge.

For both ethics and safety, the consensus group challenges the notion that prayer trials can occur without the informed consent process. In the modern research age of the Health Insurance Portability and Accountability Act (HIPAA), protected health information may not be collected without patient consent or justified waivers. One of the major arguments used in the trials that did waive informed consent is the assumption that receiving prayer therapy can do no harm. Because this idea has not yet been scientifically established, however, that argument may not carry sufficient justification for waiving informed consent. Additionally, some patients may not wish to participate in a study of prayer, may have concerns about being assigned to a group not receiving prayer, or may not wish to be prayed for by individuals of religious backgrounds other than their own. Ethically, respect for such individual preferences in addition to the potential safety issues is seen as far outweighing the theoretical concern that awareness of the study might change the spiritual landscape.

Equally important to discussing those aspects that make for a high quality clinical trial of intercessory prayer, it is imperative to consider aspects of healing prayer that may not be suitable for clinical study. Questions such as whether a deity exists or which religious modality has the best prayer or other flashpoint issues could be considered outside of the healthcare agenda. Similarly, studies that seek to replace advanced modern technological care are less likely to be considered relevant in comparison to studies that incorporate prayer as an adjunct, especially in cardiac patients. Finally, there is simply no way to test whether prayer works because of the widespread presence of healing prayer across most cultural traditions around the world.

Although healing prayer is an ancient tradition widely practiced throughout the world, the scientific literature in this area is still very young at best.[15,16] No understanding of the mechanism in how or whether prayer actually affects somatic healing has been reached. With the development and use of standardized nomenclature and definitions and clinically meaningful endpoints, study models might ultimately support the imputation of mechanistic insights and advance the field overall.

CONCLUSION

As the current literature stands today, considering concrete clinical recommendations for the use of prayer as therapy for cardiovascular disease—or any changes in practice along these lines at this time—is still premature. The trials presented above provide some intriguing "food for thought." Preliminary, suggestive findings and the intuitive appeal of a healthcare system that combines the finest of modern technology with systematic attention to the rest of the human being certainly supports the notion that further study in this area appears warranted. In addition to attention to the scientific basis of robust study designs, the purpose and intention of study in this area must be carefully scrutinized. The mission of such science cannot be to advance philosophies or defend metaphorical claims or preferences. Study designs in this area should be focused on the advance of health care, with data that yield the basis for mechanistic insights, educational curricula, practitioner certification standards and practice guidelines, or redefinition of healthcare roles commensurate with a modern—if somewhat enlightened—vision of evidence-based medical practice in cardiovascular care.

REFERENCES

1. King DE, Bushwick B: Beliefs and attitudes of hospital inpatients about faith healing and prayer, J Fam Pract 39:349-352, 1994.

2. Maugans TA, Wadland WC: Religion and family medicine: a survey of physicians and patients, J Fam Pract 32:210-213, 1991.

3. Princeton Religion Research Center: Religion in America. Princeton, NJ, 1996, The Gallop Poll. Cited in Koenig HG: Spirituality in patient care, 2002, Templeton Foundation Press.

4. Dusek JA, Astin JA, Hibberd PL, Krucoff MW: Healing prayer outcomes studies: consensus Recommendations, Alt Therap Health Med 9:A44-A53, 2003.

5. Halperin EC: Should academic medical centers conduct clinical trials of the efficacy of intercessory prayer? Acad Med 76:791-797, 2001.

6. Astin JA, Harkness E, Ernst E: The efficacy of "distant healing": a systematic review of randomized trials, Ann Intern Med 132:903-910, 2000.

7. American College of Cardiology Clinical Expert Consensus Document on Alternative Medicine. J Am Coll Cardiol. In press.

8. Byrd RC: Positive therapeutic effects of intercessory prayer in a coronary care unit population, Southern Med J 81:826-829, 1988.

9. Harris WS, Gowda M, Kolb JW et al: A randomized, controlled trial of the effects of remote, intercessory prayer on outcomes in patients admitted to the coronary care unit, Arch Intern Med 159(19):2273-2278, 1999.

10. Aviles JM, Whelan E, Hernke DA et al: Intercessory prayer and cardiovascular disease progression in a coronary care unit population: a randomized controlled trial, Mayo Clin Proc 76:1192-1198, 2001.

11. Krucoff MW, Crater SW, Green CL et al: Integrative noetic therapies as adjuncts to percutaneous intervention during unstable coronary syndromes: Monitoring and Actualization of Noetic Training (MANTRA) feasibility pilot, Am Heart J 142:760-67, 2001.

12. Kwang YC, Wirth DP, Lobo RA. Does prayer influence the success of in vitro fertilization-embryo transfer? report of a masked, randomized trial, J Reproduct Med 46(9):781-787, 2001.

13. Sicher F, Targ E, Moore D, Smith H: A randomized double-blind study of the effect of distant healing in a population with advanced AIDS, Western J Med 169:356-363, 1998.

14. Begg C, Cho M, Eastwood S et al: Improving the quality of reporting of randomized controlled trials: the CONSORT statement, JAMA 276(8):637-639, 1996.
15. Groopman J: God at the bedside. N Engl J Med 350:1176-1178, 2004.
16. McCaffrey AM, Eisenberg DM, Legedza ATR, et al: Prayer for health concerns. Arch Intern Med 164:858-862, 2004.

CHAPTER **23**

Animal-Assisted Therapy and Cardiovascular Disease

Andrew I. Wolff, MD

William H. Frishman, MD

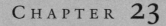

A s it has become clear that psychosocial factors play an integral role in health, particularly in influencing the progression and severity of disease, scientists have begun to identify these factors in hopes of uncovering methods to control them and thus affect the course of an illness. Some of these studies have led to the hypothesis that the presence of an animal companion is one such psychosocial factor.

This hypothesis is grounded in the significance of animals to people's lives. The household pet plays such a large role in people's lives that 99% of pet owners consider their pets to be part of their families.[1] Pets are present in 60% of households,[2] and a survey of 500 former pet-owners now in a hospital setting showed that the "thing" they missed most was their pets.[3] In the last half of the twentieth century, scientists began to wonder whether these animals have an actual physiologic effect on people's health and if so, whether they can be used as an integral part of patient care.

This interest has spurred the emergence of animal assisted therapy (AAT) in hospitals and institutions across the country. In 1996 the Delta Society, which is a leading international group that studies the human-animal bond defined AAT as a "goal-directed intervention in which an animal meeting specific criteria is an integral part of the treatment process... AAT is designed to promote improvement in human physical, social, emotional, and/or cognitive functioning. AAT is provided in a variety of settings and may be group or individual in nature."[4]

This chapter will examine the emergence of AAT and focus on its effects on the cardiovascular system.

GENERAL HISTORY OF PET-ASSISTED THERAPY

The earliest documented evidence of AAT dates back to the ninth century, when animals were used to help care for handicapped people in Belgium.[5] In 1792, physicians at a mental hospital in Great Britain used animals to help their patients learn to care for a living creature.[6] One hundred years ago, Florence Nightingale wrote that pets are perfect companions for patients that are confined to a hospital with a chronic illness.[7] More recently in the US in 1940, hospitals established programs in which veterans interacted with animals in recovery units.[8] Presently, many healthcare establishments have programs with visiting and/or residential animals.

BENEFICIAL EFFECTS OF PETS

When used in the correct situation, AAT therapy is able to aid many aspects of a person's well being. The participants of AAT should be carefully screened to ensure a positive interaction. The patient should not have a negative attitude toward animals and should be in a suitable medical condition in order to prevent any harm developing from the interaction. Katcher and Friedmann articulated nine beneficial conditions for humans that pets can help develop: "providing companionship, pleasurable activity, facilitating exercise, play and laughter, being something to care for, a source of consistency, allowing feelings of security, being a comfort to touch, and pleasurable to watch."[9] The presence of a pet provides a pleasant, nonevaluative external focus, promotes feelings of safety, and furnishes a source of comfort.[10]

AAT also improves physical health in several ways. A 10-month prospective study examined the changes induced by the acquisition of a pet in 71 subjects.[11] Dog owners were shown to have a highly significant reduction in minor health problems from the first month of ownership, with sustained effects up to the tenth month; cat owners initially reported these changes and returned to baseline after 6 months. Pet owners are shown to make fewer visits to the physician as well.[12] Many other physical and social benefits have been studied; however, they are outside the scope of this chapter.

AAT AND THE CARDIOVASCULAR SYSTEM

The importance of the affiliation between humans and dogs on its effect on the cardiovascular system dates as far back as 1929. Researchers found that stroking a dog reduced its blood pressure. Fifty years later researchers observed that the stroker's blood pressure dropped as well,[13] thus spurring the health industry to look at the effect of pet ownership on cardiovascular disease.

In 1980, Friedmann et al made a breakthrough in studying the effect pet ownership has on survival after myocardial infarction.[14] This prospective study of 92 patients admitted to the coronary care unit concluded that pet ownership is an independent predictor of 1-year survival and thus has an effect on coronary artery disease. Only 5.7% of the 53 subjects who owned pets died within 1 year after hospitalization, whereas 28.2% of the 39 subjects who were not pet-owners died in the same time period. Dog owners were not permitted to participate in the study so as to eliminate questions as to whether dog owners were in better health. The study was limited by its small sample size, its measurement techniques, and its failure to account for disease severity.

An additional study in survivors of myocardial infarction took into consideration the severity of illness.[15] Each participant's disease was assigned a severity index that allowed researchers to estimate, via discriminant analysis, the effect disease had on survival and compare it with the effects of pet ownership. Disease severity and pet ownership were independently found to affect survival (Table 23-1). Disease severity was the most important predictor, predicting 21% of the variance. In addition, the study compared the effects of pet ownership with other sources of social support. Both marital status and living situation were found not to affect survival.

The presence of a pet can also assist in preventing cardiovascular disease from developing, as researchers in Australia have shown.[16] This large epidemiological study surveyed 5741 subjects to evaluate their risk factors for cardiovascular disease, including blood pressure, cholesterol, and triglyceride levels. Male pet owners were shown to have lower systolic blood pressure, but not diastolic blood pressure. Triglyceride levels decreased by 13%, whereas cholesterol levels decreased by 2%. Only women over the age of 40 were affected significantly, as was seen by a drop in systolic blood pressure as well as triglyceride levels. Although these beneficial effects are not large, evidence has shown that even a 1% reduction in total cholesterol can create a twofold reduction in the risk of cardiovascular mortality.[17] Therefore pet-owners as a whole have been found to have lower levels of certain risk factors for cardiovascular disease, thus raising the possibility that pets may be used to prevent the development of coronary artery disease. This association, however, does not imply that the acquisition of a pet will decrease cardiovascular risk in individual people.

Table **23-1**   One-Year Survival Status According to Pet, Dog, and Cat Ownership (N = 369)[15]

Ownership status	Survived (# of subjects)	Died (# of subjects)	Chi-Square
No pets	246	16	
Pets	103	4	1.07
No dogs	263	19	
Dogs	86	1	4.05*
No cats	308	17	
Cats	41	3	0.19

From Friedmann E, Thomas SA: Pet ownership, social support, and one-year survival after acute myocardial infarction in the Cardiac Arrhythmia Suppression Trial (CAST), Am J Cardiol 76:1213-1217, 1995.
*p <0.05h

Friedmann and Thomas continued their work by examining the effect that pet ownership has on heart rate variability (HRV) in patients with healed myocardial infarcts, hypothesizing that pet owners would have an increased HRV compared to non-pet owners and thus decreased long-term cardiovascular mortality as well.[18] The measurement of HRV is a noninvasive method that can be used to help detect abnormalities of autonomic modulation of the sinus node and to provide risk assessment after a myocardial infarction. Multiple studies have shown that a depressed HRV is a strong predictor of increased mortality and of arrhythmic complications in patients after an acute myocardial infarction.[19,20] The participants of the Cardiac Arrhythmia Suppressions Trial (CAST) with healed myocardial infarctions subsequently underwent a psychosocial assessment.[18] The study showed that short and intermediate HRV indices were higher among pet owners in general, and long-term HRV indices were higher among dog owners specifically. This supports the theory that survival differences between pet owners and non–pet-owners are due to differences in cardiac autonomic modulation, thus providing long-term cardiovascular benefit and increased survival after myocardial infarction.

The previous studies demonstrate that the continued presence of a pet in a patient's life can improve his or her survival after a myocardial infarction. The use of AAT in the acute in-patient hospital setting, however, requires a brief interaction between person and animal. Although this type of therapy plays a lesser role than the chronic at-home management of a patient after myocardial infarction, it could be effective in helping patients respond to certain stressors in the hospital.

A great deal of research has focused on the ability of the human-animal interaction to attenuate a human's stress response. Allen examined the effects of various sources of social support on cardiovascular reactivity to stress.[21] Two hundred and forty married subjects, half of whom owned a pet, were subjected to mental stressors in four different social support situations: (1) alone; (2) with pet or friend; (3) with a spouse; and (4) with spouse and pet or friend. Pet-owners had significantly lower heart rates and blood pressure levels at baseline and significantly smaller reactivity from baseline during exposure to mental stress. In addition, the pet-owners were found to have the lowest reactivity and quickest return to baseline in the presence of their pets. Of note is that the duration of cardiovascular recovery after stressor exposure is a risk factor for essential hypertension.[22] Therefore the presence of a pet could be important in decreasing this risk for hypertension. The study examined healthy patients in familiar surroundings, however, and therefore inferring how patients with acute cardiac conditions in the hospital would react is difficult.

To determine the effectiveness of antihypertensive medications in limiting the blood-pressure response to mental or physical stressor, Allen examined whether social support, such as the ownership of a pet, would be more effective than ACE-inhibitor therapy in blunting the response to mental stress.[23] Forty-eight patients with hypertension were separated into two groups: one that owned pets and one that did not. Both groups were given 20 mg of lisinopril per day. Each participant's baseline blood pressure, heart rate, and plasma renin were recorded before and after exposure to certain mental stressors, such as speech and serial subtraction. The rise in blood pressure in response to mental stressors was significantly attenuated among the group who owned pets. The administration of lisinopril alone only lowered resting blood pressure without buffering the response to stress. Therefore the social support given by the ownership of a pet could be effective in buffering a person's response to stress.

The previous studies imply that the presence of an animal can have an effect on the course and severity of coronary artery disease; however, none of these studies have described an actual mechanism for this improvement. A few theories have been suggested as the mechanisms in which the cardiovascular system could benefit by the presence of a pet.[9,24] As people become stressed, they respond with the activation of their sympathetic nervous system. This fight-or-flight response induces a build-up of hormones. If nothing is done to eliminate these hormones, a gross burden is placed on the body, which eventually causes a deterioration of the cardiovascular system. By learning stress reduction techniques or by avoiding the stressor altogether, this deterioration can be avoided. Stress reduction techniques, such as stroking a pet, assist in avoiding this harmful situation.

Direct physiological evidence for the effectiveness of the human-animal interaction was shown by examining specific neurochemical plasma levels before and after a positive human-dog interaction.[25] Blood was analyzed after a decrease in the mean arterial blood pressure was noted. The study found a significant decrease in blood pressure after 5 to 24 minutes of positive dog interaction. Once the subject and dog were able to get familiar with each other, the effect was immediate. This is important in practical terms for therapy, allowing sessions to be given in repeated episodes of short duration.

The drop in blood pressure was supported by associated changes in neurochemicals. Human beta-endorphin, oxytocin, prolactin, phenylacetic acid, and dopamine increased significantly, and cortisol decreased. Oxytocin was also elevated after subjects interacted with their own dogs. The results show that the decrease in blood pressure could be an indicator of neurohumoral changes, and therefore with the absence of blood tests, blood pressure could be an accurate indicator of effectiveness of the therapy.

These studies are limited by the fact that the people studied in the presence of a pet were all pet owners and therefore have a positive attitude towards animals. It is possible that individuals who do not enjoy the presence of animals would not react the same way.

CONCLUSION

Cardiovascular disease requires much attention in the health community because of its status as the nation's leading cause of death. It is a chronic progressive disease that, if acted upon early enough, can be prevented. This possibility for prevention has prompted health professionals to research ways to influence the disease in a nontraditional manner, such as the affiliation between human and animal.

The presence of an animal can have positive effects on a person's cardiovascular system. Ownership of a pet has been shown to improve survival after a myocardial infarction, while brief interactions with animals lower one's blood pressure and buffer one's response to stress. Pet-owners may also have less mental depression, a factor associated with a higher risk of symptomatic coronary disease.[26] Although a good number of studies have shown a favorable effect of the animal-human interaction, more studies need to be devoted to researching the exact physiological mechanism behind these beneficial actions. This evidence might provide for more public support for AAT and allow for its use to be more widespread.

For now, the therapeutic use of pets in patients with cardiovascular disease should be employed only in the "correct" situation and as an adjunctive therapy, never replacing the proven medical protocol already in place.

REFERENCES

1. Voith V: Attachment of people to companion animals, Vet Clin North Amer: Small Animal Practice 15:289-295, 1985.
2. Marx MB, Stallones TF, Garrity JR, Johnson TP: Demographics of pet ownership among US adults 21-64 years of age, Anthrozoos 2(1):33-37, 1988.
3. Francis GM: Loneliness: measuring the abstract, Intl J Nurs Studies 13:153-60, 1976.
4. Delta Society: Standard of practice for animal assisted activities and therapy, Renton, WA, 1996, Delta Society.
5. Bustad LK, Hines L: Historical perspectives of the human-animal bond. In The pet connection: its influence on our health and quality of life, Minneapolis, 1984, University of Minnesota Press.
6. Jones B: The psychology of the human/companion animal bond: an annotated bibliography, Philadelphia, 1985, University of Pennsylvania Press.
7. Nightingale F: Notes on Nursing, New York, 1969, Dover Publications (originally published in 1859).
8. Kear L: Pet-facilitated therapy and the elderly, Dog World. 75(25): March 1990.
9. Katcher A, Friedmann E: Potential health value of pet ownership, Compendium of Continuing Education Prac Vet 2(2):117-21, 1980.
10. Odendaal JSJ: Animal-assisted therapy: magic or medicine? J Psychosom Res 49:275-80, 2000.
11. Serpell J: Beneficial effects of pet ownership on some aspects of human health and behavior, J R Soc Med 84(12):717-20, 1991.
12. Siegel JM: Companion animals: in sickness and in health, J Social Issues 9:157-167, 1993.
13. Cusack O, Smith E: Pets and the elderly: the therapeutic bond, New York, 1984, Haworth, 13-16.

14. Friedmann E, Katcher AH, Lynch JJ, Thomas SA: Animal companions and one-year survival of patients after discharge from a coronary care unit, Public Health Rep 95:307-312, 1980.
15. Friedmann E, Thomas S: Pet ownership, social support, and one-year survival after acute myocardial infarction in the Cardiac Arrhythmia Suppression Trial (CAST), Am J Cardiol 76:1213-1217, 1995.
16. Anderson W, Reid C, Jennings G: Pet ownership and risk factors for cardiovascular disease, Med J Aust 157:298-301, 1992.
17. Levy R: Primary prevention of coronary heart disease by lowering lipids: results and implications: Am Heart J 110:1116-1122, 1985.
18. Friedmann E, Thomas SA: Relationship between pet ownership and heart rate variability in patients with healed myocardial infarcts, Am J Cardiol 91:718-721, 2003.
19. Kleiger RE, Miller JP, Bigger JT, Moss AJ, and the Multicenter Post-Infarction Research Group: Decreased heart rate variability and its association with increased mortality after acute myocardial infarction, Am J Cardiol 59:256-262, 1987.
20. Odemuyiwa O, Malik M, Farrell T, Bashir Y, Poloniecki J, Camm J. Comparison of the predictive characteristics of heart rate variability index and left ventricular ejection fraction for all-cause mortality, arrhythmic events and sudden death after acute myocardial infarction, Am J Cardiol 68:434-439, 1991.
21. Allen K, Blascovich J, Mendes W: Cardiovascular reactivity and the presence of pets, friends, and spouses: the truth about cats and dogs, Psychosom Med 64:727-739, 2002.
22. Schuler JL, O'Brien WH: Cardiovascular recovery from stress and hypertension risk factors: a meta-analytic review, Psychophysiol 34: 649-59, 1997.
23. Allen K, Shykoff B, Izzo J: Pet ownership, but not ACE inhibitor therapy, blunts home blood pressure response to mental stress, Hypertension 38:815-820, 2001.
24. Friedmann E, Thomas SA: Health benefits of pets for families: pets and the family, Marriage and Family Review 8:191-203, 1985.
25. Odendaal JSJ: A physiologic basis for animal-facilitated psychotherapy. PhD thesis, University of Pretoria, 1999.

CHAPTER 24

Therapeutic Massage and Asian Bodywork

Elaine Calenda
Suzan Fleck

T he significance of skilled touch is most apparent when it saves lives. Manual techniques that save lives by means of open-chest heart massage to the more provocative chest compressions of cardiopulmonary resuscitation are well known. This chapter aims to inform the interested physician as to the benefits of therapeutic massage and Asian bodywork modalities for patients suffering from cardiovascular disease and how to find qualified practitioners.

Massage to increase the rate and volume of local circulation by means of pressing and rubbing is instinctual. Whether applied to self or others, touch remains the most natural and powerful medicine of all. History and folklore hold numerous accounts of the mysterious and wondrous things accomplished by human hands. Today, with the help of research, specifically aimed at exploring the effects of touch, we are discovering how much more there is to know about the power at our fingertips.

In the 1800s, clinicians and scientists performed crude experiments, primarily on animals, that showed an increased rate of circulation of fluids through the body's vessels with the use of fluoroscopic technology. The application of passive mechanical stress upon the bones, by means of pressing, shaking, and percussion may generate an electrical current or piezoelectric flow useful for bedridden patients.[1] The physiologic changes were so profound that doctors and nurses used massage for relief of many ailments in hospitals and clinics. Although the physiologic effects of various forms of manual techniques produced a positive effect on the body's systems, prolonged measures would often lead to adverse reactions. Thus a system of formalized training in the manual arts of the Western world began to crop up throughout Europe and Great Britain.[2]

Today's research is far more sophisticated than that of Goetz, who in the 1800s spent countless hours tapping the hearts of dead frogs with a blunt instrument, and tapping them back to life again and so on. It involves the treatment of human subjects in hospitals, universities, and massage training facilities. Research conducted at the University of Miami under the direction of Dr. Tiffany Field cites significant changes in blood and urine chemistry during the application of massage. The massage stimulates the release of chemicals that have a positive bearing on the immune function and reduction of anxiety.[3] This kind of evidence has reopened the doors to invite the touch therapies back into mainstream health care as well as the medical practitioners who have witnessed positive changes in their patients. The popularity of natural approaches to health is evidenced by the billions of out-of-pocket dollars spent by the public each year.[4]

In the description of the theoretical rationale for providing skilled touch to patients during bone marrow transplant, Marlaine C. Smith et al say the following:

> The theoretical framework for this study was based on Rogers science of unitary human beings and Watson's theory of transpersonal caring. Humans are energy fields in continuous mutual process with environmental energy fields. The caring intentions of the therapists expressed through touch therapies are resonant facilitators of field pattern change. These changes in field patterning may be experienced and are reflected in healing.[5]

Of course, many, if not most, physicians today still cringe when asked to indoctrinate such esoteric spouting, even when the evidence is produced. The serious-minded bodywork practitioner today has no argument with the current engagement of research, nor does he or she have difficulty with healthy skepticism. However, the preservation of the essence of all touch therapies has been accomplished, against all odds, by a few who dared to believe in healing powers that defy scientific dogma. Humans are delicate creatures who thrive on physical contact. The neglect of this vital element of survival sets the stage for the onslaught of disease. Disease is not merely the absence of health but also a singular entity that thrives on neglect and indifference to human need.[6]

In this chapter, the authors present the results of modern touch therapy research and the clinical outcomes.

HISTORY

Healing through touch is as old as the hands themselves. Written accounts of the practice of massage and other forms of manual healing date back to the earliest inscriptions. Every ancient civilization has used massage in some form to care for the ailing and to reward the victor.

The Orient has the most extensive recorded history of massage as medical treatment. The power of touch as a means of therapy has been recognized throughout the last 2 millennia. The implementation of massage as a means of affecting the functioning of the body was recorded in a Chinese medical text, *Huang Di Nei Jing Su Wen*, or *Yellow Emperor's Classic*, in the first century BCE and was the first medical text to introduce massage therapy as a means of treating disease in the body.[7]

Massage therapy remained the preeminent form of treatment throughout the Qin and Tang dynasties, when massage was a prerequisite skill to be learned by all medical students.

By the fifth century CE, the science of Oriental bodywork therapy had evolved to such a level that a doctoral degree was created at the Imperial College of Medicine in Xian, the ancient capital of the Tang Dynasty. Every Chinese medical physician was required to master *mo shou* (hand-rubbing, the common bodywork form of the time) in order to help them develop the refined palpation skills necessary for diagnostics and for the competent practice of acupuncture.[8]

The most common form of massage practiced in the Western world today is known as *Swedish massage*. The name became popular in the mid 1800s from the teachings of Per Henrik Ling of Sweden. The Swedish government hired Ling to teach self-defense to their army because he knew ways to disarm the enemy using only the hands. Ling developed medical gymnastics that consisted of active and passive exercise for treating disease and deformity. The system was known as the Swedish movement cure. Ling's work was taught in public schools in the United States in the late 1800's and early 1900's. The term *Swedish massage* evolved from the early influence of Ling's work as his movement cure blended with the manual regimen developed by Johann Mezger, a Dutch physician (1838-1909). Mezger was known for using French terms to describe different techniques used in massage.[9]

Massage had reached a peak in the United States during 1950s. Modern modalities, such as galvanic stimulation, automated traction, and other technological approaches emerged in physical medicine, and led to a steady decline in the use of massage. These technologies were somewhat effective and saved time, but a vital personal element in health care was lost.[10]

In the years that followed, massage was confined to health clubs and spas, and its practitioners were called *masseuses* and *masseurs*. In the 1950's, the term *physiotherapist* became *physical therapist* and the profession split into two factions. Physical therapists were required to attend university courses that comprised conservative sciences similar to nursing. Their skills were limited to passive and active exercise regimens, and they learned few, if any, massage techniques.[11] Few schools that offered massage training remained. These came under the auspices of vocational education. One such school was the Swedish Institute in New York City, founded in 1916. Nearly bankrupt in the 1960s, the school is thriving today because of the enormous interest in using natural approaches to healing. The program blends Asian and Western bodywork studies in a 1260-hour associate degree program. Other schools throughout the United States are developing similar programs in higher education. The Boulder College of Massage Therapy in Colorado also offers an associate degree, internships at medical centers and hospitals, and specialty certification programs in a number of modalities. These progressive schools are laying the groundwork for the resurgence of a profession that was nearly extinct.

DEFINING THE PROFESSION

Pemberton said of massage, "there is probably no other measure of equal known value in the entire armamentarium of medicine which is so inadequately understood and utilized by the profession as a whole."[12]

Massage therapy is an organized, rational, therapeutic system that involves diagnosis, assessment, prevention, and treatment of dysfunction, injury, pain and physical disorders of the soft tissue and joints of the body. It includes systematic treatment planning and ongoing evaluation of response to treatment and modification of treatment as necessary and primarily uses manual and physical techniques and modalities.[13] It is also a systematic application of massage techniques, including therapeutic exercises and other physical modalities either separately or in combination as part of a rational treatment plan for clearly identified disease, dysfunctions, or disorders, especially when performed by registered massage therapists or other healthcare providers trained in the safe and effective use of massage techniques for therapeutic purposes.

From the Greek word *massein*, "to knead," massage describes a means of touch that manipulates the skin and muscle against the bones with kneading and/or percussive action. Therapeutic massage is described as the practice of skilled touch for the purpose of reducing pain brought about by injury, disease, or prolonged stress. It includes muscular rehabilitation, passive and resistive movements, preventative care, palliative care, and general wellness styles.[9,10,11]

ASIAN BODYWORK

Oriental bodywork therapy, also called *Asian bodywork*, is defined by the professional organization the American Organization for Bodywork Therapies of Asia (AOBTA) as the following:

> The treatment of the human body, including the electromagnetic or energetic field which surrounds, infuses, and brings that body to life, by pressure and/or manipulation. This approach is based upon traditional Asian medical principles for assessing and evaluating the energetic system, and traditional Asian techniques and treatment strategies to primarily affect and balance the energetic system, for the purpose of treating the human body, emotions, mind, energy field, and spirit for the promotion, maintenance, and restoration of health.
>
> When based on appropriate education, adjunctive modalities within the scope of Asian bodywork therapy are noninvasive. They include, but are not limited to, pressure devices, application of hot or cold, external application of herbal or chemical preparations, electromagnetic treatment modalities, and education regarding appropriate principles of diet and therapeutic exercises.

CHINESE MEDICINE THEORY

Chinese medicine theory, which is the underpinning of most Asian bodywork, perceives the body as a holographic model. As in Mandelbrot sets, the gross image comprises an infinite amount of diminutive representations of itself and reflects the finer details down to the microscopic level. The parts reflect the whole. What affects one aspect of an organism affects the entire organism.[14,15] The strategy of Chinese medicine—and therefore of Asian bodywork—is to address the client's conditions as unquestionably interrelated. For the body to function properly, the symptoms are tracked back to a common root cause, which may arise from any aspect of the individual: mental, emotional, spiritual, or physical. Although a root cause exists, all levels are inextricably interwoven, thus resulting in manifestations of disease on all levels of the individual. The meridians that are conduits of the energy of the body are the means by which the physical treatment occurs, although all aspects of the individual are considered and addressed. By following the holographic model, Asian modalities treat one or more parts of the body with the understanding that these parts have direct correlation to their distal organs and tissue bodies. Auricular therapy (see Chapter 16), as well as the many other Asian bodywork forms, rely on the conductance of energy to treat disease.

ACUPUNCTURE

In recent years, acupuncture (see Chapter 15) has risen to a high level of exposure in the Western medical establishment. Recognized for its efficacy in the treatment of chronic disorders and pain and as a means to reduce anesthesia load during surgery, a growing number of physicians employ acupuncture as an adjunctive therapy. According to the American Academy of Medical Acupuncture, over 1947 physicians today pursue medical acupuncture education.

Research has related a direct correlation of disease with low energetic conductance at the location of acupuncture points. Two studies of auricular therapy showed that "there was a significantly higher frequency of reactive ear points at the Chinese heart points in the inferior concha (84%), and on the tragus (59%), for patients with myocardial infarction and angina pain than for a control group of healthy subjects (11%). There was no difference between the coronary heart disease group and the control group in the electrical reactivity of auricular points that did not represent the heart".[15,16] Given this low electrical reactivity at acupuncture/acupressure points, Asian bodywork seeks to stimulate the flow of electrical energy conducted through the meridians and thereby affect the functioning of the affected tissues and organs, thus bringing about a more homeostatic balance to the body as a whole.

Acupuncture stimulates these points and meridians with needles. Shiatsu and Asian bodywork affect the flow of the meridians via touch. Through the stimulation of meridians using a direct, stationary pressure that induces an increase in endorphin levels, as well as stretches and range of motion techniques that influence and increase the local blood and lymph circulation; shiatsu and other forms of Asian bodywork have a profound affect on a broad range of conditions, diseases, and symptoms.

ACUPRESSURE

Lesser known yet equally effective is the discipline of acupressure. Acupressure and the many forms of Shiatsu (*finger pressure*) operate under the same energetic anatomy theory as traditional Chinese medicine and acupuncture. Chinese medicine views the body as a bioelectric system. A series of channels circulate through the body affecting and influencing the functioning of all the tissues, organs and physiological responses of the body. These channels are often called *meridians* and conduct the vital life force or energy of the body. Chinese texts describe the role of this energy, or Qi, as flowing with the visible flow of the blood. Qi leads the blood. Blood leads the Qi. The blood functions as the physical aspect of nourishing fluid of the body, whereas Qi nourishes the energetic aspect. Together, the blood and Qi maintain smooth functioning throughout the body and its electrical circuits, or meridians. Research confirming these electrical circuits of the body has been ongoing since the early 1970s. Instruments that measure the conductance of meridians and their corresponding acupuncture points "provide evidence that acupuncture points and meridians have distinctive electrical properties compared with the surrounding skin...acupuncture meridians have the characteristics of electrical transmission lines".[17] The best quantified, scientific studies of acupuncture suggest that the skin's electrical properties explain the concept of acupuncture points.[16,18-23]

Each meridian correlates with the specific functioning of an organ system. Although Western medicine focuses on the physical tissue of an organ, the Eastern view perceives this organ by means of its energetic functions primarily and its physicality secondarily. This is often a point of contention when physicians and adherents to Asian/Chinese Medicine meet. It is important to recognize this energetic anatomy is an entirely different paradigm by which the body is viewed, diagnosed, and treated. The liver that an Asian bodywork therapist or acupuncturist treats may not necessarily be the liver organ considered in Western allopathic tradition.

CONSIDERATIONS FOR THE USE OF MASSAGE AND BODYWORK IN CARDIOVASCULAR CONDITIONS

The effects of therapeutic massage depend on the reflex mechanism. The effectiveness of the techniques depends on how efficiently the receptors for these reflexes are stimulated. The receptor being targeted must be accessed with the appropriate technique and intensity, so that the reflex can function appropriately.[10]

Practitioners must have proper training and knowledge of cardiac pathology to work with patients suffering from damaged hearts or compromised blood vessels. A safe and gentle protocol should be employed to elicit the relaxation response. It is common knowledge that massage and bodywork can be relaxing, but improper application of techniques can be disturbing and even damaging to the skin, muscle, internal organs, and blood vessels. Gentle massage is not always light. Too light an application can be annoying and cause the receiver to feel restless. The skilled practitioner can quickly work out the proper pressure for each individual and maintain it throughout the session. The appropriate pressure, pace, and duration of the session is paramount in achieving and maintaining the relaxation response.

THE RELAXATION RESPONSE

Relaxation, in its purest sense, is often misunderstood. One of the most common phrases uttered at the end of a bodywork session is, "I could use another hour." Another hour of stimulation, however, can leave the receiver exhausted and moody. The body's systems overcharge from prolonged massage, just as they do from too much exercise. Massage and Shiatsu are types of passive exercise; therefore limiting duration is essential for achieving a beneficial effect.[11,22]

Proper application can elicit the relaxation response. This physiologic phenomenon, activated by stimulation of the parasympathetic nervous system, is true relaxation that holds the patient in a state of rest, not sleep. It cultivates beneficial chemical releases aimed at producing the ultimate healing environment, homeostasis.[11,24]

CIRCULATORY PATHOLOGIES AND CONDITIONS

The following conditions are outlined with treatment possibilities and general guidelines for appropriate treatment. One must remember that both Chinese medicine and Asian bodywork base assessment and treatment on the individual rather than a set protocol or routine that can be applied to anyone. The skilled practitioner is able to tailor-fit a treatment specific to each client's concerns and conditions. The human system is an intricate one, and the consideration of each individual's patterns and sensitivities is integral to safe and effective treatment.

ANGINA PECTORIS

Angina is perhaps the most common cardiac condition treated by Asian bodywork. The strategy of Asian bodywork with regard to angina is to initially decrease pain, with the long-term intention of preventing future episodes. According to Shizuto Masunaga, founder and developer of Zen Shiatsu, "angina pectoralis or spasm in the coronary artery is characterized by depression, heaviness around the chest, and fear of death...[the condition of the client's meridians] imply that emotional tension and mental or physical fatigue rather than cardiac abnormality is the real cause of the problem."[25] Consideration of the emotional state of the client is taken into account, and lifestyle changes are advised. The practitioner is recommended to use steady holding techniques to calm the nervous system and thereby induce the relaxation response and avoid any heavy, deep, or thrusting techniques.

Protocols that stimulate acupressure/acupuncture points along the liver and kidney meridians for blood circulation, the bladder meridian to support the autonomic nervous system, which also incorporate the spleen meridian in order to address lack of oxygen, serve to significantly decrease the level of pain after only one treatment.[25] Similar acupuncture studies have recorded equally significant findings that indicate a reduction in the number and length/duration of attacks as well as a decrease in the necessity of drug therapy.[26]

Indeed, the effects of skillfully applied massage may have an influence on the regulation of a complex series of blood chemicals, however, the practical benefit is much more immediate and far less mysterious. With respect to angina and the autonomic phenomena of referred pain patterns, massage plays out its most primary role: to balance muscular antagonism.

Within the chest wall, there are dozens of muscles, both smooth and skeletal. Chronic pain often propagates a series of muscular contractures that prolong if not aggravate conditions of the internal organs. The heart muscle loses support when posture is poor.[27] On the anterior aspect, the pectorals and intercostals tend to shorten adaptively, whereas the antagonistic posterior muscles become weakened by stretching. The long-term effect of this loss in muscular integrity spills into the function of the ligaments of the spine leading to a collapse of the postural reflex. Moreover, the loss of the supportive role of the pericardial ligament and the respiratory muscles diminish the proper carriage of the heart within the chest cavity.[28] Regaining erect posture will require more than the absence of pain. The goal of massage in these cases will aim at working to restore proper muscle memory.[13,29] In most instances, however, the individual may have never had good posture. Proper muscle memory will therefore have to be restored by new muscle positioning until the brain—or more specifically, the proprioceptive mechanisms—are convinced that erect posture is desirable. This type of treatment marries medical massage with orthopedic massage. Orthopedic massage aims to correct musculoskeletal distress, including posture, through the restoration of proper ligamental support and reactivation of the postural reflex. Once posture has improved, even slightly, a corresponding improvement occurs in the function of the nervous system because of a reduction of physical pressure on the peripheral and autonomic nerves.[29,30]

MYOCARDIAL INFARCTION

The onset of a myocardial infarction is characterized by shooting pain beginning in the chest and radiating down the left arm to the fifth metacarpal and finger. This pain is located precisely along the heart meridian of the Asian medicine theory.

In the case of myocardial infarction, Asian bodywork defers to established medical practice during the acute phase. During the subacute phase, work specific to the meridians associated with angina pectoris is prescribed, and techniques are applied distally to proximally on the upper extremity before moving to the back and abdomen. Again, highly stimulating or deep work is contraindicated.[25] If palpitation, pain in the chest, low body temperature, or other signs of heart organ weakness persist, the client/patient must consult a physician.

HYPERTENSION

The results of a research study entitled "The Effects of Back Massage Before Diagnostic Cardiac Catheterization" shows some of the most up to date evidence of the effects of spinal massage to decrease blood pressure.[31] Patients who received a 20-minute back massage had a 20-point reduction in blood pressure. For those patients who received routine care, blood pressure dropped only 10 points.

Massage and Asian bodywork considerations for working with patients with high blood pressure are as follows:

- Obtain a complete health history including diagnosis, previous and current medical treatment, lifestyle, diet, and exercise.
- Blood pressure should be taken and recorded before and after the session in order to track changes.
- The preferred position for massage is supine and side-lying for short periods. The prone position is not always restricted but should not be prolonged.
- Massage should be applied by using moderate pressure to the extremities first, beginning with the proximal portion of the limb and working distally to avoid rushing of lymph fluid and venous blood to the torso. Pressure of the stroke is applied in layers toward the heart, but the therapist should avoid long, deep, pressure-oriented techniques or repetitive effleurage (gliding strokes) to the limbs. A sudden increase in venous return produces a comparative increase in cardiac output which raises the blood pressure.[32] Massage along the spine and the paraspinal muscles tends to decrease blood pressure. Treating the urinary bladder meridian or Shu points along the paraspinals serves to balance each organ system and tonify depleted meridian energies. Abdominal massage will temporarily increase the blood pressure, but strokes methodically directed at the intestines and along the spine, in side position, help steady blood pressure. Pressure on the digestive organs, the inferior vena cava, aorta, or respective common iliac vessels, therefore should not exceed 4 to 5 pounds per square inch. Therefore the prolonged, deep organ massage sometimes associated with various forms of Asian bodywork is not recommended.
- Massage and bodywork is applied at a pace and pressure that ensures that the patient attains the proper and proportionate autonomic nervous system response.[11,33,34]

Many forms of Asian bodywork interpret hypertension or high blood pressure as an indication that the present lifestyle is incompatible with the individual's constitution. Consideration of the levels of mental, emotional, and physical stress on the body is addressed through observation, treatment, and consultation with appropriate healthcare professionals.

From a meridian standpoint, the heart protector meridian is often involved in hypertension because of its association with the general circulation throughout the body.

THE PHYSIOLOGICAL EFFECTS OF THERAPEUTIC MASSAGE ON THE GENERAL CIRCULATION

The effect of massage on circulation can be compared to pressing a water balloon. Pressure against any one area will increase pressure throughout the entire structure. This fact must be considered more thoughtfully, therefore, when one is applying pressure against unhealthy blood vessels. The general rule is to introduce pressure gradually upon the proximal limbs, thus persuading the movement of venous blood toward the heart before proceeding to the distal limb.[29] The heart itself can benefit from pressure administered in syncopation with the pulse rate and altered respectfully to correct arrhythmic impulses, at least temporarily. This procedure begins with taking the pulse, then offering gentle compressions in rhythm with the heart beat followed by a series of 10 to 12 cupping percussions directly over the heart. The procedure is then repeated until the desired effect is achieved, but should not exceed three trials. Because the heart is self-regulating to a degree, it can respond to external as well as internal signals and adjust accordingly. To date, local heart massage is not widely taught in massage programs; however, chest and abdominal massage is, and it follows strict protocols.[10,11] Most massage programs also instill practical guidelines and contraindications, and students are encouraged to exercise caution when they are working with people with heart disease and a compromised circulation.[31,35]

The main objective of massage in these cases is to assist the action of the blood vessels thereby reducing the burden on the heart. This is accomplished by the application of strokes that simulate muscular activity in a passive environment. An adjoining benefit is experienced by the lymphatic system as the rhythmic pressure assists in the emptying of those vessels respectively, thus accelerating the amount of time excess fluid remains in the periphery where it puts undue pressure on vessels and nerves.[24] This dramatic movement of fluid though the body occurs in a relatively short time, usually 20 minutes to half an hour. Longer massage is discouraged until patients recover their resiliency, yet some touch to the body as a whole is encouraged. Local massage tends to extend the fixation patients develop regarding the problematic area.[33]

Finally, during the entire procedure, the patient maintains in the relaxation response, thus producing a healing environment in which the body can reboot its machinery. The overall benefit of therapeutic massage is not limited to physical change. During the relaxation response, stress hormone levels are low and the patient often reports feeling less anxious and more optimistic.[3,33]

POSTSURGICAL CONSIDERATIONS

Massage and bodywork can be very beneficial during a hospital stay. Many city hospitals now offer some kind of bodywork to their patients, family members, and staff. Before and after surgical procedures, touch therapy decreases anxiety levels and reduces pain and discomfort. If the physician in charge of the case permits it, gentle massage and bodywork will reactivate the body's systems and promote peristalsis. The challenge faced by the therapists is not to overdo. Deep and prolonged work must be avoided to reduce the chances of dislodging clot formations.[3,11,36] In individuals who have a history of thrombus, general massage should be postponed until the patient is cleared by a physician. The safest procedures are still touch and Asian bodywork methods that do not accelerate the rate of blood flow but still provide a great deal of comfort.

VARICOSE VEINS

In Zen Shiatsu theory, the integrity of vessel walls falls under the role of the heart protector meridian, loosely correlated with the western structure of the pericardium. The heart protector serves to physically and emotionally protect the heart organ and the circulatory system. Traditional Chinese medicine theory also attributes varicosities to the weakness of the spleen meridian, the role of which is to maintain the integrity of organs and tissues.

In the treatment of clients with varicosities, the practitioner avoids deep pressure to the site of varicosities by using light, energetic techniques or holding on or around the site to encourage flow and avoid loosening of stagnant blood that may lead to embolism.[29,31,36]

EDEMA

Edema as viewed through the Asian bodywork model is similar to Western assessment. Edema is the result of faulty water metabolism. The urinary bladder and kidney meridians govern the water (fluid) balance of the body and can be considered during treatment of common edema. When congestive heart failure is a precipitating factor, the heart and heart protector meridians may also be involved. Caution should be taken when treating severe edema or edema occurring in tandem with other conditions such as pregnancy or congestive heart failure. Avoiding deep, prolonged pressure-oriented techniques is advised. Common areas of complaint with regards to edema in both pregnancy and congestive heart failure are the legs. Pressure points in the lower extremities are contraindicated in pregnancy due to their highly stimulating effect. Light palming, brushing strokes, and holding rather than acupressure pointwork are recommended for moving fluids and stimulating the uptake of excess interstitial fluid.[10,11,24]

MODERN TREATMENT RESOURCES

A large number of textbooks on massage and bodywork have been published during the last several years. *Clinical Massage Therapy*, by Rattray and Ludwig, published in 2000, is one of the most comprehensive in its coverage of medical conditions.[11] The authors, who teach and practice in Canada, have had the advantage of cooperation from the medical establishment for decades. The text has over a thousand pages of complete information on medical and orthopedic conditions and how to use massage responsibly. A half-dozen texts like it, such as Susan Salvo's *Mosby's Pathology for Massage Therapists*, Whitney Lowe's *Orthopedic Assessment*, and Leon Chaitow's numerous texts on assessment and manual therapies cover related subject matter.

CREDENTIALING

The number of massage and shiatsu training programs has tripled in the last decade, in part because of an increasing public demand for more natural health care. Educational requirements vary from state to state. The national mean educational requirement is 500 hours in the United States and 2600 to 3200 hours in Canada. In the last 7 years, programs providing 1000 hours of training and associate degrees (equivalent to 2-year college programs) have become more common.[13,39]

Although Asian modalities generally share the same theoretical foundation, they use very diverse methods. Understanding the appropriateness or efficacy of one modality over another depends on many factors—most importantly on training and experience. As in any profession, the stronger the educational foundation of the practitioner, the more informed, effective, and safe the session. At this time, diverse offerings of education exist throughout the United States and abroad. Practitioners of Asian modalities such as Shiatsu can practice with as few hours as required in a weekend workshop and with as many as 3000 hours in programs with specialization in one particular area of study. Because of this diversity, researching the skill and depth of training of an individual practitioner is of the utmost importance.

The American Organization for Bodywork Therapies of Asia (AOBTA) provides an outline for responsible training of these professionals. Licensing varies from state to state and is often overseen by the massage licensing board of each state. In other states, Shiatsu and Asian modalities are viewed under separate conditions and are defined by licensing similar to acupuncture and chiropractics. Presently, 31 states in the United States recognize Asian bodywork and regulate it in some manner. The AOBTA and the International Shiatsu Society are professional organizations that serve as contacts for recognized schools, licensing, and member profiles.

The National Certification Board for Therapeutic Massage and Bodywork (NCBTMB) was founded in 1992. Its core purpose is to foster high standards for therapeutic massage and bodywork professionals and to advocate for the public acceptance of the value of these standards and the professionals who uphold them. Currently, there are more than 68,000 certified massage therapists and bodyworkers in the United States. NCBTMB has been an instrumental force in unifying the massage and bodywork profession by offering support to individuals, schools, and the agencies that govern the practice. By offering a national examination and recertification program, the NCBTMB has helped to standardize and elevate the massage and bodywork profession with a recognized credential.[37]

The positive response to therapeutic massage and bodywork in the last 10 years has prompted a remarkable increase in the number of training programs. The more prestigious massage and bodywork therapy programs recognize the importance of fluency in both the Western medical paradigm as well as the foundation of Asian medicine. Recognized programs emphasize the importance of various disease conditions and contraindications to treatment, as well as acknowledging the ethics of scope of practice. Today's bodywork and massage therapist serves to assist the client in seeking proper treatment under the advice of a qualified primary care provider.

SUMMARY

Although the emergence of integrative health care is a reality, some people will put more force into resisting these approaches and asking questions like "What good will touching people do?" or, worse, "I suppose it won't hurt." Until the research studies that are underway are completed, we will have to expect some skepticism, ignorance, and fear. Therapeutic massage and bodywork continues to flow into many aspects of modern life. It has become common to see people receiving seated massage at airports, malls, and in the workplace. The relief on the faces of the hospital staff as massage students do their rounds through the wards is truly remarkable. They know that the woman who has been up all night battling shoulder and back pain after gallbladder surgery will soon be asleep. The man who almost died this morning will be less afraid within the hour and will sleep like a baby. They move through the departments of oncology, cardiology, and orthopedics. Even the nurses and physicians take a few minutes to relax and regroup with a brief massage. Massage therapists have the time to spend with people in a busy world. They have the time to listen. Their approach is noninvasive. Their presence is finally welcome.

WHERE TO FIND QUALIFIED MASSAGE AND BODYWORK PRACTITIONERS

American Massage Therapy Association (AMTA)
www.amtamassage.org
American Organization of Bodywork Therapies of Asia (AOBTA)
www.aobta.org
Associated Bodywork and Massage Professionals (ABMP)
www.abmp.com
National Certification Board for Therapeutic Massage and Bodywork (NCBTMB)
www.ncbtmb.com

REFERENCES

1. Fukada E, Yasuda IL: On the piezoelectric effect of bone, J Phys Soc Japan 12:1158-1162, 1957.
2. Tappan F: *Healing massage techniques*, ed 3, Stamford, Conn., 1998, Appleton and Lange.

3. Field T, Seligman S, Scafidi F, Schanberg S: Alleviating post traumatic stress in children following hurricane Andrew, J Appl Development Psychol 17:37-50, 1996.
4. Eisenberg DM et al: Unconventional medicine in the United States: prevalence, costs, and patterns of use, N Engl J Med, 328:246-252, 1993.
5. Smith MC, Daniel L, Reeder F, Teichler L: Outcomes of touch therapies during bone marrow transplant. Altern Therap 9: 40-49, 2003.
6. Montagu A: Touching: the human significance of the skin, New York, 1978, Harper & Row.
7. Unschuld P: *Huang Di Nei Jing Su Wen,* Berkeley, 2003, University of California Press.
8. Dubitsky C, Juhan D: Bodywork shiatsu: bringing the art of finger pressure to the massage table, New York, 1997, Inner Traditions International.
9. Kellogg J: The art of massage, Brushton, NY, 1999, TEACH Services.
10. Fritz S: Fundamentals of therapeutic massage, St Louis, 1995, Mosby.
11. Rattray F, Ludwig, L: Clinical massage therapy, Toronto, 2000, Talus Incorporated.
12. Pemberton R: The physiology of massage. In American Medical Association handbook of physical medicine and rehabilitation, Philadelphia, 1950, American Medical Association.
13. Yates J: A physician's guide to therapeutic massage, ed 2, Vancouver, Massage Therapists'Association of British Columbia,1999.
14. Benoit B, Mandelbrot MS: Form, chance and dimension: the fractal geometry of nature, San Francisco, 1981, Freeman.
15. Talbot M: The holographic universe, New York, 1992, Perennial.
16. Oleson T: Electrophysiological research on the differential localization of auricular acupuncture points, Med Acupunct 11(2): Fall 1999/Winter 2000.
17. Tiller WA: What do electrodermal diagnostic acupuncture instruments really measure? Am J Acupuncture 15:18-23, 1987.
18. Reichmanis M, Marino AA, Becker RO: DC skin conductance variation at acupuncture loci, Am J Chin Med 4:69-72, 1976.
19. Becker R, Reichmanis M, Marino A: Electrophysiological correlates of acupuncture points and meridians, Psychoenergetic Systems 1:105, 1976.
20. Bergsmann O, Hart A: Differences in electrical skin conductivity between acupuncture points and adjacent skin areas, Am J Acupuncture 1:27-32, 1973.
21. Motoyama H: Electrophysiological and preliminary biochemical studies of skin properties in relation to the acupuncture meridian, Intl Assoc Religion Parapsychol 6:1-36, 1980.
22. Hu X, Wu B, Huang X, Xu J: Computerized plotting of low skin impedance points, J Tradit Chin Med 12:277-282, 1992.
23. Gunn CC: Acupuncture loci, a proposal for their classification according to their relationship to known neural structures, Am J Clin Med 4: 183-195, 1976.

24. Chikly B: Silent waves, theory and practice of lymphatic drainage therapy, Scottsdale, Ariz, 2001, IHH Publishing.
25. Masunaga S, Wataru O: Zen shiatsu: how to harmonize yin and yang for better health, New York, 1977, Japan Publications.
26. Ballegard S, Norrelund S, Smith DF: Cost benefit of combined use of acupuncture, Shiatsu and lifestyle adjustments for treatment of patients with sever angina pectoris, Acupuncture Electrotherapy Res (United States) 21(3-4):187-97, 1996.
27. Hovind N, Nielsen SL: Effect of massage on blood flow in skeletal muscle, Scand J Rehabil Med 6:74-77, 1974.
28. Severini V, Venerando A: The physiological effects of massage on the cardiovascular system, Europa Medicophys 3:165-183, 1967.
29. Travell J: Myofascial pain and dysfunction. In Johnson E, editor: The trigger point manual, upper half of the body, vol 1, Baltimore, 1983, Williams & Wilkins.
30. Barr JS, Taslitz N: The influence of back massage on autonomic functions, Phys Ther 50:1679-1691, 1970.
31. McNamara ME, Carroll D, Harten MT: Effects of back massage before diagnostic cardiac catheterization, Massage Ther J 42:80, 2003.
32. Basmajian J, Nyberg RE: Rational manual therapies, Philadelphia, 1993, Lippincott, Williams and Wilkins.
33. Bork K, Karling GW, Faust G: Serum enzyme levels after "whole body massage," Arch Dermatol Forsch 240:342-348, 1971.
34. Fraser J, Kerr JR: Psychophysiological effects of back massage on elderly institutionalized patients, J Adv Nurs 18:238-245, 1993.
35. Arkko P, Pakarinen AJ, Kari-Koskinen O: Effects of whole body massage on serum protein, electrolyte and hormone concentrations, enzyme activities and hematologic parameters, Int J Sports Med 4:265-267, 1983.
36. Alexander D: Deep vein thrombosis and massage therapy, Massage Ther J Spring 53-62, 1993.
37. National Certification Board for Therapeutic Massage and Bodywork, press release, May, 2003.

CHAPTER **25**

Magnetic Biostimulation: Energy Therapy

Michael I. Weintraub, MD
William H. Frishman, MD

Man has been fascinated with magnetism for over 4000 years. Attempts to explain this invisible force's efficacy by using unique scientific principles has generated controversy. Despite the fact that permanent magnets and electromagnetic therapies are currently riding the crest of public enthusiasm as an alternative and complementary medical treatment, the scientific community is still somewhat skeptical of the current widespread claims of benefit. With the absence of randomized, placebo-controlled trials, this is not surprising. Recently the study of magnetic fields, both static and pulsed, has evolved from being just a medical curiosity to significant and specific medical applications in diagnosis and treatment. For example, pulsed electromagnetic fields (PEMF) and transcranial magnetic stimulation (TMS) can influence biological functions and serve as therapeutic interventions for managing symptoms of epilepsy, Parkinson's disease, multiple sclerosis, aphasia, and psychiatric disease. The FDA has fully accepted PEMF as a means of stimulating and recruiting osteoblast cells at nonunion fracture sites to enhance healing. It also has been approved for the treatment of urinary incontinence. However, data regarding the use of magnetic biostimulation as a possible treatment modality for cardiovascular disease are sparse. This complementary medical therapy will be the subject of this chapter.

HISTORICAL PERSPECTIVE

Aspects of magnetic healing have been traced for more than 4000 years. According to the *Yellow Emperor's Canon of Internal Medicine*, magnetic stones (lodestones) were applied to acupressure points as a means of pain reduction. Similarly, the ancient Hindu "Vedas" ascribed therapeutic powers to Ashmana and Siktavati (instruments of stone).[1,2] Greeks and Romans used these lodestones for personal purposes and also fashioned them as magnetic rings and necklaces as well as salves to cure arthritis, pain, and various other ailments of the day. Claims and anecdotal stories persisted and led to public embracement of these "magical" devices. A major breakthrough occurred during the scientific revolution of the eighteenth century in Europe with the development of carbon-steel magnets. Father Maxmilian Hell and, later, his student, Anton Mesmer applied these magnetic devices to patients who were experiencing hysterical or psychosomatic symptomatology. In one dramatic case, Mesmer described feeding a patient iron filings and then applying specially designed magnets over the vital organs to generally stop uncontrolled seizures. His cures were not only astounding but also theatrical, and were performed in front of large groups. Claims of success forced the French Academy of Science to convene a special study in 1784 with a panel of Benjamin Franklin, JR Guillotin, and Anton Lavoisier. In a controlled set of experiments, blindfolded patients were exposed to a series of magnets or sham-magnetic objects and were asked to describe the induced sensation. The committee concluded that the efficacy of magnetic healing resided within the mind and that any healing was due to suggestion. Mesmer's theories were subsequently considered fraudulent and equated with medical quackery. This was highlighted in a scene from Mozart's 1790 comedy opera, *Cosi Fan Tutte*, in which magnets were used as a resuscitative treatment to reverse the effects of near-fatal poisoning.[3,4]

In the late nineteenth century, the benefits of magnetic healing were being reaffirmed. In 1886, the Sears Catalog advertised numerous magnetic products, such as rings, belts, caps, girdles, and so on. In the 1920s, Thacher created a mail-order catalog and advertised over 700 specific magnetic garments and devices that he described as "plain road to health without the use of medicine and was dependent on the magnetic energy of the sun." Despite the outlandish claims in the early twentieth century, standard medical texts were including galvanism and electromagnetic fields as a treatment of various neurological diseases. In 1896, D'Arsonval placed his head in a strong time-varying magnetic field that induced phosphenes (retinal stimulation), the first of many experiments with time-varying magnetic fields. Ultimately this led to the development of the first commercial magnetic stimulator in 1985. In 1979, the FDA approved the use of PEMF as a means of stimulating and recruiting osteoblast cells at fracture sites for healing. Applying coils around an orthopedic cast, PEMF would induce current flows through the fracture site, producing an 80% success rate.[5] PEMF carries a broad band of frequencies that occupy a discrete portion of the lower end of the electromagnetic spectrum. Repetition rates fall in the extremely low-frequency (ELF) range (1-100 Hz). The peak magnetic fields are typically 5 to 30 gauss at the target tissue. The presence of an "Adey window" has been proposed to explain the mechanism of actions that mediate the biological effects of weak electromagnetic forces that cannot be explained by Newtonian physics or by current laws of thermodynamics that govern ionic flux across cell membranes. This is basically at the atomic level.[6,7] Adey emphasizes the role of free radicals, which form briefly in all chemical reactions and which have essentially magnetic bonds. Thus free radical electrons have been proposed to be sensitive to both intrinsic and imposed magnetic fields. Adey specifically believed that nitric oxide (NO) and the free radicals of oxygen and nitrogen play central roles in health and disease. Thus signal transduction can arise. Low-frequency EMFs have been theorized to alter the membrane structures and ion fluxes in nerves. This essentially reduces the amplitude of nerve action potentials and makes the membrane harder to depolarize. Weintraub et al suggested that submaximal magnetic stimuli (static magnets), which penetrate only 20 mm, would preferentially activate sensory rather than motor neurons.[8,9]

CLINICAL APPLICATIONS

The FDA has accepted supra-threshold time-varying magnetic devices for investigational use in epilepsy, pain, and Parkinson disease. Recent work with spinal cord–injury patients has also shown improvement in expiratory muscle strength and colonic peristalsis with magnetic stimulation.[10,11]

The strength of static permanent magnets varies from 1 to 4000 gauss. These small devices are sold commercially and have been purported to provide the same benefit as PEMF. Weintraub et al have used a multipolar array permanent magnetic foot pad (475 gauss) to successfully treat peripheral neuropathy in diabetic patients.[8] Weintraub also noted a 50% reduction in neuropathic pain in advanced cases of carpal tunnel syndrome.[12] However, not all physicians are convinced that magnetotherapy, using static magnets, produces a therapeutic effect, and most feel that it is a placebo response. Ramey, a veterinarian, is a major critic of the use of static magnets for inducing biological effects despite the fact that the veterinary profession often uses magnetic blankets and other such devices on racehorses to improve circulation and prevent soreness.[13]

Cardiac Arrhythmias

Exposure to power lines and external electromagnetic fields has been suggested to cause adverse cardiovascular effects.[14] However, a recent animal study has provided highly suggestive evidence that low level electromagnetic fields can induce potentially beneficial alterations in heartrate and atrioventricular conduction, and favorable effects on cardiac arrhythmias, such as atrial fibrillation.[15] To be of clinical use, studies would need to focus on the noninvasive applications of magnetic fields to the heart. The ability to reduce heartrate, atrioventricular conduction and heartrate rhythm with magnets[16-18] may be of use to slow the ventricular rate in rapid atrial fibrillation or to correct ectopic rhythms. Recently, an electromagnetic cardiac pacemaker was developed.[19]

Angina Pectoris and Hypertension

A whole-body magnetic exposure in animals has been shown to increase capillary blood flow and to reduce blood pressure.[20]

Permanent magnets placed over the cervical vagosympathetic trunk may be of use in the treatment of angina and hypertension by causing enhancement of parasympathetic tone. This effect would serve to reduce blood pressure and heart rate in patients with hypertension. At New York Medical College, we are about to embark on a randomized, placebo-controlled trial that will use an external permanent magnet over the carotid bulb as a blood pressure–lowering treatment.[20a] In experimental studies, magnets have been proposed as a treatment for reducing ischemic injury and for enhancing angiogenesis.[21-23] Similarly, external application of magnets might be of use if placed over the chest to relieve refractory anginal pain or as a potential bradycardic treatment for angina if placed over the carotid bulb. We are also ready to embark on a sham-control clinical trial using magnets as an adjunct antianginal remedy.[23a]

CONCLUSION

The study of magnetic fields (static and pulsed) has recently evolved from a medical curiosity to a treatment approach for specific medical conditions. However, defining a possible clinical role in cardiology and cardiovascular disease is only at the earliest stages of development. At the same time, the efficacy of static magnets in medical treatment can only be clarified when the appropriate dosimetry component is eluciated.[24] Randomized, placebo-controlled studies using biological markers of efficacy should address the current skepticism of the scientific community regarding the clinical benefits of magnetic devices. Although some people perceive magnetic devices are safe and beneficial in promoting good health, whether this is related to a placebo effect must be determined. It is also hoped that within the next few years the potential for using magnetism for the treatment of cardiovascular disease will be elucidated.

REFERENCES

1. Rosch P: Preface: a brief historical perspective . In Rosch PJ, Markov MS, editors: Bioelectromagnetic medicine, New York, 2004, Marcel Dekker, III-VII.
2. Mourino MR: From Thales to Lauterbur, or from the lodestone to MR imaging: magnetism and medicine, Radiol 180:593-612, 1991.
3. Mackis RM: Magnetic healing, quackery and the debate about the health effects of electro-magnetic fields, Ann Intern Med 118:376-83, 1993.
4. Armstrong D, Armstrong EM: The great american medicine show, New York, 1991, Prentiss Hall.
5. Weintraub WI: Magnetotherapy: historical background with a stimulating future, Crit Rev Phys Rehab Med. In press.
6. Adey WR: Resonance and other interactions of electromagnetic fields with living organisms. Oxford, 1992, Oxford University Press.
7. Adey WR: Potential therapeutic applications of non-thermal electromagnetic fields: ensemble organization of cells in tissue as a factor

in biological field sensing. In Rosch PJ, Markov MS editors: Bioelectromagnetic medicine, New York, 2004, Marcel Dekker, 781-96.

8. Weintraub MI, Wolfe GI, Barohn RA et al: Static magnetic field therapy for symptomatic diabetic neuropathy: a randomized, double-blind, placebo-controlled trial, Arch Phys Med Rehab 84:736-46, 2003.

9. McLean MJ, Holcomb RR, Wamil AW et al: Blockade of sensory neuron action potentials by a static magnetic field in the 10 mT range, Bioelectromag 16:20-32, 1995.

10. Lin VW, Hsiao IN, Zhu E, Perkash I: Functional magnetic stimulation for conditioning of expiratory muscles in patients with spinal cord injury, Arch Phys Med Rehab 82:162-66, 2001.

11. Lin VW, Nino-Murcia M, Frost F, et al: Functional magnetic stimulation of the colon in persons with spinal cord injury, Arch Phys Med Rehab 82:167-73, 2001.

12. Weintraub MI: Neuromagnetic treatment of pain in refractory carpal tunnel syndrome, An electrophysiological and placebo analysis, J Back Musculoskel Rehab 15:77-81, 2002.

13. Ramey DW: Magnetic and electromagnetic therapy, Sci Rev Alt Med 2:13-19, 1998.

14. Jauchem JR, Merritt JH: The epidemiology of exposure to electromagnetic fields: an overview of the recent literature, J Clin Epidemiol 44:895-906, 1991.

15. Scherlag BJ, Yamanashi WS, Hou Y et al: Magnetism and cardiac arrhythmias, Cardiol Rev 12:85-91, 2004.

16. Mallioni A, Pagoni M, Lombardi F et al: Cardiovascular neural regulation explored in the frequency domain, Circulation 84: 482-92, 1991.

17. Schauerte PN, Scherlag BJ, Scherlag MA et al: Transvenous parasympathetic cardiac nerve stimulation: an approach for stable sinus rate control, J Cardiovasc Electrophysiol 10:1517-24, 1999.

18. Prystowsky EN, Nacarelli GV, Jackman WM et al: Enhanced parasympathetic tone shortens atrial refractoriness in man, Am J Cardiol 51:96-100, 1983.

19. Van Bise WL, Rauscher EA: Magnetic field impulse cardiovascular stimulation for normalizing arrhythmias and/or heart blocks, Proc Bioelectromagnet Soc Mtg, St Paul, Minn., June 10, 2001.

20. Okano H, Ohkubo C: Anti-pressor effects of whole body exposure to static magnetic field on pharmacologically induced hypertension in conscious rabbits, Bioelectromag 24:139-47, 2003.

20a. Weintraub MI, Frishman WH, Peterson S: Static magnetic stimulation of the carotid sinus in hypertension: placebo-controlled trial. Work in progress.

21. Grant G, Cadossi R, Steinberg G: Protection against focal cerebral ischemia following exposure to a pulsed electromagnetic field, Bioelectromag 15:205-16, 1994.

22. Albertini A, Zucchini P, Noera G et al: Protective effect of low frequency low energy pulsing electromagnetic fields on acute experimental myocardial infarcts in rats, Bioelectromag 20:372-77, 1999.
23. Yen-Patton GP, Patton W, Beer D et al: Endothelial cell response to pulsed electromagnetic fields: stimulation of growth rate and angiogenesis in vitro, J Cell Physiol 134:37-46, 1988.
23a. Weintraub MI, Frishman WH, Peterson S: Static magnetic stimulation pad over the heart in angina: placebo-controlled trial. Work in progress.
24. Weintraub MI: Magnetotherapy: historical background with a stimulating future. Crit Rev Phys Rehab Med 16:95-108, 2004.

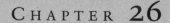

CHAPTER 26

Spinal Cord Stimulation for the Treatment of Angina Pectoris

Wilbert S. Aronow, MD

William H. Frishman, MD

P atients with refractory angina pectoris have either marked limitation of ordinary physical activity or are unable to perform any ordinary physical activity without anginal discomfort.[1] Patients with refractory angina pectoris must have objective evidence of myocardial ischemia. Objective evidence of myocardial ischemia must produce severe anginal symptoms. Anginal symptoms must continue despite maximally tolerated antianginal therapy with nitrates, beta blockers, and calcium channel blockers. Secondary causes of angina pectoris must be excluded. There must be a consensus that coronary revascularization by either percutaneous coronary intervention or by coronary artery bypass surgery is not feasible.[1]

Therapeutic options for refractory angina pectoris include enhanced external counterpulsation, transmyocardial laser revascularization (either surgical or percutaneous), percutaneous *in situ* coronary venous arterialization, gene therapy, acupuncture, electrical nerve stimulation, and spinal cord stimulation (SCS). The topic of this chapter is the treatment of refractory angina pectoris utilizing SCS.

SPINAL CORD STIMULATION

SCS, or epidural spinal electrical stimulation, has been demonstrated to have both antianginal and antiischemic effects in patients with severe angina pectoris.[2] The epidural space is punctured at the level of the fourth or sixth thoracic vertebra, and the electrode tip is placed at the level of the first or second thoracic vertebra.[1] An electrode stimulator is implanted subcutaneously in the upper left abdomen. The stimulator is switched on and off by a magnet being passed over the pulse generator, which is set by an external programmer.[3] The patient can use the magnet to switch between the two preset stimulator strengths. The strongest setting is used in the case of an established or expected anginal attack. The weaker setting is used as maintenance therapy.[3]

IMPROVEMENT IN ANGINAL SYMPTOMS

Many studies have demonstrated that SCS significantly reduces anginal symptoms and nitroglycerin consumption in patients with refractory angina pectoris.[4-14] In a prospective Italian registry of SCS implanted in 104 patients, mean age 69 years, with refractory angina pectoris, 78% had three-vessel coronary artery disease (CAD), 7% had two-vessel CAD, 10% had one-vessel CAD, and 6% had no significant CAD.[14] Mean follow-up was 13 months. Of the 104 patients, 17 (16%) died, eight (8%) due to cardiac death. In comparison to baseline, a 50% or greater reduction in weekly anginal episodes occurred in 73% of patients. Canadian Cardiovascular Society angina class increased by greater than or equal to one class in 80% of patients and by greater than or equal to two classes in 42% of patients.[14]

A placebo effect may contribute to the improvement in anginal symptoms after SCS. Unfortunately, a double-blind, randomized, sham-controlled study has not been performed to adequately evaluate the efficacy of the SCS in improving angina pectoris.

The SCS also reduced the need for acute hospital admission for chest pain in patients with refractory angina pectoris.[11,14,15] The reduction in acute hospital admission for chest pain occurred without masking of serious ischemic symptoms or unrecognized myocardial infarction.[11,14,15] The most frequent side effect was superficial infections, either at the site of puncture of electrode insertion or of the abdominal pocket. This side effect occurred in six of 104 patients (6%).[14]

EXERCISE PERFORMANCE AND MYOCARDIAL ISCHEMIA

Many studies have also demonstrated that SCS significantly increases exercise duration with an unchanged heart rate times systolic blood pressure product (HRxBP) at maximal exercise. In 13 patients with refractory angina pectoris, treadmill exercise duration significantly improved at 6 weeks after SCS implantation from 453 seconds to 533 seconds.[5] The exercise time until angina pectoris significantly increased from 250 seconds to 319 seconds. Ischemic ST-segment depression at a comparable workload significantly decreased from 0.15 mV to 0.11 mV. Ischemic ST-segment depression at maximal exercise, the HRxBP at maximal exercise, and the HRxBP at a comparable workload were not significantly changed.[5] In a 12-patient control group, none of the above variables were significantly different from the baseline period.[5]

In 10 patients with refractory angina pectoris who had a SCS implanted, with the neurostimulator on, the time to maximal treadmill exercise significantly increased from 414 seconds to 478 seconds, total ST-segment depression at maximal exercise significantly decreased from 7.1 mm to 5.6 mm, and total ST-segment depression at 90% of the maximum control heart rate significantly decreased from 3.5 mm to 2.6 mm.[6] The maximum heart rate, the systolic blood pressure at maximum exercise, and the HRxBP at maximum exercise were not significantly changed.[6]

In 10 patients with refractory angina pectoris who had an SCS implanted and the neurostimulator on, the time to maximum exercise on a bicycle ergometer significantly increased from 453 to 581 seconds, the time to angina pectoris significantly increased from 2.4 minutes to 6 minutes, the onset of ischemic ST-segment depression at a comparable workload significantly decreased from 1.9 mm to 1.3 mm, the amount of ischemic ST-segment depression at a maximum workload was not significantly changed, and the HRxBP at a maximum workload was not significantly changed.[4] In 10 patients with refractory angina pectoris, the SCS caused a significant reduction in the number of ischemic episodes during 48-hour ambulatory electrocardiographic monitoring and a significant reduction in the duration of the ischemic episodes.[7] Six of the 10 patients (60%) had no myocardial ischemia during 48-hour electrocardiographic monitoring with the SCS on.[7]

In 23 patients with refractory angina pectoris, the treadmill exercise time significantly increased from 407 seconds with the SCS off to 499 seconds with the SCS on.[8] In this study, the SCS also caused a significant reduction in the total number of ischemic episodes and in the duration of ischemic episodes observed during 48-hour ambulatory electrocardiographic monitoring.[8]

Twenty-three patients with refractory angina pectoris had an SCS implanted and were followed for 24 months.[9] Seven of the 23 patients (30%) died during follow-up. Five of these deaths were cardiac. SCS significantly increased the treadmill exercise time from 320 seconds to 410 seconds in this study.[9]

In a study of nine patients with refractory angina pectoris who had implantation of a SCS, the SCS significantly increased treadmill exercise duration from 358 seconds to 493 seconds, significantly increased the time to angina pectoris from 215 seconds to 349 seconds, and significantly reduced ischemic ST-segment depression during dipyridamole stress testing from 0.17 mV to 0.09 mV.[12] Regional myocardial blood flow as assessed by positron emission tomography before and after 6 weeks of SCS showed an unchanged total resting regional myocardial blood flow and a significant reduction in myocardial blood flow reserve at rest and after dipyridamole stress despite clinical improvement.[12]

In the Electrical Stimulation Versus Coronary Bypass Surgery (ESBY) trial, 104 patients considered at high risk for coronary artery bypass surgery were randomized to SCS (53 patients) or to coronary artery bypass surgery (51 patients).[13] At 6-month follow-up, symptom relief was excellent and similar in both treatment groups.[13] Quality of life was also similar in both treatment groups.[16] However, in comparison to the SCS group, the coronary artery bypass surgery group had a significantly higher increase in exercise capacity, significantly less ischemic ST-segment depression at both maximum and comparable workloads, and a significant increase in the HRxBP at both maximum and comparable workloads.[13]

Mortality occurred in seven of 51 patients (14%) randomized to coronary artery bypass surgery versus one of 53 patients (2%) randomized to SCS. However, three of the seven deaths in the surgical group occurred before the coronary artery bypass surgery was performed. The investigators concluded from their study that SCS may be a therapeutic alternative for patients with an increased risk of surgical complications.[13]

In 10 patients, mean age 54 years, with refractory angina pectoris, SCS abolished or improved pacing time to angina pectoris by more than 50% in 7 of 10 patients (70%).[17] After 3 to 9 months, SCS was ineffective in three of these seven patients. The clinical response to SCS was satisfactory at 5-year follow-up in four of the 10 patients (40%).[17]

In eight patients with refractory angina pectoris, SCS significantly improved exercise-induced angina pectoris and electrocardiographic signs of myocardial ischemia.[18] However, regional myocardial perfusion assessed by positron emission tomography was unchanged despite clinical improvement in this study.[18] SCS also did not change heart rate variability in 19 patients with refractory angina pectoris who had reduction of myocardial ischemia during 48-hour ambulatory electrocardiographic monitoring.[19]

A multicenter randomized study (STARTSTIM) has just been launched in 200 patients with refractory angina pectoris to compare the effects of a brief daily course of SCS (minutes) as a control to a more prolonged daily course of several hours.

MECHANISMS OF IMPROVEMENT

What are the possible mechanisms that cause clinical improvement after SCS implementation? SCS does not improve regional myocardial blood flow during exercise. Myocardial oxygen consumption, as assessed by the HRxBP at maximum exercise, is unchanged by SCS. A placebo effect may contribute to the efficacy of SCS.[18]

SCS reduces the transmission of nociceptive impulses via the spinothalamic tract because of an enhanced release of gamma aminobutyric acid (GABA) from dorsal horn interneurons.[20]

SCS-induced myocardial release of beta-endorphins could explain the beneficial effect of SCS in reducing myocardial ischemia.[21] SCS-induced myocardial release of enkephalins may also act on the presynaptic level to reduce sympathetic tone.[20,21]

CONCLUSION

SCS has been demonstrated to cause clinical improvement in patients with refractory angina pectoris in the number of anginal episodes, in nitroglycerin consumption, in maximal exercise time, in exercise time until angina, in the number of episodes of myocardial ischemia, in the duration of episodes of myocardial ischemia, and in ischemic ST-segment depression at a comparable workload. Double-blind, randomized, placebo-controlled studies have not been performed with SCS. The clinical improvement from SCS occurred despite no improvement in regional myocardial blood flow during exercise or in myocardial oxygen consumption as assessed by the HRxBP at maximal exercise. The mechanisms of clinical improvement by SCS are unclear. SCS must be considered experimental at this time, and it remains as a potential therapeutic option for the treatment of refractory angina pectoris in patients unable to have coronary revascularization or at very high risk for coronary revascularization.

REFERENCES

1. Kim MC, Kini K, Sharma SK: Refractory angina pectoris: mechanism and therapeutic options, J Am Coll Cardiol 39:923-934, 2002.
2. Bueno EA, Mamtani R, Frishman WH: Alternative approaches to the medical management of angina pectoris: acupuncture, electrical nerve stimulation, and spinal cord stimulation, Heart Dis 3:236-241, 2001.
3. Eliasson T, Augustinsson L-E, Mannheimer C: Spinal cord stimulation in severe angina pectoris: presentation of current studies, indications and clinical experience, Pain 65:169-179, 1996.
4. Mannheimer C, Augustinsson L-E, Carlsson C-A et al: Epidural pinal electrical stimulation in severe angina pectoris, Br Heart J 59:56-61, 1988.
5. Hautvast RWM, DeJongste MJL, Staal MJ et al: Spinal cord stimulation in chronic intractable angina pectoris: a randomized, controlled efficacy study, Am Heart J 136:1114-1120, 1998.
6. Sanderson JE, Brooksby P, Waterhouse D et al: Epidural spinal electrical stimulation for severe angina: a study of its effects on symptoms, exercise tolerance and degree of ischaemia, European Heart J 13:628-633, 1992.
7. DeJongste MJL, Haaksma J, Hautvast RWM et al: Effects of spinal cord stimulation on myocardial ischaemia during daily life in patients with severe coronary artery disease: a prospective ambulatory electrocardiographic study, Br Heart J 71:413-418, 1994.
8. Sanderson JE, Ibrahim B, Waterhouse D, Palmer RBG: Spinal electrical stimulation for intractable angina: long-term clinical outcome and safety, European Heart J 15:810-814, 1994.
9. Greco S, Auriti A, Fiume D et al: Spinal cord stimulation for the treatment of refractory angina pectoris: a two-year follow-up, Pacing Clin Electrophysiol 22:26-32, 1999.
10. DeJongste MJL, Hautvast RW, Hillege HL, Lie KI: Efficacy of spinal cord stimulation as adjuvant therapy for intractable angina pectoris: a prospective, randomized clinical study: Working Group on Neurocardiology, J Am Coll Cardiol 23:1592-1597, 1994.

11. TenVaarwerk IAM, Jessurun GAJ, DeJongste MJL et al: Clinical outcome of patients treated with spinal cord stimulation for therapeutically refractory angina pectoris, Heart 82:82-88, 1999.

12. Hautvast RWM, Blanksma PK, DeJongste MJL et al: Myocardial blood flow assessed by positron emission tomography in patients with refractory angina pectoris, Am J Cardiol 77:462-467, 1996.

13. Mannheimer C, Eliasson T, Augustinsson L-E et al: Electrical stimulation versus coronary artery bypass surgery in severe angina pectoris: the ESBY Study, Circulation 97:1157-1163, 1998.

14. Di Pede F, Lanza GA, Zuin G et al: Immediate and long-term clinical outcome after spinal cord stimulation for refractory stable angina pectoris, Am J Cardiol 91:951-955, 2003.

15. Murray S, Carson KGS, Ewings PD et al: Spinal cord stimulation significantly decreases the need for acute hospital admission for chest pain in patients with refractory angina pectoris, Heart 82:89-92, 1999.

16. Ekre O, Norrsell H, Wahrborg P et al: Spinal cord stimulation and coronary artery bypass grafting provide equal improvement in quality of life: data from the ESBY Study (abstract), Circulation 102(suppl II): II-432, 2000.

17. Bagger JP, Jensen BS, Johannsen G: Long-term outcome of spinal cord electrical stimulation in patients with refractory chest pain, Clin Cardiol 21:286-288, 1998.

18. De Landsheere C, Mannheimer C, Habets A et al: Effect of spinal cord stimulation on regional myocardial perfusion assessed by positron emission tomography, Am J Cardiol 69:1143-1149, 1992.

19. Hautvast RW, Brouwer J, DeJongste MJL, Lie KI: Effect of spinal cord stimulation on heart rate variability and myocardial ischemia in patients with chronic intractable angina pectoris: a prospective ambulatory electrocardiographic study, Clin Cardiol 21:33-38, 1998.

20. Latif OA, Nedelkovic SS, Warner Stevenson L: Spinal cord stimulation for chronic intractable angina pectoris: a unified theory on its mechanism, Clin Cardiol 24:533-541, 2001.

21. Eliaason T, Mannheimer C, Waagstein F et al: Myocardial turnover of endogenous opioids and calcitonin-gene-related peptide in the human heart and the effects of spinal cord stimulation on pacing-induced angina pectoris, Cardiology 89:170-177, 1998.

PART **VI**

Special Programs

CHAPTER 27

Integrative Medicine in Cardiothoracic Surgery

Traci R. Stein, MPH
Mehmet Oz, MD

C ardiac surgeons should incorporate complementary healing approaches that are equally ambitious, novel, and promising as any new technology that is offered. To achieve this goal, we must first be aware of the different perspectives that patients and physicians bring to their relationship, deepen our understanding of how patients may benefit from complementary and alternative (CAM) therapies, and better integrate these therapies into the system of conventional medicine (integrative medicine).

Focusing on unconventional approaches to healing within an academic medical center can be both challenging and rewarding. The purpose of this chapter is to provide a framework for understanding those therapies that may be beneficial and could be feasibly incorporated into conventional care. The ultimate goal is to improve the quality and humanity of the care provided and to enhance the recovery and well-being of patients undergoing heart surgery.

INTEGRATIVE MEDICINE AT COLUMBIA UNIVERSITY

The Integrative Medicine Program is housed within the Department of Surgery at Columbia University Medical Center. The aims of the program are to conduct research into the safety, efficacy, and adoptability of CAM therapies and to provide information, referrals, and selected CAM clinical services to cardiovascular service line patients. We have further broadened the definition of "integrative" to include facilitating referrals for patients and family members to resources for smoking cessation, psychotherapy, and preventive cardiology services as necessary.

The staff currently comprises a physician medical director, a research administrator, two full-time research coordinators, a clinical services coordinator/practitioner, a statistical consultant, two predoctoral fellows, and up to two undergraduate level research interns at any given time. The program also uses the services of three *per diem* complementary therapies practitioners as needed. We work collaboratively with other physicians and researchers within the university and from other institutions and host presentations by clinicians, researchers, and CAM practitioners. This rapid growth over the past few years is driven in part by both the cautiously increasing receptiveness to CAM in the medical center (evidenced in part by the growing number of inquiries and requests for services by medical staff) and the high levels of interest in and use of CAM by cardiac surgery patients. The successful development of other CAM centers at the university (the Rosenthal Center for Complementary and Alternative Medicine, which houses the NIH-funded Center for CAM Research in Aging and Women's Health; the Center for Holistic Urology; and the Integrative Therapies Program for Children with Cancer within Pediatric Oncology) has also raised the profile of integrative medicine at this institution.

CAM USE AMONG CARDIOTHORACIC SURGERY PATIENTS

Interest in CAM has increased significantly within the past decade, with an estimated 42% of the population reporting CAM therapies use in 1997.[1] Millions of patients nationally incorporate alternative medicine into their lives despite the fact that many of these services are still not covered by health insurance,[2] although this situation is changing as consumer demand encourages insurers to explore the potential cost savings of these therapies.[3] We suspected that cardiothoracic surgery patients are no exception, and this suspicion prompted us to survey 376 consecutive men and women presenting to our offices regarding their CAM therapies use in early 1998. We queried them regarding their attitudes toward healing and their roles in this process, their opinions regarding the integration of CAM with conventional medicine, and their willingness to discuss CAM therapies use with their physicians/surgeons. Seventy percent of those approached completed the questionnaire, and the sample—primarily comprised of married, white men over the age of 65, most of whom had attained at least a high school education—reported high levels of CAM use with respect to the general population. Approximately 75% of respondents reported using at least one of the 21 listed alternative treatments within the preceding 12 months (Table 27-1).[4]

Excluding vitamins (54%) and prayer (36%)—two therapies that many people do not consider alternative—we identified roughly 44% of patients as using alternative therapies, which is similar to the rate of use in the general population. The most commonly used therapies other than vitamins and prayer were some form of nutritional therapy (17%), massage (11%), chiropractic (11%), meditation (11%), and herbal supplements (9.9%). As CAM therapies have received increasing attention in the media, and because many of these therapies

Table 27-1 PATTERNS OF COMPLEMENTARY/ALTERNATIVE MEDICINE USE BY CARDIAC SURGERY PATIENTS

Therapy	Percentage of Respondents
Vitamins	53.6
Prayer	36.1
Nutritional Therapy	17.1
Massage	11.4
Herbs	9.9
Chiropractor	11.4
Meditation	11.4
Acupuncture	4.2
Homeopathy	3.0
Reflexology	2.3
Hypnosis	2.3
Yoga	2.3
Other	2.3
Energy	1.5
Imagery	1.1
Tai chi	1.5
Aromatherapy	1.5
QiGong	0.4
Ayurveda	0
Naturopathy	0.4
Chelation	0.8
Biofeedback	0.8
Acupressure	1.1

From Liu EH, Turner LM, Lin SX et al: Use of alternative medicine by patients undergoing cardiac surgery. J Thorac Cardiovasc Surg 120: 335-41, 2000.

have become more popularized within the past several years since the survey was conducted, we suspect that rates of use have increased since then. This is reflected in Ai and Bolling's survey of 225 patients by telephone the day before scheduled cardiac surgery.[5] Roughly 81% of the people in their sample confirmed that they used CAM modalities, including relaxation techniques, dietary changes, spiritual healing, imagery, massage, vitamin and herbal supplementation, and others. Being aware of patients' use of herbal therapies is of special importance, particularly in this population, because many herbs may influence the perioperative treatment course.[4,6]

We also asked patients to rate on a scale of one to 10, with one being "not at all" and 10 being "a great deal," the degree to which they felt they played a role in their own healing and to what extent, if any, the listed CAM therapies could help fight illness and maintain wellness. Users and nonusers alike felt strongly that they could influence their healing but differed significantly as to whether they felt the therapies listed could assist conventional medical treatments in fighting illness and promoting general wellness.[4]

Lastly, we asked these patients whether they discussed use of alternative therapies with their physicians or surgeons. Notably, only 17% reported having discussed the issue with their MD. More importantly, even if prompted, only 36% of patients stated that they would share this information with their physicians. Remarkably, 48% reported that they specifically *did not* wish to discuss CAM use with their medical doctor, and 16% did not answer this question. Awareness of this communication gap is critical because it will lead to problems that might otherwise be avoidable. Table 27-2[4] includes a list of commonly used herbs and vitamins that interact with widely used conventional pharmaceuticals, including digoxin, coumadin and cholesterol-reducing drugs (see Chapter 4). Many of these supplements also alter platelet adhesion and fibrinolysis. These observations have led us to insist that cardiovascular physicians restore an open dialogue with patients.

RECOMMENDED THERAPIES FOR CARDIAC SURGERY PATIENTS

Based on the available body of research and clinical observations, we recommend the following for those with cardiovascular ailments:
- Yoga
- Walking
- Guided imagery and/or other stress management techniques
- Use of other relaxing bodywork modalities, such as massage, reflexology, or acupressure/Shiatsu
- Dietary modifications and micronutrient supplementation
- Aromatherapy, energy healing, or other noninvasive CAM therapies that patients are interested in exploring

Table **27-2** POTENTIAL SIDE-EFFECTS OF SOME COMMON HERBAL MEDICINES AND DIETARY SUPPLEMENTS

Product	Effects
Echinacea	Immunosuppression
Garlic	Inhibits platelet aggregation
Ginger	Interacts with warfarin
Ginkgo	Inhibition of platelet-activating factor; interacts with warfarin
Ginseng	Inhibits platelet aggregation, increases protime; interacts with warfarin
Kava	Sedative, hepatic toxicity
St John's Wort	Inhibits cytochrome P450 enzymes; interacts with digoxin, warfarin, oral contraceptives, cyclosporin, antiviral drugs
Vitamin E	Inhibits platelet aggregation

From Liu EH, Turner LM, Lin SX et al: Use of alternative medicine by patients undergoing cardiac surgery, J Thorac Cardiovasc Surg 120:335-41, 2000.

Walking and Yoga

All patients are encouraged to walk daily because it is a low-impact exercise that most patients can begin immediately, requires no expensive purchases (such as a gym membership or equipment), and allows patients to increase exercise duration as they become more fit.

We also recommend yoga to patients because benefits can be seen on both physical and nonphysical levels. Yoga is an ancient discipline that originated thousands of years ago in India (see Chapter 9). Yoga is a spiritual practice that incorporates various exercises and is felt to enhance the link between the body and soul. Yoga is also sometimes called *moving meditation*, and the postures, or *asanas*, and breathing techniques have been shown to improve blood pressure and heart rate and increase feelings of calm and well-being.[7] Studies in the 1970s found that practicing yoga and biofeedback two to three times weekly reduced blood pressure in hypertensive individuals within 6 to 12 weeks of regular practice.[8,9] Yoga also increases lymphatic flow and may help to clear waste products and toxins from the body. This may decrease the risk of a number of cardiovascular problems.[10]

Yoga can help restore muscle strength and tone, increase flexibility, and decrease feelings of stress and anxiety. Yoga works well as both a complement to an existing exercise routine and as a primary type of exercise for those who cannot engage in more rigorous activities.

Patients and family members on the cardiac units have the option of taking part in cardiac-appropriate yoga classes. The poses are modified to prevent injury to the sternum or manubrium but still allow for stretching of the muscles unused since the surgery. It is very important to begin yoga practice with warm-up exercises. These simple movements will help to prepare for the poses to come. The warm-up exercises aid in increasing range of motion and flexibility and reducing muscular tension. All of the warm-up exercises can be done at any time of day, even at a desk at work or at the kitchen table.

Mind-Body Therapies

We recommend patients employ techniques that are associated with the *relaxation response*, the term coined by Herbert Benson to describe the feeling of "letting go," the releasing of muscle tension and calming of the mind that can be elicited using any of a variety of mind-body techniques.[11,12] The program's clinical services coordinator provides instruction in stress reduction, including diaphragmatic and other yoga-inspired breathing techniques, and all patients are encouraged to use guided imagery audiotapes before, during, and after surgery. There is strong evidence to suggest that guided imagery can affect physiology (see Chapter 5). Studies in the past few decades have found an association between use of this technique and reduced blood pressure, resting heart rate and lower cholesterol levels,[12,13] reduced anxiety,[14-16] and enhanced short-term immune cell activity.[17] Guided imagery has also been shown in recent studies to reduce depression and fatigue[14,18] as well as pain perception and need for pain medication after surgery.[15,16]

Using a 5-week program of practitioner-led group instruction and self-practice, we conducted a pilot study of guided imagery with eight heart failure patients who were awaiting transplantation. Peak oxygen consumption, 6-minute walk distance, pulmonary function, lower extremity muscle strength, dyspnea, fatigue, and quality of life were measured before and after the intervention. Minnesota Living with Heart Failure Quality of Life Score tended to improve overall (mean change = 8 ± 4 points, p = 0.06) and in the physical dimension (p = 0.02). Peak oxygen consumption, 6-minute walk distance, skeletal muscle strength, and pulmonary function were similar before and after imagery course completion. Overall, perceived dyspnea during exercise was also unchanged.

It is interesting to note that patient compliance with the guided imagery protocol was 109 ± 53% of recommended frequency (range 60% to 164%). These participants felt subjectively better, despite the fact that their responses to exercise testing demonstrated no objective benefit.[19] Physicians may argue that the latter is more important; however, many patients might prefer a better quality of life, even if longevity is not achieved.

The surgery-preparation guided-imagery audiotape we recommend to all patients, which was developed by psychotherapist Belleruth Naparstek, was compared to three other imagery audiotape programs in a placebo-controlled, double-blinded study with 335 surgery patients.[20] The Naparstek tape was the only audiotape associated with significant reductions in blood loss, length of hospital stay, and anxiety (both state and trait) levels in this trial. These findings and patient feedback prompted us to collaborate with Naparstek to develop an audiotape specifically for use by patients in the cardiac intensive care unit and later in cardiac rehabilitation. We surveyed 20 male and female patients who had undergone either bypass, valve replacement, or transplant surgery to assess whether they benefited from the audiotape. Most patients (90%) reported high levels of satisfaction with the tape, and 79% stated they would recommend it to others. Seventy-one percent thought it made their hospital stays more pleasant, and 75% reported feeling less depressed afterwards. Most (80%) reported increased feelings of relaxation from listening to the tape. Satisfaction was similar regardless of age or gender or whether they had listened to imagery before (unpublished data).

Considering the evidence of benefits from tapping into the mind-body connection and the cost-effectiveness of these interventions, we strongly encourage patients to use these health supportive audiotape programs. For those patients who request information on additional relaxation training, who are psychotic or appear to have poor reality testing or have greater anxiety or depression than could be managed with imagery or other CAM techniques, however, we provide referrals to psychologists and other specialists in this area as appropriate.

MASSAGE

Massage is a well accepted therapy in our hospital possibly because many clinicians have personally experienced comfort from this modality. We have offered massage since the inception of the Integrative Medicine Program; however, to demonstrate more than a hedonistic benefit, we have created innovative studies to assess efficacy. As in many other areas of integrative medicine research, building the model for the control group has proven difficult (see Chapter 24). We have generally used companions to speak with patients without offering a hands-on therapy, but many purists are justified in complaining about the adequacy of this approach. In a randomized study of 78 patients shortly before undergoing catheterization, we found no statistically significant reductions in subjective ratings of pain and discomfort, nor did we find reductions in analgesic and anxiolytic usage, blood pressure, heart rate, or respiration after a 10-minute massage. Although self-reported anxiety decreased in the intervention group, it was not statistically significant. However, the duration and timing of massage could be faulted as being inadequate to show a reduction in symptoms after treatment.[21]

More recently, we surveyed 54 consecutive surgery inpatients before and after receiving a complimentary massage (average duration of 15 minutes) in an effort to assess patient satisfaction with this service. This was the first ever massage for 62% of the sample. Massage techniques were customized to the needs of the patients and typically included a blend of Swedish massage, some reflexology, and occasional incorporation of acupressure/Shiatsu. Using a five-point scale, we assessed perceived pain, stress/tension, depression, fatigue, and "other symptoms" immediately before and after massage. Improvement was statistically significant on all dimensions, which may be attributed in part to the timing of the massages – which took place on postop day 1 or later, rather than immediately prior to catheterization – and the difference in setting (unpublished data). But this illustrates how a brief, relatively low-cost intervention can impact patients' subjective postoperative experiences (Figure 27-1). More research is needed to better elucidate potential mechanisms and other benefits.

Comparison of symptoms pre- and post-massage (average duration: 15 minutes)

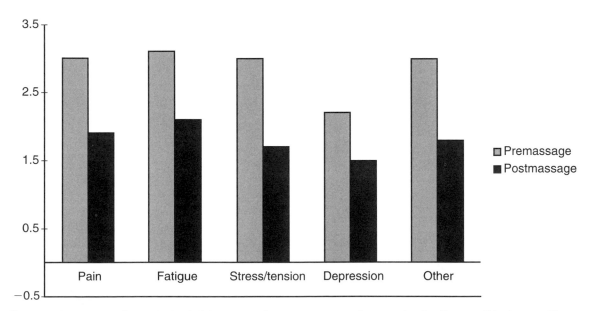

Fig 27-1. Symptoms before and after brief massage. Symptoms were rated on a scale of 1 ("not at all bothersome") to 5 ("extremely bothersome").

DIET AND MICRONUTRIENT SUPPLEMENTATION

Ample evidence recommends dietary changes and micronutrient supplementation to patients with cardiovascular disease (see Chapter 3). At minimum, we recommend patients adopt a plant-based diet that contains few or no dairy products because this diet is associated with reduced risk of obesity, coronary artery disease, hypertension, and diabetes.[22] An eating plan based primarily on whole grains, fresh fruits and vegetables, legumes, soy, and fish is certainly higher in fiber, beneficial omega-3 fatty acids[23] and phytonutrients, and lower in total and saturated fat and calories than what most patients ordinarily consume. We also encourage consumption of teas—particularly instead of other caffeinated beverages—for their polyphenol content.[24,25] Additionally, we have convinced the hospital to supply free dried fruit and nuts, which are distributed by our volunteer staff. These snacks are easy to store, relatively inexpensive, and provide the nurses a partial solution for patients who refuse to eat the hospital food.

The above dietary recommendations can be supplemented with those items found in Table 27-3.

OTHER TYPES OF HEALING THERAPIES

Energy

Energy healing is one of the more esoteric and controversial areas of CAM. Referrals to energy healing practitioners are among the most common CAM-related requests we receive, and several of our patients have asked to bring their own reiki, therapeutic touch, or other energy healers into the operating room. These therapies remain controversial even in integrative medicine because the existence of electromagnetic fields not generated by neuronal action or muscle stimulation is difficult to prove (see Chapter 25). In an effort to better understand this area of CAM, we investigated electromagnetic fields associated with biologic systems via newly available image-analysis techniques. These were used to analyze high-voltage electrophotography. Pictures were created by capturing the light emitted from corona discharges generated from the interaction of a

Table **27-3**   RECOMMENDED MICRONUTRIENTS

Supplement	Dose
Vitamin C	1000 mg daily
Vitamin E	400 IU daily
Coenzyme Q10	30 mg three times daily
L-Carnitine	500 mg two times daily
Calcium citrate	1 gram daily
Magnesium citrate	800 mg daily
Folic acid	0.4 mg daily
Vitamin B complex	50 mg daily
Supplemental pyridoxine hydrochloride	50 mg per day after determination of baseline homocysteine level

time varying high voltage electric field and the subject. Numerous investigators have reported similar corona discharges of unclear significance.[26]

If an electromagnetic field associated with biologic systems can be altered by conscious or physiologic means, then a change in images corresponding to particular electromagnetic emissions might be detectable. To this end, we performed a randomized prospectively controlled study by using five untrained controls and five self-proclaimed energy practitioners.[27] Physiologic manipulations, including biofeedback, alterations in fingertip pressure on the film, ischemia, temperature change, hyperventilation, and hypoventilation, were included to assess the variability of the corona images and seek an underlying organic explanation for observed changes. We found a correlation between change in the electromagnetic emissions for the body and the conscious desire of energy practitioners to change their states. Analyses of individual finger coronas demonstrated statistically significant differences as analyzed by overall color changes and through analysis of individual sections of the various colors dominating the field. Control subjects were unable to reproducibly affect statistically significant changes. We have not explored electrophotography as a diagnostic tool, nor do we seek a parapsychological interpretation of the resulting image; however, we have identified a phenomenon that deserves further study and may reveal additional tools for healing our patients.

AROMATHERAPY

Aromatherapy (see Chapter 18) is defined as "the art and science of utilizing naturally extracted aromatic essences from plants to balance, harmonize, and promote the health of body, mind, and spirit."[28] Typically, aromatherapy consists of the application of several drops of an essential oil (highly concentrated extracts that are distilled from a variety of aromatic plant materials) added to a carrier (often almond oil) and applied to the skin during massage. Essential oils have been described as having various properites, including antibacterial (tea tree oil), invigorating/stimulating (peppermint), and relaxing (lavender), among others.[28]

Essential oils can also be inhaled or added to bath water and are sometimes administered orally. Because of the potential toxicity of some oils, however, we recommend consulting an experienced aromatherapist before engaging in direct application of undiluted essential oils (whether to the skin or orally). Companies such as The Body Shop®, Aveda®, and Kiss My Face® also offer products that use genuine essential oils that have been diluted to safe levels.

Various studies have suggested that fragrance can reduce the physiologic responses to stress.[29-31] We evaluated how a pleasant aroma—although not one that has been associated with particular benefit—influences behavior. We based our research on the hypothesis that a pleasant aroma with no known medicinal effects can decrease cardiovascular reactivity to standard laboratory stressors.[31] Heart rate was recorded during a 5-minute resting baseline, a 5-minute Stroop task, a 5-minute interim recovery period, a 5-minute mental arithmetic task, and a 5-minute final recovery period. Seventeen subjects performed the procedure while breathing no fragrance (air alone), and 19 performed the procedure while breathing coconut fragrance. Both air and coconut fragrance were delivered via nasal cannula. Heart rate increases to stress were significantly less under the coconut fragrance than under air (F[1,29]=4.75; p < .05). For subjects exposed to coconut fragrance, heart rate increases were the following: to Stroop, 4.01 bpm +/− 3.73; to arithmetic, 2.03 bpm +/− 3.25. For subjects exposed to air, heart rate increases were the following: to Stroop, 6.05 bpm +/− 5.74; to arithmetic, 5.06 bpm +/− 4.63. However, overall, heart rate was actually somewhat higher while breathing coconut than air. During baseline and during the first stressor (Stroop task) subjects reported feeling significantly less stress while breathing coconut than while breathing air; however, this effect disappeared later in the session.

These results corroborate previous findings that breathing in pleasant fragrances while undergoing stress may reduce the physical and psychological response to that stressor; however, the finding that resting heart rate was greater during exposure to the fragrance than during exposure to air alone warrants further investigation.

PRAYER

Prayer has been increasingly researched and hotly debated during the past several years (see Chapter 22). The evidence is mixed, and many people suggest that it is neither appropriate to recommend nor study this modality.[32] The popular press has published a number of articles in which religious faith and practice have been said to promote comfort, healing, or both, and a recent report stating that 77% of hospitalized patients wanted physicians to consider their spiritual needs is consistent with this trend.[33] The purpose of this section is not to advocate for or against the use of prayer in medical settings but rather to illustrate one study that is examining the potential effects of this and other CAM therapies.

MANTRA: THE MONITORING AND ACTUALIZATION OF NOETIC TRAINING STUDY

Krucoff and others at Duke University have explored the feasibility and potential benefits of four noetic (CAM) therapies in the MANTRA pilot study.[34] The effects of the noetic therapies—stress relaxation, imagery, touch therapy, and offsite, intercessory prayer—were assessed on patients in the setting of acute coronary interventions. Eligible patients had acute coronary syndromes and invasive angiography or percutaneous interventions (PCI) and were randomized across five treatment groups: the four noetic therapies and standard care. Questionnaires completed before PCI reflected patients' religious beliefs and anxiety. Index hospitalization endpoints included post–PCI ischemia, death, myocardial infarction, heart failure, and urgent revascularization. Mortality and other clinical endpoints were gathered for 6 months after hospitalization. Of the 150 patients enrolled, 120 were assigned to a noetic therapy, and 118 (98%) of these completed their therapeutic assignments. All clinical endpoints were available for 100% of patients. Results were not statistically significant for any outcome comparisons; however, a trend toward significance was discerned. Receiving any noetic therapy was associated with a 25% to 30% absolute reduction in adverse periprocedural events in comparison to receiving standard therapy alone. Interestingly, the lowest absolute complication rates were observed in patients who received prayer from the offsite prayer groups. In patients with questionnaire scores indicating a high level of spiritual belief, a high level of personal spiritual activity, a low level of community-based religious involvement, or a high level of anxiety, noetic therapies appeared to show greater reduction in absolute in-hospital complication rates in comparison to standard therapy.[34] This prompted the MANTRA II study, a multicenter project in which Columbia is a participating site. The aim of this project was to randomize 750 patients undergoing cardiac catheterization to one of the following: prayer from the 12 different religious groups designated for this function, MIT (music, guided imagery, and healing touch—a technique similar to Therapeutic Touch), both conditions, or standard care alone. It is of note that assignment to the offsite, intercessory prayer condition is double-blinded. The data for this trial are currently being analyzed.

Although this study will not elucidate potential mechanisms for any treatment effects, this work is sure to stimulate discussion and future research in an area that is controversial, yet suggestive of benefit to patients in this setting.

We have found it helpful to have a consultative relationship with our pastoral services so that we can ally with them in managing patients who are undergoing surgery and desire spiritual support. Interestingly, we have observed that most patients actually would prefer to speak to someone who is gifted in this area, rather than talking to the heart specialist about religious or spiritual issues. Perhaps the most appropriate role for healthcare providers is not to prescribe spiritual interventions but rather to have an awareness of patients' use of this "therapy" and to honor whatever role patients perceive this to play in their healing—which may range from crucial to none whatsoever. Physicians need not function as chaplains or experts in the area of religion and spirituality but might instead serve as links to those who serve in this capacity within the medical setting for patients who prioritize this as an important component of their lives and healing.

MORBIDITY AND MORTALITY IN WOMEN AFTER CARDIAC SURGERY

Coronary artery disease is the most common cause of death for women in the United States.[35] Coronary artery bypass graft (CABG) surgery increasingly is used for women as a treatment for this disease, including for symptom control. Women now account for nearly 30% of patients undergoing CABG surgery in comparison to 11% to 15% 3 decades ago.[36] These trends are noteworthy because women, as in the case of excess myocardial infarction mortality, are reported to have higher morbidity and mortality after CABG surgery than men.[37-39]

Capdeville and colleagues[40] found that women undergoing CABG surgery with a standardized fast-track protocol have longer intubation times, ICU length of stay, and hospital length of stay than their male counterparts. In comparison to men, the onset of symptomatic coronary artery disease in women is delayed 10 to 15 years until after menopause. Therefore women are often referred for CABG surgery at an older age than men and with more comorbid conditions, such as diabetes and hypertension. But analyses looking to identify causes for the excess mortality in CABG, including comorbidities and age, have failed to explain the discrepancy adequately. Studies by Vaccarino[41] and Hogue et al[42] suggest that neither these factors nor other bias patterns as to who is referred are likely to explain the excess mortality fully. Another common explanation for women's poorer outcomes after surgery is the issue of technical difficulties due to small coronary artery size. But body size does not predict mortality;[43] women do not appear to occlude grafts more often than men; and studies are conflicting about whether they are more likely than men to have small arteries.[44,45]

EMOTIONS AND CARDIOVASCULAR DISEASE IN WOMEN

Stress, hostility, and depression, which are important risk factors for cardiovascular disease, may be responsible for much of the increase in mortality among women. A growing body of data links psychologic state with autonomic activity and with the development of coronary artery disease, which itself can be demonstrated to be linked to autonomic nervous system factors.[46-53] Mental and physical stressors produce elevations in heart rate and blood pressure and may affect blood coagulation and fibrinolysis.[54] Growing evidence suggests that psychologic states and chronic stress may increase coronary artery disease mortality.[55] Data also link depression with a risk of myocardial infarction and with an increased risk of myocardial infarction recurrence.[56-58] On average, women have rates of depression twice as high as those in men. This is possibly due in part to the interaction of occupational stress with family demands as well as socioeconomic, biological, and other emotional variables.[59]

Because of the increasing prevalence of coronary artery disease in women, amounting to nearly 1 million new cases diagnosed each year, along with the general aging of the United States population, the number of women who require cardiac surgery will likely continue to increase. Psychologic states are important pieces in the puzzle of excess mortality in women. New testable hypotheses are needed, as are interventions that would improve outcomes. Thus we should focus increasingly on understanding these factors in our research with female cardiovascular patients.

CAM INTERVENTIONS FOR WOMEN

Various states and practices of meditation and relaxation, including yoga,[7-10] have long been known to result in the lowering of heart rate and blood pressure.[60,61] More recent evidence suggests that a program of meditation or stress reduction can result in a sustained lowering of heart rate and blood pressure, well-established risk factors for coronary artery disease.[62-64] Similarly, growing evidence suggests that meditative techniques can have a positive, sustained effect on chronic pain and mood, including the reduction of depression and anxiety.[7,9,60] This has led us to study the potential for a program of CAM interventions to reduce stress and depression in women with cardiovascular disease.

This study is the result of a partnership with the Preventive Cardiology Program and the Rosenthal Center for Complementary and Alternative

Medicine, both at Columbia. This project is exploring the adoptability and potential benefits of a program of CAM therapies—yoga, guided imagery (as well as diaphragmatic breathing), and dietary modifications—with 150 women who have undergone cardiac surgery (CABG and/or valve repair or replacement) at Columbia University Medical Center. We hope these interventions will empower women to become active participants in their own healing rather than passive recipients of care, reduce the incidence and severity of stress and depression in this population, and ultimately improve outcomes.

CONCLUSIONS, RECOMMENDATIONS, AND FUTURE DIRECTIONS

Integrative cardiac medicine uses a broader view of health and healers. The following are resources and professionals we believe should ideally be part of the integrative medicine armamentarium:

- *Competent conventional care:* A skilled, conventionally trained clinician or team of healthcare providers (physician, surgeon, nurses, physician assistants, etc.)
- *Education by and referrals to nonphysician health professionals, where appropriate*: A trained health educator, preferably one who can address CAM-related questions and provide referrals where appropriate; a dietitian, preferably one who is knowledgeable about many of the dietary supplements currently available and which many patients may be taking; mental health professionals skilled in stress management/relaxation training, as well as ones trained in smoking cessation; clergy; exercise physiologists, physical therapists, or other movement therapists; and resource lists of books and other educational materials on both CAM and more conventional health-related topics.
- *CAM providers who are experts in areas relevant to patient well-being, licensed, or certified when applicable:* Massage therapists and other bodyworkers, acupuncturists, energy practitioners, yoga instructors, aromatherapists, and others.
- *Research*: To increase the comfort level of conventionally trained medical professionals with the use of CAM therapies, elucidate those therapies that are safe and effective and develop a greater awareness of those techniques that patients are already using (either on their own or concomitant with the administration of conventional care), we must conduct rigorously designed research in this area.

Ultimately, as our traditional treatment options for disease improve, we will need to remain open to the beliefs, needs, and feelings of our patients. Often, healing and patient comfort or well-being can be enhanced by using simpler techniques, many of which patients are already incorporating into their personal treatment programs. The medical community is obliged to evaluate, although not advocate, integrative approaches or we risk no longer being as valuable a resource for patients in this arena. Physicians cannot be expected to be experts in every treatment that may be of benefit to their patients. By maintaining an open dialogue with patients, being willing to serve as referral sources, and being available to discuss contraindications and treatment plans with other members of the patient's broadly defined healthcare team, however, we can ensure better delivery of optimal care.

REFERENCES

1. Eisenberg DM, Davis RB, Ettner SL et al: Trends in alternative medicine use in the United States, 1990-1997: results of a follow-up national survey, JAMA 280:1569-75, 1998.

2. Cleary-Guida MB, Okvat HA, Oz MC, Ting W: A regional survey of health insurance coverage for complementary and alternative medicine: current status and future ramifications, J Altern Complement Med 7:269-73, 2001.

3. Pelletier KR, Astin JA: Integration and reimbursement of complementary and alternative medicine by managed care and insurance providers: 2000 update and cohort analysis, Altern Ther Health Med 8:38-9, 2002.

4. Liu EH, Turner LM, Lin SX et al: Use of alternative medicine by patients undergoing cardiac surgery, J Thorac Cardiovasc Surg 120:335-41, 2000.

5. Ai AL, Bolling SF: The use of complementary and alternative therapies among middle-aged and older cardiac patients, Am J Med Qual 17:21-7, 2002.

6. Witte KA, Clark AL, Cleland JGF: Chronic heart failure and micronutrients, J Am Coll Cardiol 37:1765-74, 2001.

7. Stein TR, Fisch L, Kennedy DD, Ladas EJ: Integrative medicine for women in cardiac rehabilitation, New York, 2002, Columbia University. (Available from the Integrative Medicine Program, College of Physicians and Surgeons of Columbia University, 177 Fort Washington Avenue, MHB 7-435, New York, NY 10032. www.ColumbiaIntegrativeMedicine.org)

8. Patel CH: Yoga and bio-feedback in the management of hypertension, Lancet 2:1053-1055, 1973.

9. Patel C, North WR: Randomised controlled trial of yoga and bio-feedback in the management of hypertension, Lancet 2:93-95, 1975.

10. Lemole GM: An integrative approach to cardiac care. Minneapolis, 2000, Medtronic, Inc.

11. Hoffman JW, Benson H, Arns PA et al: Reduced sympathetic nervous system responsivity associated with the relaxation response, Science 215:190-192, 1982.

12. Beary JF, Benson H: A simple psychophysiologic technique which elicits the hypo-metabolic changes of the relaxation response, Psychosom Med 36:115-120, 1974.

13. Sharpley C: Differences between ECG and pulse when measuring heart rate and reactivity under two physical and two psychological stressors, J Behav Med 17:309-329,1994.

14. Ashton C Jr, Whitworth GC, Seldomridge JA et al: Self-hypnosis reduces anxiety following coronary artery bypass surgery: a prospective, randomized trial, J Cardiovasc Surg 38:69-75, 1997.

15. Manyande A, Berg S, Gettins D et al: Preoperative rehearsal of active coping imagery influences subjective and hormonal responses to abdominal surgery, Psychosom Med 57:177-182, 1995.

16. Lang, EV, Benotsch, EG, Fick, LJ et al: Adjunctive non-pharmacological analgesia for invasive medical procedures: a randomised trial, Lancet 355(9214):1486-1490, 2000.

17. Fawzy FI, Fawzy NW, Hyun CS et al: Malignant melanoma: effects of an early structured psychiatric intervention, coping, and affective state on recurrence and survival 6 years later, Arch Genl Psychiatry 50:681-689, 1993.

18. McKinney CH; Antoni MH, Kumar M et al: Effects of guided imagery and music (GIM) therapy on mood and cortisol in healthy adults, Health Psychology 16:390-400, 1997.

19. Klaus L, Beniaminovitz A, Choi L et al: Pilot study of guided imagery use in severe heart failure, Am J Cardiol 86:101-04, 2000.

20. Dreher, H: Mind-body interventions for surgery: evidence and exigency, Advances Mind-Body Med 14:207-222, 1998.

21. Okvat HA, Oz MC, Ting W, Namerow, PB: Massage therapy for patients undergoing cardiac catheterization, Altern Therap 8:68-75, 2002.

22. Rajaram S, Sabate J: Health benefits of a vegetarian diet, Nutrition 16:531-533, 2000.

23. Hu HB, Bronner L, Willett WC et al: Fish and omega-3 fatty acid intake and risk of coronary heart disease in women, JAMA 287:1815-1821, 2002.

24. Geleijnse JM, Launer LJ, Hofman A et al: Tea flavonoids may protect against atherosclerosis: the Rotterdam Study, Arch Intern Med 159:2170-2174, 1999.

25. Stensvold I, Tverdal A, Solvoll K, Foss OP: Tea consumption, relationship to cholesterol, blood pressure, and coronary and total mortality, Prevent Med 21:546-553, 1992.

26. Pehek JO, Kyler HJ, Faust DJ: Image modulation in corona discharge photography, Science 194:263-270, 1976.

27. Russo M, Choudhri AF, Whitworth G, et al: Quantitative analysis of reproducible changes in high-voltage electrophotography, J Altern Compl Med 7:617-627, 2001.

28. The National Association for Holistic Aromatherapy: www.naha.org.

29. Warren C, Warrenburg S: Mood benefits of fragrance. Perfumer & Flavorist 18:9-15, 1993.

30. Buckle J: Aromatherapy and cardiovascular disease. In Stein RA, Oz MC editors: Complementary and alternative cardiovascular medicine. Totowa NJ, 2004, Humana Press, 239-254.

31. Mezzacappa ES, Arumugam U, Yue SI et al: Coconut fragrance reduces heart rate reactivity to stress (abst). Psychosom Med 62:147, 2000.

32. Sloan RP, Bagiella E, VandeCreek L et al: Should physicians prescribe religious activities? N Engl J Med 342:1913-1916, 2000.

33. King DE, Bushwick B: Beliefs and attitudes of hospital inpatients about faith healing and prayer, J Family Pract 39:349-52, 1994.

34. Krukoff M, Crater SW, Green CL et al: Integrative noetic therapies as adjuncts to percutaneous intervention during unstable coronary syndromes: monitoring and actualization of noetic training (MANTRA) feasibility pilot, Am Heart J 142:760-69, 2001.
35. DelValle M, Frishman WH: Angina pectoris. In Charney P, editor: Coronary artery disease in women: what all physicians need to know, Philadelphia, 1999, American College of Physicians, 373-400.
36. American Heart Association: Statistical fact sheet: populations: women and cardiovascular diseases, www.americanheart.org. Retrieved November 15, 2003.
37. Herlitz J, Wiklund I, Sjoland H et al: Relief of symptoms and improvement of health-related quality of life five years after coronary artery bypass graft in women and men, Clin Cardiol 24:385-92, 2001.
38. Curtis AB, Cannom DS, Bigger JT et al: Baseline characteristics of patients in the Coronary Artery Bypass Graft (CABG) Patch Trial, Am Heart J 133:787-98, 1997.
39. Hogue CW, Sundt T, Barzilai B et al: Cardiac and neurologic complications identify risks for mortality for both men and women undergoing coronary artery bypass graft surgery, Anesthesiol 95: 1074-78, 2001.
40. Capdeville M, Lee JH, Taylor AL: Effect of gender on fast track recovery after coronary artery bypass graft surgery. J Cardiothorac Vasc Anesth 15: 146-51, 2001.
41. Vaccarino V, Abramson JL, Veledar E, Weintraub WS: Sex differences in hospital mortality after coronary artery bypass surgery: evidence for a higher mortality in younger women, Circulation 105:1176-81, 2002.
42. Hogue CW, Stein PK, Apostolidou I et al: Alterations in temporal patterns of heart rate variability after bypass graft surgery, Anesthesiol 81:1356-64, 1994.
43. Edwards FH, Carey JS, Grover FL et al: Impact of gender on coronary artery bypass operative mortality. Ann Thorac Surg 66:125-31, 1998.
44. Sheifer SE, Canos MR, Weinfurt KP: Sex difference in coronary artery size assessed by intravascular ultrasound, Am Heart J 139:649-53, 2000.
45. Mickleborough LL, Takagi Y, Maruyama H et al: Is sex a factor in determining operative risk for aortocoronary bypass graft surgery? Circulation 92(supp II):80-4, 1995.
46. Connerney I, Shapiro PA, McLaughlin JS et al: Relation between depression after coronary artery bypass surgery and 12-month outcome: a prospective study, Lancet 358:1766-71, 2001.
47. Booth-Kewley S, Friedman HS: Psychological predictors of heart disease: a quantitative review, Psychol Bull 101:343-362, 1987.
48. Miller TQ, Smith TW, Turner CW: A meta-analytic review of research on hostility and physical health, Psychol Bull 119:322-348, 1996.
49. Rosenman RH, Brand RJ, Jenkins CD et al: Coronary heart disease in the Western Collaborative Group Study: final follow-up experience of 8 1/2 years, JAMA 233:872-877, 1975.

50. Matthews KA, Haynes SG: Type-A behavior pattern and coronary disease risk: update and critical evaluation, Am J Epidemiol 123:923-960, 1986.

51. Barefoot JC, Larsen S, Von der Lieth L, Schroll M: Hostility, incidence of acute myocardial infarction, and mortality in a sample of older Danish men and women, Am J Epidemiol 142:477-484, 1995.

52. Mittleman MA, Maclure M, Sherwood JB et al: Triggering of acute myocardial infarction onset by episodes of anger, Circulation 92: 1720-1725, 1995.

53. Everson SA, Kauhanen J, Kaplan GA et al: Hostility and increased risk of mortality and acute myocardial infarction: The mediating role of behavioral risk factors, Am J Epidemiol 146:142-152, 1997.

54. von Kanel R, Mills JP, Fainman C, Dimsdale JE: Effects of psychological stress and psychiatric disorders on blood coagulation and fibrinolysis: a biobehavioral pathway to coronary artery disease? Psychosom Med 63:531-544, 2001.

55. Frasure-Smith N, Lesperance F, Talajic M: The impact of negative emotions on prognosis following myocardial infarction: is it more than depression? Health Psychol 14(5):388-398, 1995.

56. Barefoot JC, Helms MJ, Mark DB: Depression and long-term mortality risk in patients with coronary artery disease, Am J Cardiol 78:613-7, 1996.

57. Perlmutter JB, Frishman WH, Feinstein RE: Major depression as a risk factor for cardiovascular disease. Therapeutic implications. Heart Dis 2: 75-82, 2000.

58. Khawaja IS, Feinstein RE: Cardiovascular effects of selective serotonin reuptake inhibitors and other novel antidepressants, Heart Dis 5:153-60, 2003.

59. Krantz S, McCeney MK: Effects of psychological and social factors on organic disease: a critical assessment of research on coronary heart disease, Annu Rev Psychol 53:341-69, 2002.

60. Barrows, KA, Jacobs, BP: Mind-body medicine: an introduction and review of the literature. Med Clinics North Am 86(1):11-31, 2002.

61. Bishop SR: What do we really know about mindfulness-based stress reduction? Psychosom Med 64:71-84, 2002.

62. Barnes, VA, Treiber FA, Turner JR et al: Acute effects of transcendental meditation on hemodynamic functioning in middle-aged adults, Psychosom Med 61:525-31, 1999.

63. Schneider, RH, Staggers F, Alexander CN et al: A randomized controlled trial of stress reduction for hypertension in older African Americans, Hypertension 26:820-27, 1995.

64. Alexander CN, Schneider RH, Staggers F et al: Trial of stress reduction for hypertension in older African Americans, II: sex and risk subgroup analysis, Hypertension 28:228-237, 1996.

Index

A

AAMA. *See* American Academy of
    Medical Acupuncture
AAT. *See* Animal-assisted therapy
Abdominal cramps, 72, 109
ABMP. *See* Associated Bodywork and
    Massage Professionals
Acanthosis nigricans, 64
Acceptance, 195
ACE. *See* Angiotensin-converting
    enzymes
ACI. *See* Auriculotherapy
    Certification Institute
Aconitine, 100
Aconitum, 100
Acquired immunodeficiency
    syndrome (AIDS), 357-358
ACTH. *See* Hormones
Acupressure, 373-374, 400t, 401
Acupuncture, 113, 128. *See also*
    Auriculotherapy
    angina pectoris and, 267-269
    Asian bodywork in, 373
    auricular plastic therapy in, 284,
        284f
    CADs and, 117, 260-271, 262f,
        263b, 265t, 266t
    classical/traditional, 261-262,
        262f, 274-276
    conception vessel (CV) in, 261,
        262f
    ear/auricle in, 274-284, 275f,
        277f, 278f, 283f
    effects of, 260
    electro, 117, 264-265, 283-284
    energy fields/meridians in,
        188-189, 261-263, 262f
    gate control theory in, 263, 270

Acupuncture (*continued*)
    governing vessel (GV) in, 261, 262f
    heart channel pathway in,
        261-263, 262f
    hypertension and, 266-267
    as mind-body approach, 116-117
    needle, 282-284
    neurophysiological mechanisms
        of, 263-264
    oto, 269-270
    in pain control, 263-264
    peripheral blood flow and,
        265-266
    points, 261-263, 262f
    problems with, 271
    Qi in, 193, 261
    Qigong and, 193
    Raynaud's disease and, 266
    safety, 270-271
    SCS and, 270
    sham, 268
    in TCM, 116-117, 260-261
    TENS and, 270
    types of, 261-262
    usefulness of, 264-265, 265t
"Adequate and Well-Controlled
    Clinical Evaluations," 6-7
Adey, W.R., 385-386
ADH. *See* Hormones
Adjunct therapy, 92
Adonis microcarpa (Adonis), 89
Adonis vernalis (Adonis), 89
Aescin, 96-97
Aesculic acids, 96-97
Aesculus hippocastanum (horse
    chestnut)
    as herbal remedy, 96-97
    for venous insufficiencies, 96-97
Africa, 99
African Americans, 5, 138-139,
    144

Agency for Healthcare Research and
    Quality (AHRQ), 173
AHRQ. *See* Agency for Healthcare
    Research and Quality
AIDS. *See* Acquired
    immunodeficiency syndrome
Ajoenes, 94
Alcohol, 16, 70, 347
Allicin, 171
Alliin, 94
Alliinase, 94
Allium sativum (garlic), 300, 401t
    for atherosclerosis, 94
    Ayurveda and, 171-173
    for cholesterol, 95
    as herbal remedy, 94-95
    for hypertension, 173
Alpha Tocopherol, Beta Carotene
    (ATBC) Cancer Prevention
    Study, 59
AMA. *See* American Medical
    Association
"Amazing Grace," 328
American Academy of Medical
    Acupuncture (AAMA), 285, 373
American Board of
    Homeotherapeutics, 242, 246
American College of Cardiology, 294
American Heart Association, 118,
    294
American Institute of Homeopathy,
    234, 245
American Massage Therapy
    Association (AMTA), 381
American Medical Association
    (AMA), 20, 43-44, 128
American Organization for
    Bodywork Therapies in Asia
    (AOBTA), 372, 380, 381
American Society of Clinical
    Hypnosis, 128

Page numbers followed by f indicate
figures; t, tables; b, boxes.